Nelson

Textbook
of
Pediatrics
POCKET COMPANION

D0951732

Nelson

Textbook
of
Pediatrics

POCKET COMPANION

RICHARD E. BEHRMAN, M.D.

Managing Director
Center for the Future of Children
David and Lucile Packard Foundation

Clinical Professor of Pediatrics
Stanford University and University of California, San Francisco

Attending Physician
Lucile Salter Packard Children's Hospital
Stanford, California

Kenneth H. Webb, M.D.

Assistant Professor of Pediatrics
Stanford University

Attending Physician
Lucile Salter Packard Children's Hospital
Stanford, California

W. B. SAUNDERS COMPANY
A Division of Harcourt Brace & Company

Philadelphia, London, Toronto, Montreal, Sydney, Tokyo

W.B. SAUNDERS COMPANY
A Division of
Harcourt Brace & Company

The Curtis Center
Independence Square West
Philadelphia, PA 19106

Library of Congress Cataloging-in-Publication Data

Behrman, Richard E.,
  Nelson textbook of pediatrics pocket companion /
Richard E. Behrman.
    p.   cm.
  ISBN 0-7216-3968-2
  1. Pediatrics—Handbooks, manuals, etc. I. Nelson,
Waldo E. (Waldo Emerson). II. Nelson textbook of
pediatrics. III. Title. IV. Title: Textbook of pediatrics
pocket companion.
    [DNLM: 1. Pediatrics—handbooks. WS 39 B421n
1993]
RJ45.N4 1992 Suppl.
618.92—dc20
DNLM/DLC
for Library of Congress   93-9371
                                                     CIP

NELSON TEXTBOOK OF PEDIATRICS   ISBN 0-7216-3968-2
POCKET COMPANION   International ISBN 0-7216-4598-4

Printed in the United States of America.

Last digit is the print number:
           9   8   7   6   5   4   3   2

ACKNOWLEDGMENTS

I am very appreciative of the assistance provided by a number of pediatricians in the preparation of *Nelson Textbook of Pediatrics Pocket Companion*. For their help in preparing synopsis of individual chapters I wish to acknowledge: Doctors Louis Naumovski and Bert Glader (Chap. 14), Doctors Richard Bram and Bert Glader (Chap. 15), Doctor Rashmi Kirpekar (Chap. 16), Doctor Kathy Eckert (Chap. 17), Doctor Jim Hahn (Chap. 18), and Doctor Kenneth S. Vereschagin (Chap. 22). Doctor Kenneth Webb who was my associate in editing *The Companion* helped particularly with Chapters 10, 11, 12, 13, and 20.

PREFACE

Medical students, residents, and others in training as health professionals involved in caring for children may be overwhelmed by the quantity of medical knowledge potentially applicable to the prevention, diagnosis, and treatment of disorders that may affect children during their development from embryonic to adult life. The editors and contributors summarize this enormous amount of information and the relevant science on which it is based in *Nelson Textbook of Pediatrics* which is completely revised and updated every four years.

Because of its necessary comprehensiveness, even as a distillate of the broad field of pediatrics, *Nelson Textbook* cannot be kept in one's pocket wherever one is caring for children. Therefore, the editor has condensed the clinical portions of *Nelson* into this pocket-sized Companion Handbook. This Companion Handbook consists of brief summaries of key features of growth and development, and of the principal diseases and disorders the student or trainee is likely to encounter in caring for children.

This Companion Handbook should not and cannot be the replacement for a Textbook of Pediatrics. Each brief chapter is cross-referenced to the appropriate sections in *Nelson Textbook*, fourteenth edition. The Companion Handbook should only be used as a brief introduction to, or a reminder of, an aspect of clinical pediatrics when there is not immediate access to, or time to consult *Nelson*. Because the quantity of material presented is too brief to stand on its own, it is strongly recommended that the relevant subjects in the textbook be consulted as soon as time permits. The Handbook is a *companion* to *Nelson's Textbook*, fourteenth edition and both books should be used as a combined educational activity.

RICHARD E. BEHRMAN, M.D.
Editor

CONTENTS

GROWTH AND DEVELOPMENT

Those responsible for the care of children should be familiar with the normal patterns and milestones of growth and development and be able to recognize deviations from the normal as early as possible. Such variations are often the first clinical manifestation of underlying disorders that require attention. *Growth* refers to an increase in the size of the infant as a whole or of his or her individual parts; *development* refers to other aspects of differentiation of form and changes of function.

Physical growth and development encompasses a diverse spectrum of changes from the genetically determined activation of enzymes in the course of embryonic differentiation to the complex interaction of metabolic and clinical manifestations associated with puberty and adolescence. These changes interdigitate with, are influenced by, and have an effect on neurodevelopmental processes and cognitive and psychosocial development. Environmental factors such as available nutrition, economic considerations, and cultural and community variables play a significant role in these processes (see *Nelson Textbook*, Sec. 3.1).

EMBRYO (8–12 WEEKS) AND FETUS (12–40 WEEKS)
(*NELSON TEXTBOOK*, SEC. 3.2, CHAPS. 9 AND 15)

Embryonic movements occur by 9 wk, although they are not detected by the pregnant women until 13–14 wk. By 8 wk after conception the embryo has human form, weighs about 1 g, and is about 7.5 cm long. By 16 wk the fetus weighs about 14 g and is 17 cm long. Sex can be distinguished by the end of the 1st trimester. By the end of the 2nd trimester (28 wk) the fetus weighs about 1,000 g and is about 35 cm long. During the 3rd trimester, the increase in fetal size is primarily due to increases in subcutaneous tissue and muscle mass.

Respiratory movements occur by the 18th wk and pulmonary surfactant is detectable by the 20th wk, but alveolar development usually does not permit survival before 24 wk. By this stage a variety of other fetal systems have developed sufficiently to support life outside the uterus, independent of the placenta, if appropriate medical care is provided.

THE TERM NEWBORN INFANT
(*NELSON TEXTBOOK*, SEC. 3.3, CHAP. 9)

PHYSICAL DEVELOPMENT

Ninety five percent of term newborns weigh between 2.5 and 4.6 kg (5½–10 lb), are 45–55 cm (18–22 in) in length, and have head circumferences of 32.6–37.2 cm.

Compared to older children, in the normal newborn:

1. The external auditory canals are short and straight, the eardrums are placed more obliquely in the canal, the middle ear contains a mucoid substance that may be mistaken for an infectious exudate, and the eustachian tube is short and broad.
2. There is usually a single mastoid cell in the antrum and the sinuses are small or underdeveloped.
3. The liver and spleen are commonly palpable below the costal margins, and the kidneys are often palpable.
4. Normal infants tend to assume a posture of partial flexion.

Minor traumatic effects of labor may cause edema of the vertex or overriding of cranial bones, and orthopedic abnormalities may be caused by intrauterine posture or pressure on the growing fetus.

PHYSIOLOGY

The respiratory rate for adequate gas exchange, which is the priority at birth, ranges from 35 to 50 breaths/min. Brief variations outside this range are common. Failure to establish adequate oxygenation may lead to respiratory and metabolic acidosis and hypoxic tissue injury.

The normal heart rate ranges from 120 to 160 beats/min. Transient murmurs are common.

In response to hunger, the infant cries and turns toward a touch close to the oral area (rooting reflex). Sucking, gagging, and swallowing reflexes are active, and the infant is capable of vomiting. Hunger occurs at irregular intervals during the 1st wk and subsequently usually occurs at 2–5-hr intervals.

The first stools (*meconium*) are generally passed within 24 hr. On the 3rd–4th day, when milk feedings are established, *transitional* greenish brown stools that may contain milk curds occur. The typical brown stool occurs after a further 3–4-day interval. Stools relate to the frequency and amount of feeding; usually there are 3–5 stools/day by the end of the 1st wk. On a particular day in the 1st wk, stools may range from 0 to 7/day, particularly with breast-feeding.

The temperature of mother and infant are virtually the same at birth. The infant's temperature usually falls transiently and is restored by 4–8 hr. The caloric requirement for normal temperature and activity is about 55 kcal/kg/24 hr. By the end of the 1st wk total caloric needs are 110 kcal/kg/24 hr, half of which is used for basal metabolic needs and the remainder for growth and activity (40%), for specific dynamic action of protein (5%), and for excretory losses (5%).

The extracellular fluid compartment constitutes 35% of the newborn's body weight. During the first few days of life there is a loss of fluid that usually averages 6–10% of body weight. Excessive loss and poor intake may lead to fever and dehydration. After the 1st wk the newborn's oral water requirement ranges between 120 and 150 mL/kg/24 hr. About half of this is needed for the formation of urine and the rest for insensible and other losses.

Glomerular filtration rate (GFR) and urine output are low during the first days of life but increase rapidly in the first few weeks. During the 1st wk, proteinuria is common and the urine may contain urates, which may stain the diaper pink. The ability to concentrate urine is limited, and urea and phosphate clearance is low.

The newborn infant's hemoglobin (Hgb) ranges from 17 to 19 g/dL (30% is Hgb A and the rest Hgb F). Mild reticulocytosis and normoblastemia occur for the first 1–2 days. Leukocytes are about 10,000/mm^3 at birth and increase during the first 24 hr, with a relative neutrophilia. Counts of 25,000–35,000 may occur. After the 1st wk, the total white blood cell count is usually below 14,000 and characterized by the relative lymphocytosis of infancy and early childhood. Stress, including overwhelming infections, occasionally may be associated with little or no leukocytosis, and even leukopenia. Establishment of normal hemostatic mechanisms depends on acquisition of normal intestinal flora and production of vitamin K.

Maternal hormones transferred by the placenta may produce transient enlargement of the breasts and genital secretions (see *Nelson Textbook*, Sec. 9.9).

The gamma globulin level [immunoglobulin G or IgG] of the newborn is similar to that of the mother and protects against many viral and some bacterial infections. Maternal immunoglobulins IgM, IgA, and IgE, however, do not cross the placenta in significant amounts. IgM may be formed by the fetus in response to in utero infection.

The infant's IgG falls to a low level by about 3 mo as maternally transferred antibody disappears. Subsequently IgG rises as the infant produces his or her own immunoglobulins; it is usually normal by about 6 mo.

The infant's digestive enzymes are usually adequate for the diet, although fat is handled less well than protein or carbohydrates.

NEURODEVELOPMENT

Selected neurologic and reflex behaviors are described in Chapter 18 of this handbook and more fully in Secs. 9.3 and 20.1 of the *Nelson Textbook*. The term newborn infant has the capacity for interaction with the environment and for complex neurologic organization.

The quality of behavior that can be elicited from the newborn is highly dependent on the *behavioral state* or level of arousal of the infant: (1) deep sleep; (2) sleep with rapid eye movements (REM); (3) a drowsy state; (4) a quiet alert state; (5) an awake and active state; and (6) a state of active intense crying. In state 4 the infant is capable of engaging in the most responsive and complex interactions with the environment.

At birth, term newborn infants can fixate objects, follow movements of objects, and give preferential attention to figures of the human face. The Neonatal Behavioral Assessment Scale (NBAS) is used to assess the behavior of newborn infants in four dimensions: *interactive* processes (orientation, alertness, consolability, cuddliness); *motor* processes (muscular tone, motor maturity, defensive reactions, hand-to-mouth activity, general activity level, and reflex behavior); *control of psychological state* (habituation to bright light, a rattle, a ball, and a pin prick; self-quieting); and *response to stress* (tremulousness, lability of skin color, startle reaction).

PSYCHOSOCIAL DEVELOPMENT

The infant is born into a social milieu that begins before birth. *Bonding* consists of those emotional ties and commitments that characterize the early relationship between parents or other participants in a social event and the infant, who becomes the central figure. The infant reciprocates by *attachment* to significant persons in this environment. A host of complex interactions characterize these relationships, such as the infant's responsiveness to voices and the human face and the mother's responsiveness to the infant's cry and smell.

THE FIRST YEAR
(*NELSON TEXTBOOK*, SEC. 3.5)

Usually full-term infants regain their birth weight by 10 days of life, double their birth weight by 5 mo, and triple it by 1 yr. These full-term infants and many premature infants gain about 6–7 kg (13–15 lb) in the 1st yr. Length in term infants usually increases about 25–30 cm (10–12 in) during the 1st yr. Table 1–1 presents formulas to calculate approximate average weight and height of normal infants and children.

The anterior fontanel, which may increase in size after birth, usually decreases after 6 mo and closes between 9 and 18 mo. The posterior fontanel is generally closed to palpation by 4 mo.

The average head circumference increases from about 34–35 cm (13.4–13.8 in) at birth to 44 cm by 6 mo, and 47 cm by 1 yr (Table 1–2).

The first deciduous teeth usually erupt between 5 and 9 mo in the order: lower central incisors, upper central and then upper lateral incisors, lower lateral incisors, 1st deciduous molars, cuspids, and 2nd deciduous molars.

FIRST 3 MONTHS

Neurodevelopmental

The prone term newborn infant can turn his or her face from side to side. By 4 wk the head can be lifted above the surface

TABLE 1–1. FORMULAS FOR APPROXIMATE AVERAGE HEIGHT AND WEIGHT OF NORMAL INFANTS AND CHILDREN*

Weight	Kilograms	Pounds
(a) At birth	3.25	7
(b) 3–12 mo	$\dfrac{\text{age (mo)} + 9}{2}$	age (mo) + 11
(c) 1–6 yr	(age [yr] × 2) + 8	(age [yr] × 5) + 17
(d) 7–12 yr	$\dfrac{(\text{age [yr]} \times 7) - 5}{2}$	(age [yr] × 7) + 5

Height	Centimeters	Inches
(e) At birth	50	20
(f) At 1 yr	75	30
(g) 2–12 yr	(age [yr] × 6) + 77	(age [yr] × 2½) + 30

* From Behrman RE (ed): Nelson Textbook of Pediatrics, 14th ed. Philadelphia, WB Saunders Company, 1992, p. 19. (After Weech.)

as it is turned, the flexed posture is more relaxed, and, when the infant is supine, the head is likely to be turned to one side with the extremities extended on that side (tonic neck reflex).

At 4–8 wk the head lags when the infant is pulled from the supine to sitting position and there is no head control. By 12 wk there is some head control.

When the newborn infant is held with a hand under the trunk (Landau response), the infant will flex with the head and extremities around the supporting hand. By 1 mo of age the infant can raise the head briefly to the plane of the body, by 2 mo the infant can sustain the head in that plane, and by 3 mo the head can be raised above the plane and the legs can be extended as well.

In the first few days of life infants fixate best on objects placed close to or moved through their line of vision. They may maintain fixation with eye and head movement to nearly 90 degrees from the midline through an arc of 180 degrees.

Within 4 wk infants make contact with stationary objects

TABLE 1–2. FORMULA FOR ESTIMATING HEAD CIRCUMFERENCE IN FIRST YEAR*

Normal range of head circumference (5th–95th percentile)

$$= \left[\frac{\text{length (cm)}}{2} + 9.5\right] \pm 2.5$$

* After Dine MS, Gartside PS, Glueck CJ, et al: Relationship of head circumference to length in the first 400 days of life: A mnemonic. Pediatrics 67:506, 1981.

within their reach and exhibit reflex grasp. By 8 wk an active grasp may become evident.

Small throaty noises begin at about 4 wk. Some vowels sounds are produced by 8 wk and are usually uttered with pleasure at social contact by 12 wk.

Psychosocial Development

By 2–6 wk infants may appear more comfortable with familiar persons than strangers. Although fragmentary smiles may be manifest soon after birth, fully developed social smiles occur between 3 and 5 wk. Their absence at 8–12 wk should be investigated. Complex patterns and rhythms of feeding, sleeping, and interactions with caretaker evolve throughout this period and are highly dependent on responses of a loving, communicative, confident, nurturing mother or other caretaker.

3–6 MONTHS

Neurodevelopment

By 3 mo an infant on a firm surface can raise his or her head and chest with arms extended. By 4 mo the head can be raised to a vertical axis and turned easily side to side; when the infant is pulled from supine to sitting position, the head is brought up without lag and held steady without bobbing. By 5–6 mo the infant begins purposely to roll over.

By 3–4 mo the infant gradually abandons the tonic neck attitude as the predominant posture for one in which the head is generally maintained in the midline, the arms and legs in symmetric positions, and the hands together in the midline or at the mouth. The 4–6-mo-old infant often develops a bald spot over the occiput.

By 4 mo infants become more adept at making contact with objects of moderate size, grasping them, and bring them to the midline and to the mouth for visual and oral exploration. By 6–6½ mo most infants can grasp a large object such as a rattle and transfer it from hand to hand. With growing skills in manipulating hands and arms, infants discover the rest of their body parts.

At 5–6 mo infants can often be pulled from a sitting to a standing position and support their weight on extended legs. Often they can sit alone, leaning forward on their hands.

Psychosocial Development

By 4 mo, infants laugh aloud at pleasurable social contacts and show displeasure by changes of expression, fussing, or crying. Between 4 and 7 mo infants become increasingly responsive to the emotional tone of social contacts and develop clear preferences for those persons giving them the most care.

6–12 MONTHS

Neurodevelopment

By 7 mo prone infants can pivot in pursuit of an object. By 8–9 mo they can assume a sitting position without help and are soon able to maintain it with the back straight. By 9–10 mo most infants can creep or crawl. Between 8 and 9 mo infants are often able to stand steadily for a short time as long as their hands are held, and by 9 mo they can take a few steps similarly supported.

Between 6 and 9 mo the radial–palmar grasp evolves into movements involving the thumb and forefinger. By 12 mo many infants can pick up a small pellet with a pincer motion. Between 6 and 12 mo the infant becomes more imitative. By 9 mo they can wave bye-bye. By 12 mo infants enjoy simple games with a toy such as a ball and can extend and release objects into an offered hand.

Cognitive Development

Infants discover *object permanence* and by 9 mo are aware that covering an object does not mean that the object is not available.

Language

The infant can make repetitive vowel sounds by 6½ mo and repetitive consonant sounds (*ba-ba, ma-ma*) by 8 mo. By 8–9 mo they recognize their own name and may knowingly use a few words.

Psychosocial Development

Anxiety on separation from the regular caretaker develops between 6 and 8 mo. Children may be less willing to go to sleep and become fretful when mother leaves the room. By 9–10 mo the peek-a-boo game is played and infants usually are less dependent on the physical presence of the caretaker.

THE SECOND YEAR
(*NELSON TEXTBOOK*, SEC. 3.6)

PHYSICAL DEVELOPMENT

There is further deceleration of the growth rate, with the average child gaining about 2.5 kg (5–6 lb) in weight and about 12 cm (5 in) in length during this year. A decrease in appetite may start at about 10 mo and extend into the 2nd yr, with a loss of some subcutaneous tissue, which develops maximally by about 9 mo. With upright position, the 2nd and 3rd yr are characterized by mild lordosis and protuberant abdomen.

The growth of the brain also continues to decelerate and the head circumference increases only about 2 cm during the 2nd yr. At the end of the 1st yr the brain is two thirds and at the end of the 2nd yr four fifths of its adult size.

Eight more teeth erupt, making a total of 14–16. The order of eruption is irregular.

NEURODEVELOPMENT

By 12 mo most infants can rise independently and walk a few steps alone; by 18 mo they can run stiffly and climb stairs if one hand is held. By 20 mo the child can usually go downstairs with one hand held and climb stairs holding onto a railing. They can move quickly and need constant surveillance.

By 15 mo the child can place a pellet into a small bottle and put 1 cube on top of another. At 18 mo they can dump the pellet from the bottle and make a tower of cubes. Imitative and conceptual behavior continues to evolve with spontaneous scribbling and copying vertical lines. By 24 mo the child can imitate circular strokes and can make a horizontal line.

During this year children vigorously explore and imitatively exploit objects in their environment (e.g., empty wastebaskets, drawers, and shelves) and examine anything within reach.

COGNITIVE DEVELOPMENT

During this year children develop a sense of self separate from other persons and recognize their own capacity to initiate and choose behaviors. There is increasing concern about expectations of adults and order in daily activities.

LANGUAGE

By 18 mo vocabulary is about 10 words. However, there is wide variation and it is not unusual to have few or no sounds conveying definite meaning by this time. There may be a rich jargon of intonations and punctuations of speech that conveys no meaning. By 24 mo most children can put two or three words together.

PSYCHOSOCIAL DEVELOPMENT

Until the end of the 2nd yr, play is usually solitary. There may be contests with other children over control of objects. By 18–24 mo most children verbalize their toilet needs and can be helped to meet them with acceptable social patterns.

PRESCHOOL YEARS
(NELSON TEXTBOOK, SEC. 3.7)

PHYSICAL DEVELOPMENT

During this period gains in weight and height are steady at about 2.0 kg (4.5 lb) and 6–8 cm (2.5–3.5 in) per year. Most children are lean compared to body configuration at younger ages. The lordosis and protuberant abdomen of late infancy tend to disappear by 4 yr. By 2½ yr 20 deciduous teeth have erupted, and during this preschool period the face tends to grow proportionately more than the cranial cavity and the jaw widens.

NEURODEVELOPMENT

Alternation of feet is used to ascend stairs by 3 yr and to descend stairs by 4 yr. By 3 yr most children can stand on one foot for a short time; by 5 yr they can hop on one foot, and soon after skip.

A 3-yr-old can crudely imitate drawing a cross and when requested draw a head-and-stick-extremities person. By 4–5 yr they can make correctly proportionate copies of figures, including slanting lines. Such figures become increasingly sophisticated, with anatomic details and clothing, over this period. By 6 yr the child can translate abstract conceptions into figures and structures (e.g., sound of T into letter T).

LANGUAGE

A child puts sentences together to sustain a brief conversation during the 3rd yr, and by 5 yr language is used in social functions such as role playing. The development of language is influenced greatly by the quality and quantity of language used within the home.

PSYCHOSOCIAL DEVELOPMENT

By 3 yr most children can state their ages and whether they are boys or girls. They are increasingly aware that they are destined to become large children and adults. From 4 to 6 yr they increasingly seek adequate models and assume habits of thought, feeling, and action that represent growing perceptions or fantasies of the future (e.g., pretend to be same-sex parent).

Play activities increasingly involve other children, first in parallel and then interactively. Imaginative roles and activities also increase, and this continues into the school years. Sex play is common.

EARLY SCHOOL YEARS
(*NELSON TEXTBOOK*, SEC. 3.8)

PHYSICAL DEVELOPMENT

This is a period of relatively steady growth that ends in the preadolescent growth spurt (by about 10 yr in girls and 12 yr in boys). The average gain in weight is 3–3.5 kg (7 lb)/yr, and that in height 6 cm (2.5 in)/yr. Head circumference increases about 1 in between 5 and 12 yrs (51 cm [20 in] to 53–54 cm [21 in]), by which time the brain is about adult size. Facial bones actively develop, particularly with enlargement of nasal accessory sinuses. The frontal sinus is apparent by 7 yr.

The first permanent teeth, so-called 6-yr molars, usually erupt during the 7th yr, when shedding of deciduous teeth begins in about the same sequence as their acquisition. The 2nd permanent molars commonly erupt by the 14th yr.

During these years of vigorous physical activities, the spine becomes straighter and the body more supple. Mild degrees of knock-knees or flatfoot tend to correct themselves. Motor activities become more specialized.

Lymphatic tissue peaks in its development, exceeding in

amount that of adult years. Respiratory infections are common (6–7/yr).

COGNITIVE DEVELOPMENT

The child is increasingly capable of monitoring his or her own mental processes. Concepts of volume, mass, and perspective are achieved.

PSYCHOSOCIAL DEVELOPMENT

As children spend more time away from home, they develop greater independence and look to others in addition to family members for goals, values, and standards of behavior. During this period a sense of duty, responsibility, and realistic accomplishment are developed.

ADOLESCENCE
(*NELSON TEXTBOOK*, SEC. 3.9 AND CHAP. 10)

Adolescence is defined in terms of the stages of pubertal development because these follow a consistent pattern for individuals of each sex regardless of chronologic age. These stages (Tanner) or sex maturity ratings (SMRs) are defined in Tables 1–3 and 1–4. In females, an increase in body fat content is associated with each successive stage. In contrast, after SMR 2 males become more muscular.

TABLE 1–3. CLASSIFICATION OF SEX MATURITY STAGES IN GIRLS*

SMR Stage	Pubic Hair	Breasts
1	Preadolescent	Preadolescent
2	Sparse, lightly pigmented, straight, medial border of labia	Breast and papilla elevated as small mound; areolar diameter increased
3	Darker, beginning to curl, increased amount	Breast and areola enlarged, no contour separation
4	Coarse, curly, abundant but amount less than in adult	Areola and papilla form secondary mound
5	Adult feminine triangle, spread to medial surface of thighs	Mature; nipple projects, areola part of general breast contour

* From Behrman RE (ed): Nelson Textbook of Pediatrics, 14th ed. Philadelphia, WB Saunders Company, 1992, p. 29.
(Adapted from Tanner JM: Growth at Adolescence, 2nd ed. Oxford, Blackwell Scientific Publications, 1962.)

TABLE 1–4. CLASSIFICATION OF SEX MATURITY STAGES IN BOYS*

SMR Stage	Pubic Hair	Penis	Testes
1	None	Preadolescent	Preadolescent
2	Scanty, long, slightly pigmented	Slight enlargement	Enlarged scrotum, pink texture altered
3	Darker, starts to curl, small amount	Longer	Larger
4	Resembles adult type, but less in quantity; coarse, curly	Larger, glans and breadth increase in size	Larger, scrotum dark
5	Adult distribution, spread to medial surface of thighs	Adult size	Adult size

* From Behrman RE (ed): Nelson Textbook of Pediatrics, 14th ed. Philadelphia, WB Saunders Company, 1992, p. 30. (Adapted from Tanner JM: Growth at Adolescence, 2nd ed. Oxford, Blackwell Scientific Publications, 1962.)

EARLY ADOLESCENCE

This refers to the first stage of puberty (SMR 2), which ranges (±2SD) in age of onset from 10.5 to 14 yr in boys and from 10 to 13 yr in girls. The duration in boys is 0.5 to 2 yr and in girls 0.2 to 1.2 yr.

Physical Development

In females, follicle-stimulating hormone (FSH) stimulates growth of the ovaries in late SMR 1, which increases estrogens that produce the breast bud development of SMR 2; thickening of the vaginal mucosa; increased pigmentation, vascularization, and eroticization of the labia majora; slight enlargement of the clitoris and uterus; and development of the endometrium and myometrium.

In males, the testes enlarge as a result of an increase in the size of the seminiferous tubules and number of Leydig and Sertoli cells. The abundant increased secretion of testosterone causes enlargement of the epididymis, seminal vesicles, and prostate. The scrotum thins and becomes hypervascular. Enlargement of the penis begins shortly thereafter. In 3–5% of males there also may be some, usually mild, breast development (gynecomastia).

In both sexes adrenal androgen secretion is responsible for initiation of growth of pubic and axillary hair and increase in size and secretion of sebacious follicles. Ejaculation in males usually occurs approximately 1 yr following the onset of testicular growth at the time of appearance of pubic hair.

Dentition

The cuspids and first molars are shed and the permanent 1st and 2nd premolars and molars erupt.

Neurodevelopment

There should be mature responses.

Cognitive Development

A broad range of cognitive achievement occurs among children who are in SMR 2.

Psychosocial Development

Initiation of strivings for independence conflict with desires for limit setting. There is also a desire for privacy and distancing from physical affection by parents of the opposite sex. There is a turning toward same-sex peer groups for friendships. Synchrony of pubertal development with that of the peer group is particularly important.

MIDDLE ADOLESCENCE

This is defined as SMR 2 and 3. The age of onset is normally 12.5 to 15 yr in boys and 12 to 14 yr in girls. It lasts 0.5 to 2 yr in boys and 0.9 to 3 yr (pubic hair) or 7 yr (breasts) in girls. It is a period of acceleration of upright and linear growth as well as further development of secondary sex characteristics. The bulk of fat tissue in females and muscle tissue in males is deposited.

Physical Development

Females average an 8-cm/yr increment in height at 12 yr; males average 10 cm/yr at 14 yr. Skeletal growth progresses from distal to proximal parts of the body. The longer arms and legs of males, relative to their total body length, results from the later onset of their growth spurt compared to females. Elongation of the trunk and increase in anterior–posterior diameter of the chest are late manifestations of the growth spurt.

Although the changes in secondary sex characteristics of SMR 3 and 4 characterize this period, the onset of menarche is the most dramatic event and its timing is related to these changes. In the United States menarche occurs at a mean of 12.5 yr. Sixty percent of females are SMR 4 at menarche, but a variety of genetic, nutritional, and other factors influence this timing.

Circumanal hair growth antedates axillary and facial hair, which appear about when pubic hair reaches SMR 4. Body odor parallels development of axillary hairs as a result of androgenic stimulation of apocrine sweat glands.

Gynecomastia occurs in many males during this period.

Neurodevelopment

This is completed.

Cognitive Development

This continues the trends set in early adolescence.

Psychosocial Development

School and peer groups gain in importance and sex differences in peer relationships become more apparent. Needs for achievement, independence, interpersonal skills, loyalty, intimacy of shared information, and development of self-image dominate this period. Interaction between parents and children changes during this period.

Dating behavior goes through a progression of increasing sexual activity during middle adolescence, with increased risk of sexually transmitted disease and pregnancy.

Vocational and educational decisions are of primary concern.

LATE ADOLESCENCE

This usually has its onset from 14 to 16 yr in boys and 14 to 17 yr in girls. The end of these changes is generally reached between the ages of 17 and 21 yr.

Physical Development

The body approximates young adult size and proportions. Little additional linear growth occurs after the growth spurt of middle adolescence, and the remaining epiphyses become fused. In addition to the changes in secondary sex characteristics, which characterize SMR 5, there is a deepening of the male voice and a relative enlargement of the uterine fundus.

Psychosocial Development

Cognitive, social, and moral development continue to evolve through the rest of life. The ability to dialogue with parents and to engage in empathetic intimate relationships with others increases.

ASSESSMENT OF GROWTH AND DEVELOPMENT
(NELSON TEXTBOOK, SEC. 3.10)

The determination of whether or not the growth and development of a particular child is normal should be based on accurate information and, when possible, serial observations over months or years.

HEAD CIRCUMFERENCE, LENGTH (STATURE), WEIGHT

Standard reference charts depict patterns of normal growth of these measurements, with indications of their variability (percentiles). These should be used to compare a patient to other children of the same age and are particularly useful when serial measurements are available. Children whose height, weight, or head circumference at any given time in relation to other children of the same age is above or below the 10th percentile may deserve further consideration. Sequential measurements, family patterns, and SMRs are particularly important in such evaluations.

Reference data relating to the distribution of relationships between weight and length (height or stature) regardless of age are also available. In general, children whose weights are less than the 5th percentile or over the 95th percentile for their actual heights should receive further evaluation. The combination of these reference standards and those relating a given measurement to age may be particularly useful; for example, children with low heights for age who have acceptable weight for height may have experienced nutritional growth failure in the past, whereas if both height for age and weight for height are strikingly low, both past and current growth failure may be suspected. In contrast, children with normal height for age who have conspicuously low weight for height are likely to have either relatively acute nutritional or growth problems or variant physiques.

BODY PROPORTIONS AND ORGAN SYSTEMS

In addition to changes in body proportions, variations in body forms of normal children may be expressed as differences in physique:

1. Ectomorph, characterized by relative linearity, light bone structure, and small mass relative to length.

TABLE 1–5. APPROXIMATION OF SURFACE AREA TO WEIGHT*

Weight Range†	Approximate Surface Area
1–5 kg	$m^2 = (0.05 \times kg) + 0.05$
6–10 kg	$m^2 = (0.04 \times kg) + 0.10$
11–20 kg	$m^2 = (0.03 \times kg) + 0.20$
21–40 kg	$m^2 = (0.02 \times kg) + 0.40$

* From Behrman RE (ed): Nelson Textbook of Pediatrics, 14th ed. Philadelphia, WB Saunders Company, 1992, p. 40.
† The figures 5, 10, 20, and 40 are given in italics to indicate a simple mnemonic. The formula $m^2 = (0.02 \times kg) + 0.40$ gives reasonable estimates from 21 to 70 kg.

2. Endomorph, characterized by relatively stocky build, with large amounts of soft tissue;
3. Mesomorph, in between 1 and 2 and often relatively muscular.

Other variations in body proportions depend on different rates of growth of body parts; for example, the size of the brain and cranial cavity approach adult proportions more rapidly than the size of the face or length of the legs. Alterations in proportionate sizes of trunk, extremities, and head are characteristic of certain growth disturbances and underlying pathophysiologic processes. Several body systems also show distinct variations in growth that often correlate closely with function; for example, the lymphoid tissue, including thymus and spleen, of the school-age child exceeds that of an adult, and subcutaneous tissue is greatest at about 9 mo.

Ossification of the skeleton and dental development have distinct patterns that must be considered in assessing possible abnormalities.

Functional changes are also relevant to the assessment of growth and development. For example, there is a pubertal growth in heart size that parallels the general growth spurt and relates to changes in heart rate and blood pressure. Calorie needs increase with growth in size but maintain a relatively constant relationship to body surface area, which appears to be relatively closely correlated with the body's mass of metabolically active tissue (Table 1–5).

PSYCHOSOCIAL DIMENSIONS OF PEDIATRICS
(*NELSON TEXTBOOK*, SECS. 3.13–3.21)

This section deals with the *psychic* (internal) and *social* (external) dimensions of the activities, functions, and behaviors of children. The former consist of feelings, attitude, thoughts, fantasies, memory, judgment, values, and self-image. The latter encompass relationships with the environment, people, and circumstances in which the child lives. The psychosocial perspective considers the child's emotional and social development and its deviations and disturbances in terms of interactions between the child and the environment. It includes the integration of cognitive and affective processes and the formation of conscience and its exercise. Various theories are helpful in partially understanding the complex nature of psychosocial development (medical or physiologic, psychoanalytic, cognitive, behavioral).

SPECIAL SOCIAL ISSUES

Adoption

This issue is managed successfully by most adopted children and their families. Ideally placement should be made as soon after birth as possible to foster attachment and bonding. Adoptions of older children or across racial or religious lines or by single parents present increased adjustment risks. Adopted children should be informed of the adoption as soon as they have reasonably good verbal facility and comprehension, usually by 3–4 yr. There is current controversy about providing adopted children access to information about their biologic parents.

Foster Care

Placement is typically provided by local welfare agencies for abandonment, severe neglect, or abuse. Children of substance-abusing women present a growing problem. Frequent changes in foster parents, fragmented social, education, and health services, and decreased access to needed services may exacerbate the problems of children in foster care.

Family Mobility

Changes in residence may create significant direct and indirect stress on children. Children should be appropriately prepared in advance of a move and may require special attention during a transition period of resettling.

Separation and Death

Enduring and frequent separations may cause significant sequellae and even brief separations may present minor untoward transient effects. Manifestations depend on the child's age and stage of development. Reactions to reunions may also be problematic. For some the effects of divorce are long lasting. The mourning process after the death of a parent is not typical of that experienced by a mourning adult, is highly dependent on the child's developmental stage, and requires sensitive attention to the details of a given child's reactions to the death. In general, children should participate appropriately in the rituals that surround the death and burial of a parent.

PSYCHOSOCIAL PROBLEMS
(*NELSON TEXTBOOK*, SECS. 3.22–3.50)

Psychiatric Sequelae of Central Nervous System Injury

Children with brain damage, epilepsy, and mental retardation have an increased frequency of behavioral disorders.

Those with hydrocephalus, motor deficits, and encephalitis also have a greater than average incidence of psychiatric disorders. Low intelligence, language disorders, and bilaterality of motor handicaps increase the incidence of psychiatric disturbances. No specific type of disturbance is encountered, and, when problems of impulse or anger control, aggressiveness, hyperactivity, or other emotional reactions occur, they do not differ in quality from those of children with intact nervous systems who have the same disturbances. The most significant factor in a child's adjustment to a chronic handicapping organic condition is the capacity of his or her parents to adjust and cope. Therefore, understanding a family's psychosocial supports is critical to management. Neuroleptic drugs may also be helpful for some children.

Psychosomatic Disorders

In these disorders psychological conflict significantly alters somatic function. Any kind of emotional distress may be associated with any kind of disorder.

Conversion disorders (reactions), the loss or alteration of physical functioning without a demonstrable organic illness (e.g., gait disturbance, paralysis, blindness), usually start suddenly and often can be traced to a precipitating environmental event. The manifestations often end abruptly after a short period and are more common during adolescence.

Hypochondriasis refers to a preoccupation with the fear of having a serious illness and the use of multiple somatic complaints to assuage inner tension. This is most common in older children and adolescents, and often there is an adult role model with similar complaints.

Psychophysiologic disorders are characterized by chronic anxiety that produces functional abnormalities within the autonomic nervous system, leading to structural changes within organ systems (e.g., some cases of eczema, asthma, ulcerative colitis, and peptic ulcer).

Treatment of these disorders requires awareness that symptoms are not within conscious control, early psychiatric assessment, parental acceptance of the emotional basis of the problem, and psychotherapy.

Rumination

Repeated regurgitation of food without nausea or associated gastrointestinal illness may rarely lead to weight loss or failure to gain weight. The disorder appears between 3 and 14 mo, is potentially fatal, and often, but not invariably, is associated with a disturbed parent–child relationship. *Treatment* involves positively reinforcing correct eating behavior, negatively reinforcing rumination, adverse conditioning, and family counseling and therapy.

Pica

This refers to chronic ingestion of nonnutrient substances (e.g., plastic, paint, earth) usually at 1–2 yr of age. It may be a symptom of family disorganization, poor supervision, and affectional neglect. There is an increased risk of lead poisoning and parasitic infection.

Enuresis (Bedwetting)

The involuntary discharge of urine after the age at which bladder control should have been established is a common problem, more frequent in boys than girls. When the child has never been dry at night, bedwetting is often related to inadequate or inappropriate toilet training. When bedwetting occurs in a child who had previously been dry at night, it is often precipitated by stressful environmental events, intermittent, transitory, and more easy to manage. Very infrequently there is organic pathology.

Treatment consists of enlisting the cooperation of the child and instituting an appropriate reward system, requiring older children to launder soiled bedclothes and pajamas, withholding liquids after dinner, and voiding before bedtime. Occasionally conditioning devices (alarms) may be useful. Imipramine (Tofranil) administration usually has only a brief effect and symptoms may exacerbate after its discontinuance.

Encopresis

This refers to defecation into inappropriate places at any age after bowel control should have been established. Organic defects are rarely found. Chronic soiling is often associated with chronic constipation, fecal impaction, and overflow incontinence. It may progress to psychogenic megacolon. This symptom often represents the child's unconscious anger and defiance.

Supportive *treatment* similar to that used in enuresis may be helpful, including judicious use of mineral oil, high-fiber diet, sitting on the toilet 10–15 min after each meal, and rewards. However, psychotherapy is usually required.

Sleep Disorders

These are common in childhood, and separation anxiety often contributes to the problem. They are usually adequately managed by parental support, reassurance, encouragement, and the adoption of a calm, understanding, but firm attitude. A quiet period before bedtime and regular bedtime hours are important.

Night terrors, consisting of an acute arousal with confusion, anxiety, disorientation, and autonomic activity, may occur in the preschool years. They are usually self-limited and respond to parental reassurance.

Habit Disorders

At different development stages children may manifest various patterns of repetitive movement (habits). When these patterns interfere with the child's physical, emotional, or social functioning, they are considered disorders.

Teeth grinding may result in dental occlusion. It may be relieved by making bedtime more relaxed and enjoyable, relieving anxiety, and providing emotional support.

Thumbsucking, normal in early infancy, makes the older child appear immature and may interfere with normal alignment of the teeth. Parents should ignore the thumbsucking but give attention to more positive aspects of the child's behavior and provide praise and encouragement for the child who tries to restrain thumbsucking.

Tics are repetitive movements that appear to represent discharges of tension. Undue parental attention can reinforce tics, and ignoring them often decreases their occurrence. Siezures must be distinguished from tics.

Stuttering usually resolves spontaneously, but if it does not respond to time and emotional support, a speech therapist should be consulted.

Anxiety Disorders

When anxieties, which are a normal aspect of development, become detached from specific situations, or become socially disabling, they constitute disorders requiring treatment.

School phobias, in which, for various reasons, a child will not attend school, occur in 1–2% of children and are often associated with depression as well as anxiety. Management involves treatment of underlying psychiatric problems, family therapy, and liaison work with the child's school.

Separation anxiety disorders are characterized by unrealistic and persistent worries of possible harm befalling primary caregivers, reluctance to go to school or to sleep without being near parents, avoidance of being alone, nightmares involving separation themes, somatic symptoms, and complaints of subjective distress. Supportive child and family psychotherapy, and parent training are usually effective. Antidepressant and antianxiety medicines may be necessary as adjunctive treatment.

Obsessive–compulsive disorders are characterized by repetitive thoughts that invade consciousness and repetitive rituals or behaviors that interfere with normal functioning. Treatment includes overexposure to the situations that lead to the symptoms and anxiety and pharmacotherapy with clomipramine, fluoxetine, and fluvoxamine.

Affective Disorders

Major depression in infancy is characterized by separation from the primary caregiver after 6–7 mo of age, leading to crying, searching, panic-like behavior, and hypermobility. Subsequently these infants become apathetic, hypotonic, and inactive, cry silently, stare into space, and have a sad expression. Therapy consists of reestablishment of a nurturing environment with a constant caring adult. In school-age children this disorder develops over a period of days or weeks and presents with a variety of symptoms, including sad facial expression, easy tears, irritability, withdrawal, and eating and sleeping disturbances. Adolescents typically present with impulsivity, fatigue, depression, and suicidal ideation. They may develop hallucinations and delusions. Treatment includes tricyclic antidepressants and psychotherapy.

Dysthymic disorder is characterized by more intermittent periods of a normal mode, lasting days to weeks, than in major depression. The course is less intense but more chronic, lasting up to several years. Disruptions in important relationships may start as early as infancy. There is often a history of depressive illness in both parents. Some present the picture of helpless, passive, clinging, dependent, lonely children; others become hardened, aloof, and negativistic. Antidepressive pharmacotherapy may be useful, especially in those with vegetative symptoms of depression. When symptoms are secondary to an underlying disorder (e.g., substance abuse, physical illness, anorexia), these problems also need to be treated.

Manic–depressive bipolar disorder usually occurs after puberty and initially presents as a major depressive disorder in some adolescents. Manic symptoms include overactivity, loquaciousness, insomnia, and paranoid delusions. Lithium carbonate is effective in treating bipolar illness and manic symptoms. Individual and family psychotherapy are important.

Suicide and Attempted Suicide

This is a major problem in adolescence, and the incidence is rising in children under 15 yr. Completed suicides are associated with preceding suicide attempts, depression, general psychopathologic factors, family history of suicidal behavior or depression or drug use, suicidal ideation, preoccupation with death and dying, wish to die, feelings of hopelessness or worthlessness, hostility and the notion of revenge, and substance abuse.

Treatment of threats and attempts at suicide should be managed:

1. Take threat seriously and admit to a hospital.
2. Explore in detail the child's life during the preceding 48–72 hr to identify precipitating events, risk factors, and the degree of premeditation or impulsivity.
3. Try to determine whether the patient intended to stop or to be discovered and whether the behavior prior to, or subsequent to, the attempt promoted or impeded the patient's being discovered before or after the attempt. The choice of method used or proposed and closeness or remoteness of help are important in making this judgment
4. Arrange for social service and psychiatric evaluation to aid in a decision about subsequent disposition.

Disruptive Behavioral Disorders

Numerous behaviors considered appropriate at certain developmental stages (e.g., lying, breath-holding, defiance, and temper tantrums, which frequently occur at 2–4 yr) are obviously pathologic when present at later ages. Others are never developmentally appropriate (e.g., truancy, runaway behavior, fire-setting).

Breath-holding may be severe enough to result in loss of consciousness or seizures. There are no sequellae, and parents are best advised to ignore the behavior and leave the room because without sufficient reinforcement the behavior soon disappears.

Defiance, oppositionalism, and temper tantrums should be dealt with by acknowledging verbally to the child that the reasons for his or her frustration are understandable but the particular response is unacceptable. The child should be given time and space to recover. If the child is unable to give up the behavior, parents should nonemotionally impose time out or room restrictions. Choices of acceptable activity should, where possible, be given to the child.

Lying in a 2–4-yr-old may represent playing with language, fantasy, or a way of delaying an unpleasant confrontation. In school-age children it often represents an attempt to avoid the pain of a loss of self-esteem. Many adolescents lie to avoid parental disapproval. Regardless of age, when lying becomes a frequent way of managing conflict and anxiety, intervention is warranted. Parents should confront the child and give a clear message of what is acceptable coupled with support and sensitivity to avoid shaming the child. Psychotherapy is indicated if the problem is unresponsive to such measures.

Aggressive behavior and conduct disorders may be manifest in a variety of antisocial activities. Conduct disorder is a severe entity manifested by a combination of several of the following over a period of at least 6 mo: stealing, lying, fire-setting, truancy, property destruction, cruelty to animals, rape, use of a weapon while fighting, armed robbery, cruelty to others, and repeated runaway attempts. Treatment of aggressive behavior may necessitate a variety of individual, group, and family psychotherapeutic approaches when parents and others are unable to cope with the child's behavior.

Sexual Behavior and Its Variations

Children establish *gender identity*—identify themselves as boys or girls—by about 18 mo and understand that boys become men and girls become women by 18–30 mo. By 30 mo gender usually is firmly established and resistant to change. During adolescence the final decision about same- or different-sex gender object choice is often made.

Transsexualism is the conviction by a person biologically of one gender that he or she is a member of the other gender. *Transvestism* (cross-dressing) may occur transiently as an isolated behavior, more commonly in boys than girls, or may be chronic, associated with other sexual behaviors that suggest gender role confusion. Persistent distress of a child or parents about gender identity or behavior requires sensitive expert counseling.

Psychosis

Infantile autism is characterized by qualitative impairment in verbal and nonverbal communication, in imaginative activity, and in reciprocal social interactions. It occurs before 30 mo. Psychotherapy and psychopharmacology are of limited benefit.

Children may have *pervasive developmental disorders* involving social interaction and communication not qualifying for the diagnosis of autism. The psychotic reactions of older children tend to resemble adult disorders and require evaluation and management by pediatric psychiatrists.

Psychological Reactions to Stress in Children

Acute and chronic physical illnesses, hospitalization, or procedures may result in a variety of untoward behaviors in children that require various degrees of supportive psychotherapy for the child and family in order to avoid or ameliorate longer term psychological illness.

ABUSE AND NEGLECT OF CHILDREN
(*NELSON TEXTBOOK*, SECS. 3.51–3.53)

This encompasses any maltreatment of children or adolescents by those responsible for caring for them. Physician's responsibilities to these children include detection, reporting, prevention, and treatment. Neglect includes failure to seek adequate medical care for a child or to provide food, shelter, clothes, appropriate hygiene, and other necessities.

PHYSICAL ABUSE

About 70% of abused children suffer from physical injuries; two thirds of these children are under 6 yr of age. The abuser is a related caretaker or friend of the mother in 95% of cases. Abusing parents are often lonely, unhappy adults under stress who respond with anger to some misbehavior of the child. The event usually is related to a family crisis.

This diagnosis should be suspected when:

1. Medical findings are unexplained or inconsistent with the offered history.
2. The child suggests the injury was caused by an adult.
3. There are pathognomonic bruises, burns, scars, or injuries—for example, bruises of buttocks and lower back, finger and thumb prints on extremities, human bite marks, characteristic cigarette burns, lash and choke marks, subdural hematomas, metaphyseal fractures, multiple bony injuries at different stages of healing, and circular burns from hot water emersion.

A child suspected of being abused must be reported to a Child Protective Services (CPS) agency immediately and cannot be legally discharged from a clinic or office without consulting this agency. A safe caretaking arrangement must be established. Hospitalization may be indicated for ongoing medical care or if the diagnosis is unclear. The risk for serious reabuse, including death, is significant. Treatment usually requires multiple medical and social services.

SEXUAL ABUSE

This includes *molestation* (touching or fondling of the child's genitalia or asking the child to fondle the adult's genitals or forced exposure to sexual acts or pornography); *sexual intercourse* (vaginal, oral, or rectal penetration or attempted penetration on a nonassaultive basis); and *rape* (forced or assaultive intercourse). Sexual abuse by family members (incest) is the most common form, abuse by friends or acquaintances next most frequent, and that by strangers least common.

Diagnosis usually depends on the graphic history offered by the victim, often preceded by disclosure to the mother or a friend. Physical examination may be corroborative but often is not helpful. Associated conditions or behavior include genital or urinary tract infections, genital or anal trauma, recurrent urethritis, enuresis, encopresis, inappropriate sexual behavior, runaway behavior, substance abuse, suicide attempt, pregnancy, or signs of physical abuse.

Evaluation and management is similar to, but more complex than, that of physical abuse. All sexual abuse is a criminal offense and must be investigated by the police. Psychological support is essential. Treatment of sexually transmitted disease and to prevent pregnancy are also indicated.

NONORGANIC FAILURE TO THRIVE (FTT)

Neglectful failure to provide sufficient food is a form of abuse usually seen in children under 2 yr of age, but may occur in older children who are confined or deliberately starved. Emotional deprivation is concurrent. Unintentional errors in feeding techniques or formula preparation may also occur. These infants usually exhibit thin extremities, narrow face, prominent ribs, and wasted buttocks. Rashes are common, and these children are often dirty. In addition to reporting these children to CPS and providing other management appropriate to abused and neglected children, intensive nutritional support is required.

NEURODEVELOPMENTAL DYSFUNCTION IN THE SCHOOL-AGE CHILD (Learning Disorders)

These impairments of development are often associated with academic underachievement, behavioral difficulties, problems of social adjustment, and considerable distress of the affected child and his or her parents. The cause usually cannot be determined, but an association between learning disorders and a broad variety of problems has been suggested (e.g., from abnormal chromosome patterns and low-level lead intoxication to low birth weight, head trauma, and sociocultural deprivation).

Clinical manifestations vary widely, involving functions such as attention, memory, language, visual–spatial ordering, temporal–sequential ordering, neuromotor function, higher order cognition, and social cognition. Usually more than one function is involved. There is special confusion and disagreement about the definitions and terminology to be applied to deficits in attention (e.g., attention deficit hyperactivity disorder [ADHD] vs. attention deficit disorder [ADD] vs. hyperactivity vs. hyperkenetic impulse disorder vs. minimal brain dysfunction). This issue is significant because, in addition to psychosocial and educational therapy, stimulant medications (methylphenidate, dextroamphetamine, magnesium pemoline) may moderate dysfunctions in some children with certain disorders.

MENTAL RETARDATION

This is one of the most common chronic illnesses of childhood and is characterized by limitations in performance that results from significant impairments in measured intellectual and adaptive behavior. It is the prototype *developmental disability*. Others include cerebral palsy, specific learning disabilities, autism, and visual or hearing impairments.

TABLE 1–6. LEVELS OF SEVERITY OF MENTAL RETARDATION*

Category	Descriptive Features
Borderline (IQ 68–83)	Strictly speaking, children with IQ scores above 69 do not meet the criteria for mental retardation, but they are vulnerable to educational problems. Many such children are able to function adequately with special help in regular classes. Most achieve independent social and vocational adjustment
Mild (IQ 52–67)	This group includes almost 90% of children formally classified as mentally retarded. Most need at least some special class placement, although mainstreaming should be considered, and some can achieve 4th–6th grade reading levels. Those who have well-developed adaptive skills may be able to function independently as adults.
Moderate (IQ 36–51)	Educational goals for children in this group focus primarily on gaining maximal self-care and perhaps some academic skills up to a 2nd-grade level. Those who are well adjusted may be able to function semi-independently in supervised living and sheltered workshop settings.
Severe (IQ 20–35)	Children in this group can learn minimal self-care and simple conversational skills. They need much supervision throughout their lives.
Profound (IQ below 20)	Children in this group require total supervision. Very minimal self-care skills are possible, and few individuals are toilet trained. Language development generally is minimal.

* From Behrman RE (ed): Nelson Textbook of Pediatrics, 14th ed. Philadelphia, WB Saunders Company, 1992, p. 96.

TABLE 1–7. ATYPICAL PHYSICAL FEATURES THAT MAY BE ASSOCIATED WITH INCREASED INCIDENCE OF MENTAL RETARDATION*

Hair
  Double whorl
  Fine, friable, prematurely
    gray or white locks
  Sparse or absent hair
Eyes
  Microphthalmia
  Hypertelorism
  Hypotelorism
  Upward-and-outward or
    downward-and-outward
    slant
  Inner or outer epicanthal
    folds
  Coloboma of iris or retina
  Brushfield spots
  Eccentrically placed pupil
  Nystagmus
Ears
  Low-set pinna
  Simple or abnormal helix
    formation
Nose
  Flattened bridge
  Small size
  Upturned nares
Face
  Increased length of philtrum
  Hypoplasia of maxilla or
    mandible
Mouth
  Inverted V shape of upper lip
  Wide or high-arched palate

Head
  Microcrania
  Macrocrania
Hands
  Short 4th or 5th metacarpals
  Short, stubby fingers
  Long, thin tapered fingers
  Broad thumbs
  Clinodactyly
  Abnormal dermatoglyphics
    (e.g., distal triradius)
  Transverse palmar crease
  Abnormal nails
Feet
  Short 4th or 5th metatarsals
  Overlap of toes
  Short, stubby toes
  Broad, large big toes
  Deep crease leading from
    angle of 1st and 2nd toes
  Abnormal dermatoglyphics
Genitalia
  Ambiguous genitalia
  Micropenis
  Large testicles
Skin
  Café-au-lait spots
  Depigmented nevi
Teeth
  Evidence of abnormal
    enamelogenesis
  Abnormal odontogenesis

* From Behrman RE (ed): Nelson Textbook of Pediatrics, 14th ed. Philadelphia, WB Saunders Company, 1992, p. 96.

The etiology and pathogenesis of mental retardation is diverse. Levels of severity and atypical physical features that may be associated are indicated in Tables 1–6 and 1–7. Treatment should be individualized and may be multidimensional, tailored to the child's developmental level and the etiology, when determined.

2

NUTRITION AND NUTRITIONAL DISORDERS

NUTRITIONAL REQUIREMENTS
(NELSON TEXTBOOK, SECS. 4.1–4.8)

The goal of nutrition is appropriate growth and development and avoidance of deficiency states. Requirements vary with stages of development and genetic and metabolic differences among individuals. Good nutrition helps to prevent illness and to develop physical and mental potential.

Appropriate dietary allowances that prevent deficiency states in most individuals have been identified, but because some essential substances have not been identified, a varied diet after infancy may be the only way of providing them. Only human milk provides all the essentials for a prolonged time.

WATER

The need for water is related to caloric consumption, insensible loss, and specific gravity of urine. The infant, whose water content is higher than the adult's, must consume larger amounts of water per unit body weight compared to the adult; when calculated per unit of caloric intake, the amounts required are almost identical. The range of water requirements of children of different ages under ordinary conditions are presented in Table 2–1.

CALORIES

The unit of heat in metabolism, one large calorie (Cal) or kilocalorie (kcal), refers to the energy content of food. The average calorie requirement in infants is about 45–55 kcal/lb/24 hr (80–120 kcal/kg/24 hr); it decreases to 25 kcal/lb/24 hr at maturity. A child's daily requirement, which depends on the growth pattern, sense of well-being, and satiety, is about 80–120 kcal/kg for the 1st yr of life, with subsequent decreases of about 10 kcal/kg for each succeeding 3-yr period. Puberty requires increased caloric consumption.

PROTEINS

Although there are 24 amino acids, only 9 are essential to new tissue formation; the absence of any one of these results in negative nitrogen balance. The quantity and distribution of these amino acids determines the *biologic value* of proteins.

TABLE 2–1. RANGE OF AVERAGE WATER REQUIREMENTS OF CHILDREN AT DIFFERENT AGES UNDER ORDINARY CONDITIONS*

Age	Average Body Weight (kg)	Total Water in 24 hr (mL)	Water per kg Body Weight in 24 hr (mL)
3 days	3.0	250–300	80–100
10 days	3.2	400–500	125–150
3 mo	5.4	750–850	140–160
6 mo	7.3	950–1100	130–155
9 mo	8.6	1,100–1,250	125–145
1 yr	9.5	1,150–1,300	120–135
2 yr	11.8	1,350–1,500	115–125
4 yr	16.2	1,600–1,800	100–110
6 yr	20.0	1,800–2,000	90–100
10 yr	28.7	2,000–2,500	70–85
14 yr	45.0	2,200–2,700	50–60
18 yr	54.0	2,200–2,700	40–50

* From Behrman RE (ed): Nelson Textbook of Pediatrics, 14th ed. Philadelphia, WB Saunders Company, 1992, p. 107.

CARBOHYDRATES

These supply the bulk of the diet and most of the body's energy needs. Most absorbed sugar is converted to glycogen in the liver; some is directly oxidized in the brain, heart, and elsewhere.

FATS

Fats or their metabolic products are important parts of cell membranes, efficient stores of energy, and vehicles for fat-soluble vitamins (A, D, E, and K). Humans do not synthesize linoleic or linolenic fatty acids, which must be supplied in the diet.

FEEDING OF INFANTS
(*NELSON TEXTBOOK*, SECS. 4.9–4.12)

Cooperation between a mother and her infant is required for successful feeding. The mother's feelings are readily transmitted to the infant and are a large determinant in a pleasurable and effective feeding experience.

Most term infants may start feeding by 6 hr of life, but feedings should be withheld if there is any question about the infant's tolerance of feeding. Mothers who wish to initiate breast-feeding in the delivery room and continue on a demand basis thereafter should be supported. Artificially fed infants should receive sterile water for the first feeding. Formula or breast-feeding is usually provided every 2–4 hr/24 hr.

By the end of the 1st mo 90% of infants have established

a regular schedule. By the end of the 1st wk most term infants want 6–9 feedings/24 hr and have increased their intake from 30 mL to 80–90 mL every 3–4 hr. Feeding is progressing satisfactorily if the infant is no longer losing weight by 4–5 days and is gaining weight by 12–14 days. Individual feeding patterns are highly variable during the first months of life.

Infants cry for many reasons aside from hunger, such as being uncomfortably hot or cold, soiled, wet, or ill. They also cry to gain attention and nurture, which are important to their development.

BREAST-FEEDING

Human milk is the most appropriate of all available milks for the human infant. It is fresh, free of bacteria, and readily available at the proper temperature. It reduces chances of gastrointestinal disturbance secondary to unsanitary conditions or to artificial milk allergy or intolerance. Ingested maternal antibodies and macrophages in colostrum and human milk also provide protection against some infections. If the mother's diet is sufficient and balanced, her milk supplies the necessary nutrients for the infant except for fluoride and, after several months, vitamin D.

Maternal contraindications to breast-feeding include acute maternal infection if the infant does not have the same infection, septicemia, nephritis, eclampsia, profuse hemorrhage, active tuberculosis, typhoid fever, malaria, chronic poor nutrition, substance abuse, AIDS, and severe psychological disturbances. *Infant contraindications* include birth weight less than 2,000 g with a growth rate that requires higher caloric intake than available in breast milk and a weak or debilitated infant who may require gavage feeding of breast milk.

Breast-feeding should be initiated as soon after delivery as the condition of the mother and infant permits. Regular and complete emptying of the breasts is the most satisfactory stimulus to secretion of human milk. The infant should be allowed to empty the breast frequently during the time when only colostrum is being formed in order to facilitate lactation. Once lactation is well established, mothers are capable of producing more milk than their infant needs. Hospital routines and physicians' and nurses' attitudes should be supportive. Appropriate care for tender nipples, a happy relaxed state of mind, avoidance of fatigue, a good diet, appropriate hygiene, and adequate instruction in the technique of breast-feeding, and eventually in weaning, are very important.

FORMULA FEEDING

Whole cow's milk or a modified commercial form of it is the basis of most formulas. Other animal milks and milk substitutes are available for infants who cannot tolerate cow's milk. Sterilization, refrigeration, and processing of formula make it more digestible and reduce the risk of gastrointestinal infections. Infants who do not have an underlying disorder can grow and develop normally if they receive adequate formula feedings. Cow's milk has a higher protein

TABLE 2–2. AVERAGE NUMBER OF FEEDINGS PER 24 HOURS*

Age	Average No. of Feedings in 24 Hours
Birth–1 wk	6–10
1 wk–1 mo	6–8
1–3 mo	5–6
3–7 mo	4–5
4–9 mo	3–4
8–12 mo	3

* From Behrman RE (ed): Nelson Textbook of Pediatrics, 14th ed. Philadelphia, WB Saunders Company, 1992, p. 126.

content than human milk. Commercial formulas modify cow's milk to bring the protein and ash content closer to that of human milk, replace saturated with unsaturated fats, and add vitamins.

Homogenized milk has smaller fat globules and a smaller, less tough protein curd.

Evaporated milk can be kept without refrigeration for long periods of time in unopened cans. The casein–fat curd is smaller and softer than that of boiled whole milk and the lactalbumen is less allergenic. Each fluid ounce contains 44 kcal. Vitamin D is usually added.

Commercially prepared modified milks are usually derived from cow's milk, simulate human milk, contain 20–22 kcal/oz, and are available in liquid and powdered forms. They are fortified with vitamin D, other vitamins, and sometimes iron.

Milk substitutes and hypoallergenic milks include goat's milk, milks consisting of amino acid mixtures or proteins derived from soybeans, and those not containing lactose.

Formulas combine milk, sugar, and water, are modified to produce a smaller curd, and should usually contain 20 kcal/oz. The average number of feedings per 24 hr and the average quantity of each feeding during the first year of life are presented in Table 2–2 and 2–3, respectively. The inter-

TABLE 2–3. AVERAGE QUANTITY OF FEEDINGS*

Age	Average Quantity Taken in Individual Feedings
1st and 2nd wk	2–3 oz (60–90 mL)
3 wk–2 mo	4–5 oz (120–150 mL)
2–3 mo	5–6 oz (150–180 mL)
3–4 mo	6–7 oz (180–210 mL)
5–12 mo	7–8 oz (210–240 mL)

* From Behrman RE (ed): Nelson Textbook of Pediatrics, 14th ed. Philadelphia, WB Saunders Company, 1992, p. 126.

TABLE 2–4. REPRESENTATIVE FORMULAS[*][†]

	1–3 Days	Cal	4–10 Days	Cal	10 Days	Cal
Evaporated milk	6 oz	240	7 oz	280	13 oz	520
Sugar	1 tbsp	60	1 tbsp	60	3 tbsp	180
Water	14 oz		14 oz		17 oz	
	20 oz	300	21 oz	340	30 oz	700
Cal/oz		14		16		22
Cal/100 mL		47		56		70
Whole milk	12 oz	240	14 oz	280	26 oz	520
Sugar	1 tbsp	60	1 tbsp	60	3 tbsp	180
Water	8 oz		7 oz		6 oz	
	20 oz	300	21 oz	340	32 oz	700

[*] From Behrman RE (ed): Nelson Textbook of Pediatrics, 14th ed. Philadelphia, WB Saunders Company, 1992. p. 126.
[†] Total volume is divided into six bottles, and the total intake is regulated by the infant.

val between feedings ranges from 3 to 5 hr. For the first months feedings may be demanded throughout a 24-hr period. Each infant should be primarily responsible for determining the quantity of intake and its timing. These should gradually adjust to the needs of the parent as well as the infant. Representative formulas for the first 10 days of life are presented in Table 2–4. Subsequent adjustments of milk, water, and glucose should be made in accordance with an infant's activity and growth curves.

SOLID FOODS

The introduction of solid foods to the diet before 4–6 mo of age does not contribute significantly to the health of the normal infant, although this may be helpful in extending the interval between nighttime feedings. Usually various precooked cereals are introduced first.

FIRST YEAR FEEDING PROBLEMS
(NELSON TEXTBOOK, SEC. 4.13)

Underfeeding is suggested by restlessness, crying, failure to gain weight adequately, failure to sleep, constipation, and irritability. It may also result from the infant's failure to take a sufficient quantity of food even when offered. It may be caused by inadequate technique, abnormal "bonding," or systemic disease. Treatment consists of increasing fluid and caloric intake and appropriate attention to the cause.

Overfeeding frequently results in regurgitation and vomiting, but may also result in excessive weight gain. Diet adjustment is indicated.

Regurgitation, return of a small amount of swallowed food during or shortly after eating, is common and may be reduced to negligible amounts by improved feeding and handling techniques. *Vomiting*, or more complete emptying of the stomach, is also a common symptom that may be associated with a variety of both trivial and serious disturbances (see *Nelson Textbook*, Secs. 13.13, 13.14, and 13.16).

Loose or mildly diarrheal stools may be secondary to dietary disturbance rather than infection (see *Nelson Textbook*, Secs. 12.10 and 13.59–133.61). Stools of breast-fed infants tend to be softer than those of artificially fed infants, but loose stools also may result from artificial feeding, overfeeding, formulas with high sugar content, or contamination.

Constipation or obstipation is uncommon, especially in breast-fed infants. Insufficient food or fluid, anal fissures, high fat or protein diet, and aganglionic megacolon may be causes.

Colic is a frequent symptom complex consisting of sudden onset of paroxysmal abdominal pain and severe crying, occurring in infants under 3 mo of age and rarely persisting beyond this age. The abdomen is tense and the legs are drawn up on it. A paroxysm may persist for several hours. Supportive management is important.

FEEDING DURING THE SECOND YEAR
(*NELSON TEXTBOOK*, SEC. 4.14)

Most infants adapt to a schedule of three meals each day by the end of the 1st yr of life. Because of the constantly decelerating growth rate, there is a gradual reduction of the infant's caloric intake per unit of body weight toward the end of the 1st yr and during the 2nd yr. Children, including infants, tend to select diets that, over several days, are balanced. Thus, their strong likes or dislikes for particular foods should be respected when possible and practical, as should their decisions about the quantity of intake.

Before 1 yr infants should be allowed to participate in the act of feeding, and they should increasingly be allowed to feed themselves during the 2nd yr. Eating habits formed during this period will affect eating patterns in subsequent years. Nutritious snacks may be given in either or both of the between-meal periods.

NUTRITIONAL DISORDERS
(*NELSON TEXTBOOK*, SECS. 4.15–4.33)

MARASMUS

Severe infantile malnutrition results from inadequate caloric intake and is common in areas where there is insufficient food, inadequate knowledge of feeding techniques, or disturbed parent–child relations. Failure to gain weight is followed by loss of weight, resulting in emaciation. Subcutaneous fat disappears, resulting in wrinkled, loose skin, loss of skin turgor, wizened facial appearance, constipation, flat or distended abdomen, fretfulness, muscle atrophy, and hypotonia. Eventually there may be edema, listlessness, and small mucous stools. Treatment focuses on nutritional and fluid support.

PROTEIN MALNUTRITION (Kwashiorkor)

This syndrome, which is the most serious and prevalent form of malnutrition worldwide, results from a severe deficiency of protein and an inadequate caloric intake. It may become evident from infancy through 5 yr of age, usually after weaning from the breast.

Clinical manifestations initially include lethargy or irritability. Advanced malnutrition results in inadequate growth, lack of stamina, loss of muscle tone, secondary immunodeficiencies and susceptibility to infections, edema, dermatitis, sparse thin red- or grey-streaked hair, and ultimately stupor, coma, and death.

Treatment includes acute management of shock, infection, and organ failure, and fluid and electrolyte replacement. This is followed by nutritional replacement and maintenance.

OBESITY

This disorder is most commonly caused by excess intake of food. It is most frequent in the 1st yr of life, at 5–6 yr of age, and during adolescence. The child whose obesity is due to excess caloric intake usually is not only heavier but taller, with advanced bone age. Psychological disturbances are common. Diet and activity are usually the appropriate treatments, and they are very dependent on motivation.

VITAMINS

Vitamin A Deficiencies

This dietary deficiency usually causes disease by 2–3 yr of age. The disease also may result from chronic malabsorption, including fats. Ocular lesions develop insidiously, initially with impaired night vision and subsequently with drying of the conjunctiva and cornea, photophobia, impaired vision, mental and physical retardation, apathy, and anemia. *Prevention* requires at least 500 mg daily and *treatment* requires oral and intramuscular daily vitamin A until recovery occurs.

Hypervitaminosis A

Acute ingestion of 100,000 mg or more of vitamin A may result in nausea, vomiting, drowsiness, bulging of the fontanel, diplopia, papilledema, cranial nerve palsies, and other symptoms suggesting a brain tumor. Chronic ingestion may result in the insidious onset of anorexia, pruritus, lack of weight gain, irritability, limitation of motion, tender swelling of bones, seborrheic lesions, and eventually the acute clinical manifestations. *Treatment* consists of discontinuation of the excessive intake.

Thiamine (Vitamin B_1) Deficiency (Beriberi)

This water-soluble factor found in cow's milk, vegetables, cereals, fruits, and eggs functions as a coenzyme in carbohydrate metabolism, and deficiency results in impaired nerve condition. Absorption decreases with gastrointestinal or liver disease. *Clinical manifestations* of deficiency include fatigue, apathy, irritability, depression, drowsiness, anorexia, nausea, and abdominal discomfort. Progression results in peripheral neuritis, congestive heart failure, cranial nerve signs, and psychic disturbances. **Wernicke encephalopathy** is characterized by irritability, somnolence, ocular signs, mental confusion, and ataxia. *Diagnosis* is based on response to thiamine. *Treatment* with 10–50 mg of thiamine daily is sufficient, but because other B complex deficiencies may be present, all the other vitamins of the B complex should be administered.

Niacin Deficiency (Pellagra)

Clinical manifestations may initially be vague, consisting of anorexia, lassitude, weakness, burning sensations, numbness, and dizziness. Chronic deficiency is characterized by dermatitis, diarrhea, and dementia. Intense sunlight may exacerbate cutaneous manifestations. Stomatitis, glossitis, vomiting, diarrhea, and nervous symptoms may occur. Evidence of other deficiencies is common. Therefore, the entire B complex should be administered during *treatment*. Sun exposure should be avoided. Liver, lean pork, salmon, poultry, and red meat are good natural sources.

Pyridoxine (Vitamin B₆) Deficiency and Dependency

Etiologies include destruction of pyridoxine by heat processing of cow's milk and cereals, malabsorption syndromes, drug antagonists (e.g., isoniazid), and metabolic errors in enzyme structure or function.

Clinical manifestations of deficiency include:

irritability and seizures in infants fed deficient formulas for 1–6 mo
peripheral neuropathy
skin lesions (cheilosis, glossitis, and seborrhea around the eyes, nose, and mouth)
anemia

Dependency convulsions may occur immediately after birth or months later. Microcytic, hypochronic anemia may also result.

Diagnosis is based on:

ruling out common causes of seizures
response to treatment with pyridoxine
xanthurenic acid in urine after administration of 100 mg/kg of tryptophan

Treatment consists of a single dose of 100 mg pyridoxine IM for deficiency convulsions and 10–100 mg of oral pyridoxine daily for dependency states. Sensory neuropathy may result from excess intake.

Vitamin B₁₂ Deficiency (see chap. 16)

Vitamin C (Ascorbic Acid) Deficiency (Scurvy)

This potent reducing agent is essential in a number of enzymatic activities and in the formation of normal collagen. *Clin-*

ical manifestations usually occur in 6–24-mo-old infants and when fully developed include pain, pseudoparalysis, edematous swelling along shafts of legs, subperiosteal hemorrhage, prominent costochondral junctions, petechial hemorrhages of skin and mucous membranes, and anemia.

Diagnosis is based on:

history of poor intake of vitamin C
characteristic clinical picture
roentgenographic changes in long bones (especially distal ends): loss of trabecula and ground glass appearance

Treatment consists of 100–200 mg/day of ascorbic acid or 3–4 oz of orange or tomato juice daily.

Vitamin D Deficiency (Rickets)

This results in failure of mineralization of growing bone or osteoid tissue, leading to early roentgenographic changes of demineralization in the ends and then the shafts of long bones.

Etiology is related to:

inadequate intake (breast-feeding without vitamin D prophylactic supplementation or unfortified cow's milk)
inadequate exposure to ultraviolet rays of sunlight
clinical conditions that interfere with metabolic conversion (hepatic, renal) or activation of vitamin D or disrupt calcium and phosphorus hemostasis
rapid growth (premature infants)
malabsorption
drugs that interfere with metabolism (anticonvulsants)

Clinical manifestations progress from early osseous signs such as craniotabes, enlargement of costochondral junctions, and thickening of the wrists and ankles to advanced skeletal abnormalities. The latter include enlarged anterior fontanel, box-like and enlarged head, delayed dentition, prominent costochondral junctions, pigeon breast deformity, scoliosis, kyphosis, pelvic deformities, bowlegs, knock-knees, reduced stature, and poor muscle tone. Tetany may also occur.

Diagnosis is based on:

history of inadequate intake or exposure to sunlight, or the presence of a disease state (hepatic, renal, etc.)
physical signs
roentgenographic examination: widened, concave, frayed distal ends of ulna and radius with increased distance from the ends to the metacarpal bones.
abnormal serum findings: normal or low calcium; phosphorus below 4 mg/dL; elevated alkaline phosphatase

Prevention is achieved by providing 10 mg (400 IU) of vitamin D daily and adequate sunlight.

Treatment consists of daily administration of 50–150 mg of vitamin D_3 or 0.5–2 mg of 1,25-dihydroxycholecalciferol. Healing usually is demonstrated in 2–4 wk. A single dose of 15,000 mg of vitamin D also may be used. Tetany secondary to calcium levels less than 7–7.5 mg/dL should be treated by calcium chloride or calcium gluconate administration.

Hypervitaminosis D

Ingestion of excessive amounts of vitamin D may result in hypotonia, anorexia, irritability, constipation, polydipsia, polyuria, pallor, hypercalcemia, and hypercalciuria. Dehydration usually occurs. Vomiting and hypertension also may occur. Renal damage, metastatic calcification, and osteoporosis may result from chronic excessive intake.

Vitamin E Deficiency

Decreased intake, malabsorption, increased requirements resulting from high unsaturated fatty acid diet in prematures, and excess iron administration may produce signs of deficiency.

Clinical manifestations may include muscle weakness, anemia, retinopathy, and a degenerative neurologic syndrome.

Prevention is usually accomplished by a diet of 0.7 mg vitamin E/g of unsaturated fat in the diet. Large doses may be required to prevent neurologic damage from malabsorption, such as occurs with biliary atresia.

Vitamin K Deficiency

Although dietary deficiency may occur, childhood deficiency is usually due to factors affecting absorption (diarrhea) or utilization of fat or factors limiting intestinal bacterial synthesis (antibiotic administration) or the administration of drugs such as dicumarol. Hypoprothrombinemia results.

Clinical manifestations relate to hemorrhage.

Treatment of mild prothrombin deficiency with 1–2 mg vitamin K/day orally is effective in infancy. Severe hypoprothrombinemia with hemorrhagic manifestations requires 5 mg/day of vitamin K_1 parenterally. In hypoprothrombinemia resulting from liver damage, vitamin K usually is not effective.

3

PREVENTIVE PEDIATRICS

Preventive pediatrics aims to avoid rather than cure disease and disability. The remarkable improvements in child health that have occurred in the United States and other developed countries since the turn of this century have mainly been the result of social and economic changes and public health measures, including preventive pediatrics.

PRIMARY PREVENTION
(NELSON TEXTBOOK, SEC. 5.1)

This includes a broad range of activities directed at avoiding disorders before they begin.

COMMUNITY PRIMARY PREVENTION

Programs of major importance that have been universally adopted include sewage disposal, water sanitation, improved housing, hygienic control of food (including milk pasteurization), and mosquito control measures. Other important programs that can have a significant effect on preventing pediatric morbidity and mortality include fluoridation of water; measures to prevent accidents, poisonings, suicides, and homicides; adolescent pregnancy and AIDS prevention programs; and measures to prevent substance abuse.

PEDIATRIC AMBULATORY PRIMARY PREVENTION

The purpose of regularly scheduled child health maintenance visits is to facilitate normal growth and development by evaluating each child's progress, anticipating and ameliorating problems, and preventing disease.

Prenatal discussions with prospective parents may relieve their anxiety, promote understanding of early developmental issues, establish the basis for the future physician–patient–parent relationship, and provide the pediatrician with historical information relevant to anticipating newborn problems.

Newborn care includes physical examinations, prophylaxis for gonococcal eye infection (silver nitrate drops) and hemorrhage disease of the newborn (IM vitamin K), screening tests for phenylketonuria and hypothyroidism, and collection and storage of 15 mL of cord blood for blood typing and other tests, if needed. The general condition of the infant, information about home care and follow-up visits, and reassurance about the availability of a pediatrician for questions should be provided before discharge. A telephone call to the parents is indicated after the baby has been home 1–2 wk. Follow-up visits should depend on the infant's status and parents' previous experience, but an office visit at 3–4 wk after birth usually is indicated to ensure feeding is going well, solve minor problems, and reassure parents.

Schedules for evaluation and preventive measures, including immunizations, are provided in Tables 3–1A and 3–1B. Special considerations in regard to routine immunizations are as follows.

DPT (Diphtheria and Tetanus Toxoids and Pertussis

Three major *contraindications* are:

an acute febrile illness
an evolving or suspected neurologic disease
a severe reaction to a prior dose of DPT

Adverse reactions after DPT include:

local swelling and tenderness at the injection site, slight fever, and irritability (common and minor)
excessive somnolence, protracted inconsolable crying, and an unusual shock-like syndrome (uncommon)
convulsions or manifestations of encephalopathy (rare)

Poliovirus Vaccines

Two types of vaccines are licensed in the United States and are equally protective: (1) OPV, a live, attenuated, trivalent poliovirus vaccine (Sabin); and (2) IPV, an inactivated or killed trivalent poliovirus vaccine (Salk).

OPV should not be given to:

individuals known to be or suspected of being immuno-compromised
household contacts of immunocompromised individuals
subsequent siblings of a child with congenital immunode-ficiency, until the younger children have been shown to be normal

Adults and children traveling to areas where poliomyelitis is endemic should be fully immunized.

MMR (Measles–Mumps–Rubella) Vaccine, Combined

Contraindications include:

pregnancy
immunodeficiency
therapeutic immunosuppression
acute febrile illness
anaphylaxis to egg ingestion

Adverse reactions to MMR include:

transient rashes and fever 6–11 days after immunization to the measles component
transient arthralgias, rare arthritis, and paresthetic pains to the rubella component

TABLE 3–1A. EVALUATION AT SPECIFIC AGES*,†

Procedure	Months							Years									
	2	4	6	9	12	15	18	2	3	4	5	6	8	10	12	14	16
Interview																	
Family history	+																
Pregnancy and delivery	+																+
Neonatal course	+											+					
Other past history	+																
Development evaluation (see Nelson Textbook Sec. 3.11)	+	+	+	+	+	+	+	+	+	+	+	+	+	+	+	+	+
Hearing, vision	+	+	+	+	+	+	+	+	+	+	+	+	+	+	+	+	+
Gastrointestinal (defecation, etc.)	+		+	+	+	+	+	+	+	+	+	+	+	+	+	+	+
Urinary	+				+			+									
Dental care									+	+	+	+	+				
Drugs, alcohol, tobacco														+	+	+	+
Pica														+	+		
Sexual behavior															+	+	+

38

Examination																		
Physical examination	+	+	+	+	+	+	+	+	+	+	+	+	+	+	+	+	+	+
Height and weight	+	+	+	+	+	+	+	+	+	+	+	+	+	+	+	+	+	+
Head circumference	+	+	+	+	+	+	+	+	+									
Blood pressure										+	+	+	+	+	+	+	+	+
Vision																		
Fixes eyes	+																	
Red reflex	+																	
Fundus			+	+														
Strabismus			+	+		+												
Snellen chart										+	+	+	+	+	+	+	+	+
Hearing																		
Gross	+	+	+															
Audiometer										+	+	+	+	+	+	+	+	+
Speech					+		+		+									
Hip dislocation	+	+	+															
Gait				+		+		+										
Scoliosis											+	+	+	+	+	+	+	+
Pubertal development														+	+	+	+	+
Laboratory																		
Hgb or Hct			+	+				+					+	+	+		+	+
Urinalysis			+										+				+	+
Urine culture (girls)											+			+	+	+	+	+
Tuberculin								+					+	+	+	+	+	+

* From Behrman RE (ed): Nelson Textbook of Pediatrics, 14th ed. Philadelphia, WB Saunders Company, 1992, p. 152.
† Note: Interval history and dietary and sleep patterns should be included in each routine visit and are not listed on the table. Items not previously performed, as with an older child who is a new patient, should be carried out at the initial visit.

TABLE 3–1B. PREVENTIVE MEASURES AT SPECIFIC AGES*

Procedure	Months						Years							
	2	4	6	9	12	15	18	2	3	4	5	6	8	10	12	14	16
Immunizations																	
DTP	+	+	+			+†											
Td											+‡						+
OPV	+	+	±	(optional)		+†											
MMR	+	+	+			+	+				+						
Haemophilus influenzae type b	+	+			+					(+)§							
Influenza viral (high risk only)									Annually hereafter							(+)‖	
Pneumococcal (high risk only)								+									

Counseling (for special attention)									
Diet	+	+	+	+	+	+	+	+	+ +
Sleep	+	+	+	+	+	+	+	+	+ +
Toilet training			+	+	+				
Accidents (see Nelson Textbook Sec 6.31)					+				
Day care						+			
School problems						+	+	+	+ +
Puberty and sexuality						+	+	+	+ +
Substance abuse								+	+ +

* From Behrman RE (ed): Nelson Textbook of Pediatrics, 14th ed. Philadelphia, WB Saunders Company, 1992, p. 153.
† The 4th dose of DTP and the 3rd dose of OPV may be given simultaneously with the MMR at 15 mo, or DTP and OPV may be deferred until 18 mo.
‡ Immunization should be on entry to school at 4–6 years.
§ AAP recommends second dose of MMR at 5 yr of age.
‖ United States Public Health Service recommends 2nd dose of MMR at 12 yr of age.

Haemophilus influenzae b (Hib) Vaccine

A conjugated vaccine (HbOC) should be given simultaneously with DTP and OPV at 2, 4, and 6 mo of age, but at a different site; a 4th dose should be given at 15 mo. Alternatively, PRP-OMP conjugated vaccine may be given in two doses, 2 mo apart at 2–6 mo, with a 3rd dose at 12 mo of age.

If Hib is not administered within the first 6 mo, doses are recommended at 7, 11, and 15 mo.

These vaccines do not interfere with DTP, OVP, or MMR.

Delayed immunization of DTP, OVP, and MMR

Unimmunized infants between 2 and 14 mo should be started on the same sequence of immunizations and intervals as younger infants. Children 14 mo to 7 yr also require immunization as indicated in the *Nelson Textbook*, Sec. 5.1.

Special Vaccines

Annual immunization of normal children against viral influenza disease is not indicated. These vaccines are indicated for certain groups of children at high risk from lower respiratory tract infections.

The 23-valent pneumococcal vaccine is not recommended for routine use in children, but is recommended for those over 2 yrs of age with functional or anatomic asplenia.

Newborn infants should be immunized with hepatitis B vaccine and those born to carrier mothers should also receive hepatitis immune globulin (HBIG).

Tuberculin Tests

These should be performed early in the 2nd yr, before school entry, and in early adolescence.

SECONDARY AND TERTIARY PREVENTION
(*NELSON TEXTBOOK*, SEC. 5.2)

These measures involve recognizing and eliminating precursors of disease (screening of blood lipid levels) or efforts to identify and reverse diseases in early stages (scoliosis screening) and measures to ameliorate disabilities arising from established diseases (physiotherapy for contractures), respectively. Many measures listed in Tables 3–1A and 3–1B are secondary preventive efforts. A great deal of the care for chronic illness and disability in childhood represents tertiary prevention.

CHILD HEALTH IN THE DEVELOPING WORLD
(*NELSON TEXTBOOK*, SEC. 5.4)

The health problems that affect very large numbers of children in these areas are:

low birth weight (LBW)

- 27 million of the 137 million infants born annually weigh less than 2,500 g

– LBW infants have 2–3-fold higher mortality than normal-weight infant
– high morbidity is associated with LBW

malnutrition

– aggravated by LBW and infections
– high mortality
– abnormal growth and development

enteric diseases

– high frequency of diarrhea as a result of unsanitary water and food handling
– breast feeding important to prevention
– oral rehydration therapy important to treatment

immunization—preventable diseases

– focus on measles, neonatal tetanus, pertussis, and polio

CHILDREN AT SPECIAL RISK
(NELSON TEXTBOOK, SEC. 5.5)

Socioculturally disadvantaged children in the United States have an increased incidence of health and developmental problems.

- Native Americans, Eskimos, Aleuts

    high poverty rates
    increased LBW, neonatal, and postneonatal infant mortality rates
    accidental deaths, suicide, and homicide increased
    recurrent otitis media increased
    psychosocial problems such as depression, alcoholism, drug abuse, teenage pregnancy, child abuse and neglect, school failure

- Migrant farm worker's children

    increased infections, trauma, poor nutrition, dental problems, developmental delays
    poor school attendance

- Children of immigrants

    great variation among groups
    growth retardation
    nutritional deficiencies
    hepatitis and parasitic diseases
    psychosocial stress

- Homeless children

    increased frequency of intestinal infections, anemia, neurologic disorders, mental illness, dental problems, trauma, substance abuse
    developmental delays, severe depression, and learning disorders common
    poverty

- Runaway youth

    poverty
    psychopathology and school failure common

TABLE 3–2. MORBIDITY ASSOCIATED WITH LOW INCOME STATUS*

Increased frequency of:
  Low birth weight
  Cytomegalic inclusion disease
  Iron-deficiency anemia
  Lead poisoning
  Poor vision
  Hearing disorders
  Psychological problems

More disability days:
  More hospital days/yr
  Longer average length of stay in hospitals
  Lower survival when ill with leukemia
  More likely to be unable to attend regular school because of a chronic condition

---

* From Behrman RE (ed): Nelson Textbook of Pediatrics, 14th ed. Philadelphia, WB Saunders Company, 1992, p. 163.
  (After Starfield B: Family income, ill health, and medical care of U.S. children. J Publ Health Policy 3:244–259, 1982.)

      criminal activity (esp. prostitution)
      high increase of physical and sexual abuse
      sexually transmitted diseases common
  • Foster children

      increase in poverty, substance abuse, child abuse and neglect; increasing numbers of children are in foster care
      chronic health problems, especially psychoeducational ones, increased
  • Children in poverty

      22% of all children and 40% of all poor
      associated morbidity (Table 3–2)

VULNERABLE CHILDREN: STRENGTHS AND INTERVENTIONS

   success associated with accepting temperament
   avoidance of additional social risks important
   poor prognosis associated with multiple social, educational, and physical problems
   social supports beneficial
   intensive, comprehensive, flexible team management needed
   one caring person often important

HEALTH ADVICE FOR TRAVELING CHILDREN
(*NELSON TEXTBOOK*, SEC. 5.6)

GENERAL RECOMMENDATIONS

1. Seek consultation about specific areas well in advance of departure.
2. Discuss eating and drinking habits because most problems occur through ingestion.

3. Focus on common problems related to travel, such as jet lag, altitude sickness, and environmental exposures (esp. insects as vectors).
4. Discuss HIV risk for adolescents and adults.
5. Preexisting medical problems require special arrangement.

IMMUNIZATIONS

see recommended modification of routine schedule (Table 3–3)

available special vaccines are indicated in Table 3–4

TABLE 3–3. MODIFICATION OF ROUTINE IMMUNIZATION SCHEDULES FOR TRAVELING CHILDREN*

Vaccine†	Modified Schedule
MMR	Children younger than 6 mo of age should not be vaccinated because of maternal antibodies. Children ages 6–12 mo should receive one dose of measles vaccine before departure and revaccination with MMR at 15 mo of age or at 12 mo if remaining in a high-risk area. If the child is 12–14 mo of age, MMR should be given and revaccination should be considered when the child starts school. Older children who were previously immunized with measles vaccine before 1980 should be revaccinated.
OPV	Children should receive at least three doses at intervals of 6 wk when time permits. When traveling infants are less than 6 wk old, an initial dose should be given and three additional doses at 6, 10, and 14 wk should be administered if remaining in the endemic areas. Children traveling to endemic areas who have received a first or second dose of the primary series should receive their second/third doses 4 wk after their prior dose. Children who have received less than the primary series and who remain in endemic areas should complete the primary series within the endemic area with doses at 4-wk intervals.
HbCV	See Table 4–1B and text in Nelson Textbook.
DTP	Young infants should receive three doses, the first no sooner than 6 wk and the next two doses at intervals of no less than 4 wk. Children less than 7 yr old who have received fewer than three doses and who will remain in endemic areas should complete their remaining doses at 4-wk intervals.

* From Behrman RE (ed): Nelson Textbook of Pediatrics, 14th ed. Philadelphia, WB Saunders Company, 1992, p. 166.
† DTP = diphtheria and tetanus toxoids and pertussis vaccine; HbCV = Haemophilus influenzae type B conjugated vaccine; MMR = measles, mumps, rubella; OPV = oral polio vaccine.

TABLE 3–4. IMMUNIZATION FOR TRAVELING CHILDREN*

Live Attenuated Virus Vaccines[†]	Inactivated Vaccines	Toxoids	Immunoglobulins
Measles[‡] Mumps[‡] Rubella[‡] OPV Yellow fever[§]	Cholera[§] HbCV IPV Hepatitis B Japanese encephalitis[∥] Meningococcal Pertussis[∥] Plague Rabies Typhoid[#]	Diphtheria[∥] Tetanus[¶]	Immune globulin Rabies immune globulin

* From Behrman RE (ed): Nelson Textbook of Pediatrics, 14th ed. Philadelphia, WB Saunders Company, 1992, p. 166.
[†] Generally contraindicated in immunodeficient children. An exception is measles vaccination, which is recommended for both asymptomatic and symptomatic HIV-infected children. Live vaccines should be given simultatneously or at least 30 days apart. Live, attenuated immunization should not be coadministered with immune globulin (OPV and yellow fever are exceptions); administer these vaccines at least 3 mo after immune globulin use. Immune globulin should be administered no sooner than 2–4 wk after a live virus vaccine is given.
[‡] Administered together as MMR or separately.
[§] May be required for entry into certain countries.
[∥] Administered together at DTP or DT.
[¶] Not available in the United States. May be obtained in endemic areas for high-risk individuals.
[#] A new licensed oral live attenuated typhoid vaccine (Vivotef, Ty21a) can be given to immunocompetent children >6 yr of age.
HbCV = *Haemophilus influenzae* type B conjugate vaccine; IPV = injectable polio vaccine (enhanced); OPV = oral polio vaccine.

TRAVELER'S DIARRHEA

high frequency

E. coli most common cause, but great variety of potentially responsible agents depending on country

prevention by careful selection and preparation of food, water, and especially formula

chemoprophylactic agents usually not indicated for children

antimicrobial treatment should be done in consultation with physician

dehydration greatest threat to children

MALARIA CHEMOPROPHYLAXIS

malaria is major and increasing problem
measures to reduce mosquito contact critical
prophylactic medication is very effective

– chloroquine is primary drug for children in most endemic areas because *P. vivax, P. ovale, P. malariae,* and

other species remain sensitive; start 1–2 wk before departure and continued for 4–6 wk after leaving endemic area
- chloroquine-resistant *P. falciparum* and other species require prophylaxis and treatment with other drugs; specifics depend on age of child

4

GENERAL CONSIDERATIONS IN THE CARE OF SICK CHILDREN

CLINICAL EVALUATION
(*NELSON TEXTBOOK*, SECS. 3.21 AND 6.1)

DEVELOPMENTAL DIMENSIONS

Observations, history, and physical examination are greatly influenced by the child's developmental stage. This relates both to the child's overall state of well-being or functional status and to specific organ systems.

THE CLINICAL INTERVIEW (History)

This is a major means of engaging the child and/or his or her parents in the active management of the child's care. Because no single encounter can accomplish everything that is needed to complete a clinical assessment, the clinician must set, define, and state priorities. Keep in mind that children attend to and interpret nonverbal communication before they understand the meaning of words. They also need to know what is happening and what is going to happen to them in the immediate future.

Because information must be obtained from parents before the child reaches later developmental stages when he or she can contribute information, it is important to ask questions of the parents in terms of the way in which the child's signs and symptoms would present to an observer. When the child also is able to contribute information directly, his or her observations and interpretations as well as reactions to the interview will be related to his or her developmental stage.

PHYSICAL EXAMINATION

The child should be in a comfortable position; usually for the younger child this is on the parent's lap. Observations of the child–parent interaction may be as important as observations of the child. The clinician must be patient and flexible in making observations and performing the physical examination of a child.

Those portions of the physical examination that require optimal cooperation should be done first (e.g., blood pressure measurement, pulmonary and cardiac examinations, evaluation of eyes and central nervous system [CNS]). The clinician should then proceed to those parts of the examination that usually are more bothersome to the child. The abdominal examination requires the child to be on the examination table. The most intrusive portions of the examination should be done last (e.g., examination of the eye, ear canals, and oropharynx).

OTHER SOURCES OF INFORMATION

It may be necessary to consult other agencies or institutions to obtain psychological testing, as well as obtain laboratory studies, and other consultations to complete fully an evaluation.

WELL CHILD EVALUATION

Well child visits are recommended prenatally, in the newborn period, at 2 wk, at 2, 4, 6, 9, 15, 18, and 24 mo, annually between 3 and 6 yr, and every 2 yr thereafter (see Table 3–1). Each visit should include, in addition to appropriate observation, history, examination, screening, and preventive measures:

> developmental evaluation
> feeding and diet discussions
> accident prevention counseling
> growth measurements
> assessment of family and social relations
> anticipatory guidance about health and related issues appropriate to developmental stages before next visit

SICK CHILD EVALUATION

There are many reasons for such visits, but intercurrent infection, and often a febrile child, is the most common. In addition to a history and physical examination, selected observations correlate well with serious illness in febrile children after 3 mo of life and may be helpful in assessing acute illness in general (Table 4–1). Normal is scored as 1, moderate impairment as 3, and severe impairment as 5. The chance of serious illness is 1–2% if the total score is ≤10 and increases at least 10-fold with higher scores.

The child's developmental stage has a significant impact on the manifestation of illness and, thus, on all the components of the clinical evaluation, resulting in approximately 90% sensitivity for serious illness. In general, the younger the child the less the sensitivity of observation, history, and physical examination. Screening laboratory tests may be helpful in further improving the sensitivity of diagnosis.

PATHOPHYSIOLOGY OF BODY FLUIDS
(*NELSON TEXTBOOK*, SEC. 6.2)

Understanding the physiologic regulation of body fluids depends on an appreciation of: (1) the total amounts of water

TABLE 4–1. OBSERVATIONAL SCALE FOR PREDICTION OF SERIOUS ILLNESS OF BACTERIAL AND NONBACTERIAL ORIGIN*

Observation Item	1 Normal	3 Moderate Impairment	5 Severe Impairment
Quality of cry	Strong with normal tone OR Content and not crying	Whimpering OR Sobbing	Weak OR Moaning OR High-pitched continual cry Hardly responds
Reaction to parent stimulation	Cries briefly then stops OR Content and not crying	Cries off and on	
State variation	If awake → stays awake OR If asleep and stimulated → wakes up quickly	Eyes close briefly → awake OR Awakes with prolonged stimulation	Falls to sleep OR Will not rouse
Color	Pink	Pale extremities OR Acrocyanosis	Pale OR Cyanotic OR Mottled OR Ashen
Hydration	Skin normal, eyes normal AND Mucous membranes moist	Skin, eyes normal AND Mouth slightly dry	Skin doughy OR tented AND Dry mucous membranes AND/OR Sunken eyes
Response (talk, smile) to social overtures	Smiles OR Alerts (≤2 mo)	Brief smile OR Alerts briefly (≤2 mo)	No smile Face anxious, dull, expressionless OR No alerting (≤2 mo)

* From McCarthy P, Sharpe MR, Spiesel SZ, et al: Observation scales to identify serious illness in febrile children. Pediatrics 70:802, 1982.

and solute present in the body as a whole, which depends on the balance between intake and output; (2) the distribution of water and solutes in the various compartments of the body and the maintenance of a steady state equilibrium for most substances; and (3) the concentration of the solutes within each compartment and the changes that occur in response to altering the content of solute and/or water.

Regulatory mechanisms are designed to prevent large changes in solute concentrations and rapid changes in volume that can lead to profound functional alterations.

WATER
(NELSON TEXTBOOK, SEC. 6.3)

Total body water (TBW) constitutes 78% of body weight at birth and decreases to the adult level of 60% by 1 yr of age. TBW is linearly related to weight, but fat is low in water content so the percentage is smaller in obese than in normal-weight individuals.

TBW consists of several compartments whose relative sizes change significantly from conception through the first 9 mo of postnatal life:

Extracellular fluid (ECF) decreases from fetal life to constitute 20–25% of body weight in the older child and is made up of plasma water (5%), interstitial water (15%), and transcellular water (1–3%).

Transcellular water is composed primarily of gastrointestinal secretions and cerebrospinal, intracellular, pleural, peritoneal, and synovial fluids.

Intracellular fluid (ICF) approximates 30–40% of body weight, consisting of the sum of fluids in cells from various tissues throughout the body.

Regulation of Water

Plasma osmolality is maintained at 285–295 mOsm/kg H_2O by balancing water intake and production from oxidation against losses from kidneys, lungs, skin, and gastrointestinal tract.

Intake is normally stimulated and primarily regulated by thirst. Volume restoration usually takes priority over tonicity. Disorders of the thirst mechanism may occur with CNS disease, potassium deficiency, and malnutrition.

Absorption in the gastrointestinal tract is by passive diffusion in response to active transport of solutes such as sodium. Inhibition of solute transport leads to large volumes of intraintestinal water.

Excretion encompasses obligatory losses due to evaporation from the lungs and skin, renal losses necessitated by solute excretion, and losses of free water as a result of varying the rate and diluteness of urine flow. Evaporative losses relate to surface area of the body, temperature, rate of respiration, humidity, and sweating. Renal losses are affected by antidiuretic hormone (ADH), diet, glomerular filtration rate (GFR), state of renal tubular epithelium, and concentration of plasma adrenal steroids.

ADH is primarily regulated by the effective osmotic pressure of ECF (especially Na^+ and Cl^-) and acts by increasing the permeability of the renal collecting ducts to water, resulting in water conservation and concentrated urine. Decreased production of ADH by the supraoptic hypophyseal system or decreased responsiveness in the renal collection ducts leads to *diabetes insipidus* and water loss in a dilute urine. ADH release may be stimulated by pain, trauma, surgery, burns, and various drugs such as demerol and morphine, and may be inhibited by emotional factors, alcohol, and other drugs such as diphenylhydantoin.

Distribution of fluid volumes within the body among ECF and ICF spaces is determined by active transport of potassium into and sodium out of cells, through energy-requiring processes operating across cell membranes that are freely permeable to water. A rise or decrease in ECF osmolality results in a decrease or increase in cell water volume, respectively.

The fluid volume of the *intravascular space* (plasma water) depends on the balance between filtration pressure (hydrostatic) and oncotic forces (albumin and other molecules) at the capillary level. Thus *interstitial space* volume may be increased by decreased plasma protein concentration, increased capillary permeability, or increased venous pressure and may be observed clinically as *edema*.

Osmolalities in the fluid compartments of the body are comparable, although individual solute concentrations within the compartments vary. However, the water content of different body fluids normally differs, and variations from normal values can be clinically significant (e.g., displacement of serum water by lipids in diabetes mellitus).

SODIUM
(*NELSON TEXTBOOK*, SEC. 6.4)

This is the principal osmotically active solute responsible for the maintenance of intravascular and interstitial volumes.

Regulation

Intake may respond to large changes in body composition, but usually it is determined by cultural customs. Infant intake is high because of high sodium in cow's milk.

Excretion is primarily by renal mechanisms but also through sweat and fecal loss.

Regulation of excretion depends on a balance between renal GFR and tubular reabsorption, resulting in less than 1% of filtered sodium being excreted under normal circumstances despite wide fluctuations in intake and GFR. The proximal tubule is the major site of reabsorption, but the loop of Henle plays a significant role and is central to the countercurrent multiplier system essential for water balance and concentration of urine; fine regulation occurs in the distal nephron. This system has substantial capacity to prevent positive or negative sodium balance, but it takes about 3 days to achieve a new steady state after marked alterations in intake.

Distribution is primarily extracellular, although cell membranes are permeable to sodium. Adenosine triphosphatase (ATPase) systems extrude cell sodium, maintaining a 10–140 mEq/L ICF-to-ECF gradient.

Influence of Disease States

Disease states may affect regulation and usually result in changes in volume rather than sodium concentration. Thus, edema often results from retention of sodium with compensatory water retention, and ECF volume contraction is common with ECF sodium loss and hyponatremia as a result of compensatory loss of water.

Patients with chronic renal disease usually can modify their rate of sodium excretion, but the upper and lower limits of sodium tolerance are generally limited. Tubular disease is associated with more limited ability to conserve sodium.

Intravascular changes in sodium concentration—hyponatremia and hypernatremia—usually reflect an abnormal handling of water with relatively more or less water present in the ECF, respectively.

POTASSIUM
(*NELSON TEXTBOOK*, SEC. 6.5)

This is the major intracellular cation and, thus, its body content is an index of cellular mass at different ages.

Regulation

Intake may vary widely, and *absorption* in the upper gastrointestinal tract is relatively complete; exchange with sodium occurs in the lower bowel.

The kidney maintains chronic balance and can adjust *excretion* over a wide range to compensate for broad fluctuations in intake. Urinary potassium is more dependent on tubular secretion than glomerular filtration. Factors affecting distal nephron potassium excretion include mineralocorticoid activity, dietary potassium, acid–base status, distal tubular flow rate, and sodium delivery to the distal tubule. Aldosterone increases urinary excretion of potassium and decreases sodium excretion by altering permeability of the luminal membrane to sodium, allowing exchange with intracellular potassium. Plasma potassium also exchanges with sodium in colonic contents and can be excreted in sweat.

Intracellular uptake of potassium, a first-line defense against toxicity from potassium load, is enhanced by insulin, epinephrine, and alkalosis. Systemic acidosis moves potassium out of cells.

Imbalance

Hypokalemia may result from prolonged decreased intake, increased excretion (e.g., diuretics), renal tubular acidosis, Cushing syndrome, thyrotoxicosis, diabetic ketoacidosis, extrarenal losses (e.g., diarrhea, frequent enemas or cathartics, protracted vomiting, enterocutaneous fistulas), and rapid intracellular uptake (e.g., correction of acidosis). Hypokalemia may produce untoward functional changes in skeletal muscle (weakness), smooth muscle (ileus), and the heart (arrhythmias) as a result of changes in transmembrane electrical potential. Potassium deficiency, if severe, may lead to intracellular acidosis and systemic alkalosis as a result of increased aciduria. If prolonged, renal injury may also occur.

Hyperkalemia may result from small increases in total body potassium, usually secondary to impaired renal excretion (e.g., acute or chronic renal failure, adrenal insufficiency, potassium-sparing diuretics); transiently from acute increases in intake (e.g., potassium salts of penicillin); acute tissue breakdown (e.g., trauma, major surgery); and redistribution (e.g., metabolic acidosis, succinylcholine, digitalis overdose). Neuromuscular effects of hyperkalemia are due to changes in transmembrane potential and include paresthesias, weakness, paralysis, and arrhythmias.

CALCIUM
(*NELSON TEXTBOOK*, SEC. 6.6)

The bones of infants are less densely mineralized than those of adults, although at all ages 99% of body calcium is in bone.

Regulation

The gastrointestinal tract plays the primary role, and dairy products are the most important source.

Absorption occurs along the small intestine and is enhanced by 1,25-dihydroxy vitamin D_3 produced in response to hypocalcemia, parathyroid hormone (PTH) release, and renal conversion of 25-hydroxy vitamin D_3. Absorption is increased by low intake, depleted stores, growth, and administration of vitamin D and PTH. Decrease occurs in the presence of gastrointestinal phytate, oxalate, and citrate; increased gastric motility; or decreased bowel length.

Excretion is diurnal, through renal mechanisms. It is decreased by 1,25-dihydroxy vitamin D_3 and increased by PTH, expanded ECF, osmotic diuretics, furosemide, thiazides, growth and thyroid hormones, physical inactivity, metabolic acidosis, prolonged fasting, and increased serum phosphate level.

Calcium is bound to serum protein, especially albumin, and the amount of ionized calcium is physiologically important.

Imbalance

Hypocalcemia due to reduced ionized calcium may result from vitamin D deficiency, disorders causing hypoparathyroidism, hyperphosphatemia, magnesium deficiency, pancreatitis, alkalosis, or rapid correction of acidosis.

Hypercalcemia may be caused by hyperparathyroidism, hyperthyroidism, vitamin D intoxication, excess calcium intake, immobilization, malignancies, thiazide diuretics, low-phosphate diet, milk–alkali syndrome, and other disorders.

MAGNESIUM
(*NELSON TEXTBOOK*, SEC. 6.7)

This cation plays a major role in cellular enzymatic activity.

Regulation

Sixty percent is in bone, with most of the remainder found intracellularly in muscle and liver. Growth requires high intake.

Absorption occurs in the upper gastrointestinal tract, and is enhanced by vitamin D, PTH, and increased sodium absorption. Absorption is decreased by calcium, phosphorus, and increased intestinal motility. Two thirds of intake is lost in feces.

Balance depends primarily on urinary excretion; serum concentration depends on mobilization from bone and can be maintained normally despite large changes in intake and excretion.

Imbalance

Hypomagnesemia may result from malabsorption syndromes, hypoparathyroidism, diuretics, hypercalcemia, renal tubular acidosis, prolonged intravenous fluid therapy without supplements, and neonatal tetany. Manifestations include tetany, seizure, tremors, personality change, nausea, anorexia, and arrhythmia.

Hypermagnesemia may be due to decreased renal functions, magnesium-containing laxatives, enemas, intravenous fluid load, magnesium sulfate treatment for preeclampsia, and asphyxia. Manifestations include hyporeflexia, respiratory depression, drowsiness, and coma.

HYDROGEN ION (Acid–Base Balance)
(*NELSON TEXTBOOK*, SEC. 6.8)

Terminology

Hydrogen ion or proton: a hydrogen atom with the neutralizing electron removed

pH: the negative logarithm of the concentration of hydrogen ions

Acid: the hydrogen ion or proton donor

Base: the hydrogen ion or proton acceptor

Buffer: a substance that reduces the change in hydrogen ion concentration of a solution on the addition of an acid or base

Regulating Mechanisms

Hydrogen ion concentrations of body fluids are maintained in relatively narrow ranges by the presence of buffers. Buffers are the first line of defense against change but cannot maintain acid–base balance without compensatory and corrective physiologic changes in the lungs and kidneys.

Major buffer systems include:

Bicarbonate–carbonic acid system (extracellular)

$$pH = 6.1\,k + \log \frac{\text{bicarbonate}}{\text{carbonic acid}}$$

proteins and organic phosphates (intracellular)
mono- and dihydrogen phosphate system (urine)

In response to increases or decreases in plasma carbon dioxide (CO_2) levels, *ventilation* is increased (lowering P_{CO_2}, by excreting CO_2 and increasing pH) or is decreased (raising P_{CO_2}, by retaining CO_2 and decreasing pH), respectively. This process alters the ratio of carbonic acid to bicarbonate, but does not cause loss or gain in hydrogen ions.

Renal mechanisms are responsible for eliminating (or retaining) hydrogen ions by generating (or excreting) bicarbonate in response to changes in plasma bicarbonate buffer levels. This is accomplished by: (1) reclaiming nearly all filtered bicarbonate in the proximal tubule, and (2) generating new bicarbonate in the distal segment of the nephron, resulting in net excretion of hydrogen ions (by phosphate buffering and ammonia production) needed to maintain hydrogen ion balance under most circumstances.

Usual Acid–Base Balance

The equivalent of the net amount of hydrogen ions produced from the diet and incomplete catabolism of carbohydrates, fats, and organic acids, after initial buffering and respiratory compensation, is excreted by the kidneys to maintain balance and a blood pH of 7.35–7.45.

Disturbances of Acid–Base Balance

METABOLIC ACIDOSIS.   May result from:
increased production of H^+ (e.g., diabetic ketoacidosis)
inadequate excretion of H^+ (e.g., renal insufficiency)
loss of bicarbonate in urine (e.g., renal tubular acidosis) or stools (e.g., diarrhea)
expansion of ECF by bicarbonate-free solution

- Manifestations

    decreased serum bicarbonate, pH
    increased P_{CO_2} with fall in P_{CO_2} and carbonic acid
    deep, rapid respirations (Kussmaul)
    decreased peripheral vascular resistance and cardiac function

- Compensatory mechanisms

    buffering by bicarbonate, hemoglobin, plasma proteins, and phosphate
    respiratory CO_2 excretion
    increased renal ammonia production and hydrogen ion excretion in urine, leading to bicarbonate generation

METABOLIC ALKOLOSIS.   May result from:
excessive loss of H^+ (persistent vomiting)
addition of bicarbonate to ECF (IV administration)
contraction of ECF

- Manifestations

    increased pH and plasma bicarbonate
    depressed respirations with increased P_{CO_2}
    increased urine pH (increased bicarbonate)
    hypochloremia and hypokalemia
    cramps and weak feeling

- Compensatory mechanisms

     buffering by bicarbonate, hemoglobin, plasma proteins, and phosphates
     decreased ventilation
     renal threshold for bicarbonate exceeded (increased renal bicarbonate absorption and aciduria if volume depletion and hypokalemia)

RESPIRATORY ACIDOSIS.   Due to inadequate pulmonary excretion of CO_2.

- Manifestations

     increased pH, P_{CO_2}, and bicarbonate
     respiratory distress with decreased ventilation
     hypoxia often coincident
     vasodilation
     headaches
     cerebral depression

- Compensatory mechanisms

     buffering by nonbicarbonate systems
     increased renal H^+ excretion with bicarbonate generation

RESPIRATORY ALKALOSIS.   Due to excessive pulmonary excretion of CO_2 (hyperventilation).

- Manifestations

     decreased plasma P_{CO_2} and bicarbonate
     increased pH
     neuromuscular irritability
     paresthesias due to decreased Ca^{++}

- Compensatory mechanisms

     buffering primarily by intracellular systems to release H^+
     increased renal excretion of bicarbonate

MIXED DISORDERS.   May result in profound changes:

     severe acidosis due to respiratory plus metabolic acidosis (e.g., respiratory distress syndrome)
     respiratory acidosis and metabolic alkalosis (e.g., congestive heart failure treated with excessive diuretics)
     metabolic acidosis and respiratory alkalosis (e.g., hepatic failure)

Clinical Assessment of Acid–Base Disorders

Clinical assessment is based on measurement of serum pH, P_{CO_2}, and bicarbonate (Fig. 4–1). If P_{CO_2} and bicarbonate do not vary in the same direction, mixed disorder should be considered. Arterial and venous samples are often needed to evaluate patients with critical hemodynamic compromise.

CHLORIDE
(*NELSON TEXTBOOK*, SEC. 6.9)

The intake, output, and blood concentration of this major anion of ECF usually parallel those of sodium.

	PH	PCO_2	BICARBONATE
Simple disorders			
Metabolic acidosis	↓	↓	↓
Metabolic alkalosis	↑	↑	↑
Respiratory acidosis	↓	↑	↑
Respiratory alkalosis	↑	↓	↓
Mixed disorders			
Metabolic acidosis with respiratory acidosis	↓ ↓	↑ ,N, ↓	↑ ,N, ↓
Metabolic alkalosis with respiratory acidosis	↑ ,N, ↓	↑	↑
Metabolic acidosis with respiratory alkalosis	↑ ,N, ↓	↓	↓
Metabolic alkalosis with respiratory alkalosis	↑ ↑	↑ ,N, ↓	↑ ,N, ↓

Figure 4–1. Typical serum findings in clinical disturbances of acid–base balance. In the simple disorders it has been assumed that the primary acid–base disturbance has been compensated (see text for details). (↑ = increased from normal; ↓ = decreased from normal; N = normal.) (From Behrman RE [ed]: Nelson Textbook of Pediatrics, 14th ed. Philadelphia, WB Saunders Company, 1992, p. 192.)

Imbalances

Hypochloremia results from chloride loss in excess of sodium loss (e.g., vomiting, correction of metabolic acidosis, potassium deficiency) and inadequate intake. Manifestations include metabolic alkalosis with hypokalemia, anorexia, failure to thrive, muscle weakness, and lethargy.

Hyperchloremia results from renal chloride conservation in excess of sodium and potassium (e.g., correction of alkalosis) and excessive intake (e.g., inappropriate parenteral alimentation).

The *anion gap* is the difference in concentrations between sodium and chloride plus bicarbonate. Normally this is 8–16 mEq/L as a result of unmeasured anions (e.g., phosphate, sulfate, proteins, organic acids) exceeding unmeasured cations (K^+, Ca^{2+}, Mg^{2+}). The anion gap:

increases in renal failure, diabetic ketoacidosis, salicylate poisoning, etc.
decreases in nephrotic syndrome

PHOSPHORUS
(*NELSON TEXTBOOK*, SEC. 6.10)

Phosphorus body content increases throughout childhood, 80% in bone, as result of intake of dairy products and meat. Phosphorus is primarily in the form of phospholipids in plasma (which are high in infancy) and phosphoglycerides and sphingolipids in cell membranes and organelles. Inorganic phosphorus is a major urinary buffer.

The kidney is the major site of *regulation*, where PTH reduces tubular reabsorption and results in phosphaturia. ECF and bone exchange also influence plasma levels.

Imbalances

Hyperphosphatemia may result in hypocalcemia and may be due to hypoparathyroidism, renal insufficiency, excessive intake, and cytolysis.

Hypophosphatemia is usually asymptomatic and may result from low intake (e.g., malnutrition, malabsorption), redistribution into cells (e.g., during correction of diabetic ketoacidosis), renal losses (e.g., diuretics, renal tubular defects), vitamin D deficiency, and rapid growth in LBW infants.

PARENTERAL FLUID THERAPY
(*NELSON TEXTBOOK*, SEC. 6.11)

Infants and young children are especially susceptible to conditions that affect fluid balance.

MAINTENANCE THERAPY
(*NELSON TEXTBOOK*, SECS. 6.12–6.14)

Replacement

Normal losses of basal amounts of fluids and electrolytes from lungs, urine, sweat, and feces must be replaced.

TABLE 4–2. STANDARD BASAL CALORIC OUTPUT*,†

Weight (kg)	Output (kcal/24 hr)		
	Male	Male and Female	Female
3		140	
5		270	
7		400	
9		500	
11		600	
13		650	
15		710	
17		780	
19		830	
21		880	
25	1,020		960
29	1,120		1,040
33	1,210		1,120
37	1,300		1,190
41	1,350		1,260
45	1,410		1,320
49	1,470		1,380
53	1,530		1,440
57	1,590		1,500
61	1,640		1,560

* From Behrman RE (ed): Nelson Textbook of Pediatrics, 14th ed. Philadelphia, WB Saunders Company, 1992, p. 196.
† *Increments or decrements:*
  1. Add or subtract 12% of above for each degree C (8% for each degree F) above or below rectal temperature of 37.8°C (100°F).
  2. Add 0–30% increments for activity.
  3. For neonate of 3–5 days use 50 kcal/kg.

CALCULATION. Based on metabolic rate because requirements of fluid and electrolytes relate directly to catabolism of fuels (water of oxidation, renal solute excretion, and heat production; see Table 4–2).

Requirements	IV	Milk Feeding
Water	115 mL/100 kcal	140 mL/100 kcal
Sodium	3 mEq/100 kcal	3 mEq/100 kcal
Potassium	2.5 mEq/100 kcal	2.5 mEq/100 kcal

Modification Due to Disease

- Decreased requirements with:

    anuria or extreme oliguria
    meningitis, due to excessive ADH release
    high-humidity atmosphere
- Increased requirements with:

    gastrointestinal losses
    heat stress
    hyperventilation
    third spacing
    adrenal insufficiency, cystic fibrosis
    loss of renal concentrating capacity

Route

Replace fluids orally if possible, or intravenously.

Caloric Intake

5% dextrose solutions usual for short duration
intravenous alimentation for long duration; infectious and
  metabolic complications are associated

DEFICIT THERAPY
(*NELSON TEXTBOOK*, SECS. 6.15–6.18)

Children with deficits in body water and electrolytes resulting from many different causes can be successfully treated in
a similar manner because the deficits reflect the physiologic
readjustment of the patient, not only the results of direct
losses. Management is dictated more by the severity and
type of defect than by its underlying cause. The *severity of
clinical disturbances* depends on the magnitude of deficit in
relation to body reserves and the rate at which it develops.
The *type of deficit* depends on the relationship between the
magnitude of losses of water and that of losses of electrolytes, principally sodium.

   Severity of a deficit is gauged from changes in body weight
that represent a disproportionately greater loss in body
water than solute:

	Infants	Older Children
Mild	5%	3%
Moderate	5–10%	6%
Severe	10–15%	9%

Types of Dehydration

Isonatremic: proportional losses of water and sodium

– serum sodium 130–150 mEq/L

Hyponatremic: greater loss of sodium than water

– serum sodium less than 130 mEq/L
– ECF loss from body exacerbated due to loss into ICF

Hypernatremic: greater loss of water than sodium

– serum sodium greater than 150 mEq/L
– ECF loss from body ameliorated as a result of water
  movement out of ICF into ECF

Estimation of Magnitude and Type of Deficit

Table 4–3 indicates important historical information that
should be elicited, and Table 4–4 summarizes the findings
with various degrees of severity. Most infants and children
appear ill when dehydrated, and signs of circulatory failure
appear with increasing degrees of dehydration.

   Table 4–5 indicates the effects of various types of dehydration on physical signs. The risk of shock is greatest for the
same degree of severity when there is hyponatremic dehydration because of exacerbation of ECF losses.

TABLE 4-3. HISTORICAL DATA REQUIRED IN ESTIMATING MAGNITUDE AND TYPES OF DEFICIT AND IN PLANNING DEFICIT THERAPY*

Intake (during period of illness)
  Quantity and how given
  Type: water, electrolyte, protein, drugs
Output (during period of illness)
  Quantity
  Type: urine, vomiting, diarrhea, sweat, drainage
Balance
  Weight change
General medical
  Age
  Cardiovascular, respiratory, renal, or central nervous system disease

* From Behrman RE (ed): Nelson Textbook of Pediatrics, 14th ed. Philadelphia, WB Saunders Company, 1992, p. 199.

Serial laboratory measurements of electrolytes, acid–base balance, hematocrit, hemoglobin, plasma proteins, blood urea nitrogen, and creatinine and urinalysis are helpful in evaluating the changing severity, response to therapy, and complications. Variations in specific ions may be associated with specific physical manifestations, but not invariably.

PRINCIPLES OF THERAPY
(*NELSON TEXTBOOK*, SEC. 6.18)

Emergency management may be required for some patients, such as those in shock. *Oral rehydration* may be appropriate for some patients with mild to moderate dehydration. *Parenteral rehydration* is usually indicated for patients having severe dehydration, vomiting, and profound ongoing losses.

Initial Parenteral Therapy

goal is to prevent or treat shock by rapidly expanding ECF, especially plasma
20–30 mL/kg isotonic NaCl and 5% glucose (no K^+)
bicarbonate, lactate, or acetate used to partially replace NaCl when acidosis is present
infusion rate depends on circulatory status, and repeated infusions and blood are required if shock is not reversed

Subsequent Parenteral Therapy

goal is to completely replace remaining deficit and replace ongoing abnormal and obligatory losses
monitor response to treatment

• Isotonic dehydration

replace two thirds of ECF loss in first 24 hr because some ECF sodium exchanges with ICF potassium
complete replacement of losses plus maintenance and ongoing losses in 1–2 days and K^+ in 3–4 days

TABLE 4–4. CLINICAL ASSESSMENT OF SEVERITY OF DEHYDRATION*

Signs and Symptoms	Mild Dehydration	Moderate Dehydration	Severe Dehydration
General appearance and condition:			
Infants and young children	Thirsty; alert; restless	Thirsty; restless or lethargic but irritable to touch or drowsy	Drowsy; limp, cold, sweaty, cyanotic extremities; may be comatose
Older children and adults	Thirsty; alert; restless	Thirsty; alert; postural hypotension	Usually conscious; apprehensive; cold, sweaty, cyanotic extremities; wrinkled skin of fingers and toes; muscle cramps
Radial pulse	Normal rate and strength	Rapid and weak	Rapid, feeble, sometimes impalpable
Respiration	Normal	Deep, may be rapid	Deep and rapid
Anterior fontanel	Normal	Sunken	Very sunken
Systolic blood pressure	Normal	Normal or low	Less than 90 mm Hg, may be unrecordable
Skin elasticity	Pinch retracts immediately	Pinch retracts slowly	Pinch retracts very slowly (>2 sec)
Eyes	Normal	Sunken (detectable)	Grossly sunken
Tears	Present	Absent	Absent
Mucous membranes	Moist	Dry	Very dry
Urine flow	Normal	Reduced amount and dark	None passed for several hours; empty bladder
Body weight loss (%)	4–5	6–9	10 or more
Estimated fluid deficit (mL/kg)	40–50	60–90	100–110

* From Behrman RE (ed): Nelson Textbook of Pediatrics, 14th ed. Philadelphia, WB Saunders Company, 1992, p. 200. (Modified from World Health Organization guide.)

TABLE 4–5. EFFECTS OF TYPE OF DEHYDRATION ON PHYSICAL SIGNS*

Parameter	Isonatremic Dehydration (Proportionate Loss of Water and Sodium)	Hyponatremic Dehydration (Loss of Sodium in Excess of Water)	Hypernatremic Dehydration (Loss of Water in Excess of Sodium)
ECF volume†	Markedly decreased	Severely decreased	Decreased
ICF volume†	Maintained	Increased	Decreased
Physical signs			
Skin			
Color‡	Gray	Gray	Gray
Temperature	Cold	Cold	Cold or hot
Turgor§	Poor	Very poor	Fair
Feel	Dry	Clammy	Thickened, doughy
Mucous membranes	Dry	Slightly moist	Parched‖
Eyeball	Sunken and soft	Sunken and soft	Sunken
Fontanel	Sunken	Sunken	Sunken
Psyche	Lethargic	Coma	Hyperirritable
Pulse‡	Rapid	Rapid	Moderately rapid
Blood pressure‡	Low	Very low	Moderately low

* From Behrman RE (ed): Nelson Textbook of Pediatrics, 14th ed. Philadelphia, WB Saunders Company, 1992, p. 200.
† ECF, extracellular fluid; ICF, intracellular fluid.
‡ Signs of shock rather than of dehydration itself.
§ Reflects magnitude of fluid loss from ECF.
‖ Tongue often has shriveled appearance because of loss of cellular fluid.

- Hyponatremic dehydration

    similar to isonatremic except extra sodium loss must be replaced over several days

    Na^+ loss [mEq] = (135 − measured serum sodium) × total body water [L] (50–55% of admission weight)

    3% NaCl used only for convulsions or other manifestation of water intoxication

- Hypernatremic dehydration

    increased risk of CNS injury from hyperosmolality or its treatment

    sodium and ECF deficits are small

    administer 60–75 mL/kg/24 hr of 5% dextrose containing 25 mEq/L sodium as a combination of bicarbonate and chloride

    reduce maintenance 25% because of high ADH

If parenteral therapy is prolonged, nutrition is needed.

THERAPY FOR SPECIFIC DISEASE STATES
(*NELSON TEXTBOOK*, SECS. 6.19–6.26)

Acute Diarrhea with Dehydration

Dehydration is isonatremic in 70%, hypernatremic in 20%, and hyponatremic in 10% of cases.

When *oral rehydration* is indicated for losses, treat as per Table 4–6 with 50 mL/kg within 4 hr if dehydration is mild and 100 mL/kg over 6 hr if dehydration is moderate, contraindications for oral hydration include:

    shock
    severe dehydration
    uncontrolled vomiting
    chronic diarrhea
    diarrhea exceeding 100 mL/kg/hr
    inability to drink
    serious complications

TABLE 4–6. COMPARISON OF COMPOSITION OF ORAL SOLUTIONS (mmol/L)*

Component	WHO (ORS)[†]	Traditional Solution[‡]	Reformulated Solution[‡,§]
Sodium	90	30	50
Potassium	20	25	25
Chloride	80	25	45
Bicarbonate	30	36	30
Glucose	111	28[‖]	28[‖]

* From Behrman RE (ed): Nelson Textbook of Pediatrics, 14th ed. Philadelphia, WB Saunders, 1992, p. 204.
  [†] World Health Organization oral rehydration solution composed of (g/L water): NaCl, 3.5; NaHCO3, 2.5; KCl, 1.5; glucose 20.0.
  [‡] Bicarbonate usually present as a precursor, such as citrate. Also contains (mEq/L): Ca, 4; Mg, 4; SO4, 4; PO4, 5.
  [§] Lytren (Mead Johnson). Other solutions are similar except for sodium and chloride concentrations, which range from 45 to 75 mEq/L.
  [‖] Additional sugars provided as corn syrup to total carbohydrate content of 77 g/L.

For *maintenance oral rehydration,* use 100 mL oral rehydration solution (ORS)/kg/24 hr until mild diarrhea stops; for severe diarrhea, the amount of ORS ingested should equal stool volume (est. 10–15 mL ORS/kg/hr).

During treatment, continue oral intake of nutrients. Usually stools decrease within 48 hr of intravenous treatment in fasted patients, and oral caloric feedings can be initiated and gradually increased.

Diarrhea in Dehydrated Chronically Malnourished Children

Fluid composition disturbances include overexpanded ICF, ECF and ICF hypo-osmolality, and low serum protein. Cardiovascular instability is common, and low urinary osmolality may exist. Nutritional and ECF resuscitation are critical.

Pyloric Stenosis and Dehydration

Metabolic alkalosis from excessive loss of HCl, NaCl, and K^+ often can be corrected within 12 hr. More Na^+ and K^+ (as soon as the child is voiding) replacement is given as chloride salt than in other forms of dehydration. Severe K^+ deficit is indicated by acid urine.

Fasting and Thirsting Dehydration

Parenteral therapy usually is required if dehydration is prolonged, especially in infants, who often vomit oral intake. Isonatremic solutions produce rapid, safe expansion of ECF and improve renal function. Older children with less ECF should receive one fourth to one third less fluids per kilogram for the same degree of dehydration.

Hyponatremia in CNS Disorders

Large urinary sodium losses may result from surgical or traumatic brain damage, encephalitis, and cerebral hemorrhage or tumors and may require large amounts of NaCl and limitation of water intake in order to avoid dehydration, shock, and azoturia.

Asymptomatic hyponatremia may occur in tuberculous meningitis.

Acute CNS infections may result in water intoxication and convulsions as a result of water retention, requiring fluid restriction and occasionally hypertonic saline infusion.

Preoperative, Intraoperative, and Postoperative Fluids

Preoperatively, patients who have no deficit should receive carbohydrate to assure adequate liver glycogen and usual maintenance of water and electrolytes. Newborns are at special risk from deficits and aspiration.

Overhydration is the primary risk of parenteral fluid administration, particularly glucose and water without low maintenance sodium.

Postoperative fluid should be limited for 24 hr and not exceed 85 mL/100 kcal

Isolated Electrolyte Disturbances

- Acidosis

    treat CO_2 retention with improved ventilation

    treat underlying cause of metabolic acidosis, but also may need to administer bicarbonate*:

    required mEq* bicarbonate = serum bicarbonate (desired − existing) × body wt [kg] × 0.5–0.6 (apparent distribution)

- Alkalosis

    treat underlying causes of overventilation (salicylate intoxication, CNS disease, anxiety, respirator, etc.)

    - increased risk of tetany

    treat underlying metabolic causes

    - decrease excess administration of alkali
    - volume contraction responds to ECF expansion and replacement of lost Cl^- + K^+ (e.g., vomiting, gastric suctioning, diuretic administration)
    - decrease H^+ (e.g., vomiting) or K^+ (e.g., Bartter syndrome) loss

- Hyponatremia

    cause is sodium depletion resulting from:

    - excess water administration or retention (inappropriate secretion of ADH)
    - redistribution of water to plasma (severe or terminal illness)
    - artifact due to increased lipids and decreased water in plasma (e.g., diabetic ketoacidosis) or to laboratory error

    treat with water restriction (asymptomatic) alone or with hypertonic saline (symptomatic)

    symptomatic (e.g., convulsions, shock) plasma levels usually less than 120 mEq/L

    required mEq Na^+ (for symptomatic hyponatremia) = serum Na^+ (desired − existing) × body wt [kg] × 0.6–0.7 (apparent distribution)

- Hypernatremia

    cause is excessive intake (e.g., faulty formula preparation)

    associated severe acidosis and cerebral hemorrhage intermittent peritoneal dialysis may be needed

- Hypokalemia (other than dehydration)

    causes

    - urinary loss (e.g., hyperaldosteronism, Bartter syndrome)
    - congenital gastrointestinal alkalosis from loss of Cl^- and K^+ in stools
    - diuretics

---

* Rarely necessary to increase more than 15 mEq/L.

  manifestations

  - muscle weakness
  - ileus
  - dilute urine and renal damage

  treat with K^+

- Hyperkalemia (other than dehydration)

  causes

  - renal failure
  - excessive administration
  - error in handling or measuring blood

  manifestation: cardiac arrythmia
  treatment

  - discontinue intake
  - administer bicarbonate, glucose, and insulin
  - Kayexalate resin administration

- Hypomagnesemia

  causes

  - chronic intestinal losses (e.g., chronic diarrhea)
  - prolonged parenteral fluids
  - hyperaldosteronism
  - infantile tetany

  manifestations

  - tetany
  - convulsions
  - disorientation

  treat with magnesium

- Hypermagnesemia

  causes

  - renal failure
  - Addison disease
  - excess intake (e.g. Mg^{2+} treatment of hypertension)

  manifestations

  - loss of deep tender reflexes
  - drowsiness and coma
  - respiratory depression
  - cardiac arrhythmias

  treatment: IV calcium gluconate

TETANY
(NELSON TEXTBOOK, SECS. 6.27–6.29)

This hyperexcitable state of the central and peripheral nervous systems results from an abnormal concentration of ions in the fluid bathing nerve cells.

  Manifest tetany: carpopedal spasm, laryngospasm, paresthesias, irritability, muscle twitching, seizures
  Latent tetany: ischemia, mechanical (Chvostek sign), or electrical (Erb sign) stimulation needed to produce manifestations of tetany

Alkalotic tetany: hyperventilation (often psychogenic) or overventilation (respirators, exacerbated by low Ca^{++}, correction of metabolic acidosis)

Hypocalcemic Tetany

Hypocalcemic tetany (serum calcium below 7 mg/dL) is caused by:

Parathyroid function disorders of the newborn (neonatal hypocalcemia)

may be associated with refractory target cells and increased thyrocalcitonin
early (1st 36 hr of life) associated with LBW, intrauterine growth retardation (IUGR), infants of diabetic mothers, hypoxia
late follows feeding of high-phosphate (cow's) milk, with elevated serum phosphate depressing calcium without compensatory PTH release
treatment

- asymptomatic infants may respond to oral calcium gluconate
- symptomatic infants require IV calcium gluconate (10%), 2 mL/Kg given slowly while monitoring electrocardiogram (ECG) (bradycardia, arrhythmias)
- reduce serum phosphate in late form by increasing calcium intake

Congenital absence of parathyroids (e.g., DiGeorge syndrome)—requires dihydrotachysterol
Vitamin D deficiency and metabolic abnormalities

vitamin D is critical to normal maintenance of serum calcium
tetany onset from nutritional deficiency is usually at 3–6 mo
liver and renal disorders or drugs (diphenylhydantoin) may disrupt vitamin D metabolism

Hypomagnesemic Tetany

Hypomagnesemic tetany may require specific treatment.

FAILURE TO THRIVE
(*NELSON TEXTBOOK*, SEC. 6.30)

Etiology is most commonly environmental and psychosocial circumstances (nonorganic):

inadequate nutrient intake
emotional deprivation and disruption
anorexia nervosa/bulimia
abuse and neglect
secondary to impact of organic disease

Organic disorders may involve any system. It is especially common with chronic diarrhea and malabsorption, CNS abnormalities, chronic pulmonary and renal disorders, and infection.

Diagnosis and treatment often are facilitated by initial trial of hospitalization with adequate diet for growth and observation of social interactions.

ACCIDENTAL INJURY
(*NELSON TEXTBOOK*, SEC. 6.31)

This is the major cause of death and morbidity in children 1–14 yr of age in the United States. Motor vehicle accidents are the leading cause of mortality for individuals 1–25 yr of age, but significant numbers of serious accidents also occur at home, in school, and on the farm. Social stress factors correlate with the risk of accidental injury.

EMERGENCY MEDICAL SERVICES
(*NELSON TEXTBOOK*, SEC. 6.32)

PREHOSPITAL CARE

Cardiopulmonary resuscitation (CPR) success rates for arrest are low, especially for infants, but there is substantial opportunity to decrease mortality and morbidity from trauma.

Rapid transport to a hospital is the highest priority and is dependent on rapid assessment of vital functions (Table 4–7) and often minimal intervention (e.g., load-and-go versus stabilization).

HOSPITAL-BASED EMERGENCY ROOM (ER) CARE

Children constitute 26% of ER visits and 5% of ER admissions. A high proportion of ER visits are by poor children. The ratio of medical to surgical visits is 2:1.

High-predictive-value diagnostic tests that facilitate rapid treatment decisions must be used.

MAJOR TRAUMA IN THE ER

88% is blunt, with high incidence of acute injury
Two thirds of pediatric victims have isolated head injury
15% of pediatric trauma involves major head injury

TABLE 4–7. PREHOSPITAL PRIMARY SURVEY (ABCDs)*

Airway	Breath sounds
Breathing	Work of breathing; color; respiratory rate
Circulation	Strength of peripheral pulses; color and temperature of extremities; heart rate; blood pressure
Disability	Modified Glasgow Coma Scale (see Table 4–8); pupillary responses; fontanel tension

rman RE (ed): Nelson Textbook of Pediatrics, 14th ed. Philadelphia, s Company, 1992, p. 220.

Management

1. Stabilize cervical spine using neutral position.
2. Assess (Table 4–7) and maintain:

   Airway (intubate under direct visualization when needed)
   Breathing (oxygen, relief of gastric distention)
   Circulation (anticipate shock)

3. Evaluate and manage Disabilities (CNS; see Table 4–8) and treat elevated intracranial pressure (ICP).
4. Do complete evaluation.

TABLE 4–8. MODIFIED GLASGOW COMA SCALE*

	Eyes Opening	
Score	>1 Yr	<1 Yr
4	Spontaneously	Spontaneously
3	To verbal command	To shout
2	To pain	To pain
1	No response	No response

	Best Motor Response	
Score	>1 Yr	<1 Yr
6	Obeys	Spontaneous
5	Localizes pain	Localizes pain
4	Flexion—withdrawal	Flexion—withdrawal
3	Flexion—abnormal (decorticate rigidity)	Flexion—abnormal (decerebrate rigidity)
2	Extension (decerebrate rigidity)	Extension (decerebrate rigidity)
1	No response	No response

	Best Verbal Response		
Score	>5 Yr	2–5 Yr	0–23 Mo
5	Oriented and converses	Appropriate words and phrases	Smiles, coos appropriately
4	Disoriented and converses	Inappropriate words	Cries, consolable
3	Inappropriate words	Persistent cries or screams	Persistent inappropriate crying or screaming
2	Incomprehensible sounds	Grunts	Grunts, agitated or restless
1	No response	No response	No response

* From Behrman RE (ed): Nelson Textbook of Pediatrics, 14th ed. Philadelphia, WB Saunders Company, 1992, p. 221.

CARE OF THE CRITICALLY ILL CHILD
(*NELSON TEXTBOOK*, SECS. 6.33–6.35)

In general,

be alert to early signs of serious illness (see Table 4–7)

alterations in mental status and musculoskeletal positioning are highly significant (see Table 4–8)

poor capillary perfusion (refill longer than 3 sec) may present as depressed consciousness or urine output or cyanosis before onset of shock

hypoxia can occur without cyanosis

respiratory insufficiency may be manifest by noisy, difficult breathing; retractions, flaring, grunting; tachypnea for age; deep, irregular, or seesaw respirations

- CPR

    indicated for life-threatening cardiopulmonary insufficiency

    primary goal is to avoid brain hypoxia or ischemia

    ABCD's may include closed-chest cardiac massage, ventilation, and drugs

    prognosis is generally poor

- ICP

    treatment directed at decreasing volume of intracranial contents:

    - raising head above heart
    - hyperventilation (decrease flow)
    - remove cerebrospinal fluid (CSF)
    - administer osmotic agents IV (to remove brain water)
    - use drugs to decrease ICP (barbiturates, corticosteroids) and control seizures

- Cardiovascular problems

    management includes:

    - drugs for treatment of dysrhythmias, poor contractility, and afterload and preload abnormalities
    - fluid infusion to alter preload
    - defibrillation
    - mechanical devices to support circulation

- Respiratory failure

    treatment includes:

    - airway management
    - respiratory support (oxygen; pressure applied to airway, such as continuous positive airway pressure (CPAP), mechanical ventilation)
    - extracorporeal membrane oxygenation (ECMO)

- Acute liver failure

    treated by:

    - fluid management
    - protein restriction
    - elimination of gastrointestinal blood
    - bowel sterilization

- Renal failure

  treatment includes:
  - fluid restriction and electrolyte management
  - dialysis
  - continuous arteriovenous hemofiltration
  - venovenous hemofiltration

Monitoring of organ systems is essential in caring for critically ill children.

PATTERNS OF PRESENTATION IN CRITICAL CARE

Other patterns of presentation in critical care requiring immediate response include:

Coma—requires assessment of other threats to life (e.g., airway obstruction, shock, apnea, dysrhythmias) in addition to evaluation of CNS

Herniation—may be indicated by depressed consciousness, abnormal pupil responses or ocular movements, unusual respiratory patterns, and abnormal gross movements

Status epilepticus, or continual repetitive convulsions—should be terminated but may precipitate need for life support

Shock—requires aggressive treatment with fluids and, depending on etiology, with antibiotics, cardiovascular support drugs, and support of organ system dysfunction

- hypotension may occur late
- administration of boluses of 10 mL/kg of colloid or 20 mL/kg of crystalloid solutions

Metabolic collapse—may be caused by many insults but usually presents with alteration of vital signs and often acidosis

DROWNING AND NEAR-DROWNING
(*NELSON TEXTBOOK*, SEC. 6.36)

EPIDEMIOLOGY

A high proportion of the 7,000 drowning deaths/yr are children, especially 1–4-yr-olds (20% in bathtubs).

PATHOPHYSIOLOGY

The degree of hypoxemia is related to duration of submersion, content and temperature of water, pulmonary aspiration volume, and the individual's responses. Hypothermic patients may have a good prognosis.

CLINICAL MANIFESTATIONS

Successful resuscitation usually is not followed by cardiac or renal problems unless there is prolonged submersion with severe hypoxia and metabolic acidosis. Pulmonary edema and infection associated with aspiration are common. CNS dysfunction is the major problem.

TREATMENT

Resuscitation should be initiated immediately after rescue at site, unless contraindicated by special circumstances, and includes:

mouth-to-mouth ventilation, followed by
positive pressure as soon as possible
closed-chest massage

CPR should be continued during transport.

Routine ER measures include bicarbonate administration because acidosis is common.

All patients with history of submersion are admitted because of risk of pulmonary and CNS problems. Respiratory and circulatory support should be tailored to the patient's condition. Multiple organ system failure may occur.

PROGNOSIS

The death rate is about 20%, and CNS morbidity is very variable.

BURN INJURIES
(*NELSON TEXTBOOK*, SEC. 6.37)

DEFINITIONS

1st degree: involves epithelium and is characterized only by pain and redness

2nd degree: involves epithelium and part of corneum, sparing appendages from which re-epithelialization occurs

3rd degree: involves entire thickness of dermis, and healing can occur only by ingrowth from margins or grafting

4th degree: extends to subjacent tissues

Mild: less than 10% of body surface

Moderate: 10–30% of body surface

Severe: greater than 30% of body surface

EPIDEMIOLOGY

Burns are the second leading cause of nonvehicular accidental deaths (7,800/yr), and 30% occur in children. Most children's burns occur at home during waking hours and are preventable.

PATHOPHYSIOLOGY

Hemodynamic (e.g., losses of H_2O, electrolytes, plasma), autonomic, cardiopulmonary (e.g., decreased cardiac output), renal (e.g., oliguria), and metabolic disturbances occur rapidly after severe burns.

EMERGENCY MANAGEMENT OF SEVERE BURNS (see Table 4–9)

First 24 Hours

goal is to restore volume and electrolyte hemostasis and minimize organ dysfunction and edema from initial loss of albumin

volume of fluids needed:

- 2,000 mL/m^2 of body surface/24 hr plus
- 5,000 mL/m^2 of body surface burned/24 hr
- one half in 8 hr; one half in next 16 hr
- estimate surface burned from Fig. 4–2

administer IV isotonic salt solution containing albumin, lactate or bicarbonate, and 5% glucose (e.g., add 12.5 g [50 mL of 25%] human serum albumin to 950 mL lactated Ringer's in 5% dextrose)

monitor hydration therapy closely

Second and Subsequent Days

goal is to replace continuing loss of fluid and electrolyte from burn exudate and evaporation

volume of fluids needed:

- 1,500 mL/m^2 of body surface/24 hr plus
- 3,750 mL/m^2 of body surface burned/24 hr

sodium requirements decrease after 48 hr and fluids can be administered orally or IV, with a sodium concentration of 50 mEq/L for children 1 yr or more (35–40 mEq/L for those less than 1 yr) and 30–40 mEq K$^+$/L

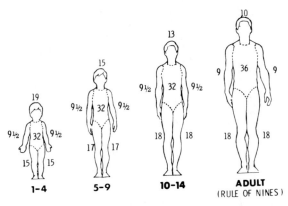

Figure 4–2. Burn assessment chart. Numbers under the figures indicate age; the others indicate the percentage of body surface. (From Behrman RE [ed]: Nelson Textbook of Pediatrics, 14th ed. Philadelphia, WB Saunders Company, 1992, p. 235. Body proportions modified from Lund CL, Brower NC: The estimation of areas of burns. Surg Gynecol Obstet 79:352, 1944.)

TABLE 4-9. PRIORITIES OF MEDICAL PROCEDURES IN THE EMERGENCY PHASE OF BURN INJURIES*

Procedure	Indication	Comment
Establish an adequate airway	Burns of the face	Avoid emergency tracheostomy
	Laryngeal edema	
	Smoke inhalation	
Examine for trauma to head, skeleton, or nervous system	Explosions	Remove clothing; radiologic examination helpful
Begin intravenous infusion	To prevent intravascular dehydration	Use isotonic fluids
Empty stomach through a nasogastric tube	To prevent gastric dilation, vomiting, or aspiration	Antacids may be helpful
Insert an indwelling urinary catheter	To monitor hourly urine output	Use a closed drainage system
Examine the burn wound	To estimate depth and extent	Use burn charts corrected for age
Clean, débride, and dress the burn area	To minimize microbial colonization	Use topical antimicrobial therapy
Administer medications	To treat infections; to prevent tetanus; for sedation	Use intravenous route for sedation
Begin fluid, electrolyte, and protein replacement	To correct antecedent deficits and concurrent losses	Use appropriate formula to estimate requirements

* From Behrman RE (ed): Nelson Textbook of Pediatrics, 14th ed. Philadelphia, WB Saunders Company, 1992, p. 234.

transition to oral hourly intake usual after 24 hr

wound management and physiologic monitoring are critical

hypermetabolism, increased glucose requirement, and severe protein and fat wasting require:

– 1,800 kcal/m^2 of body surface/24 hr plus
– 2,200 kcal/m^2 of body surface burned/24 hr

complications include cardiac dysfunction, respiratory problems, oliguria and renal failure, and sepsis and endotoxemia

rehabilitation program should be started early

TRANSPLANTATION MEDICINE
(*NELSON TEXTBOOK*, SECS. 6.38–6.47)

Organ and tissue transplants may be used to treat end-stage organ failure, benign tumors, and systemic and localized malignancies and to correct inborn errors of metabolism.

IMMUNOLOGY

The recipient's recognition of alloantigens of the human major histocompatibility complex (MHC), the human leukocyte antigen (HLA) complex, on donor cells initiates graft rejection by host T lymphocytes. Other minor histocompatibility antigens also may play a role in rejection and graft-versus-host disease (GVHD). The HLA complex includes class I (HLA-A, HLA-B, HLA-C) and class II (HLA-DP, HLA-DQ, and HLA-DR) molecules, which determine recognition by host lymphocytes. Matching of antigens is important for graft acceptance.

GVHD

Engraftment by donor lymphocytes in an immunocompromised host results in donor T cell activation against host MHC antigens (e.g., in skin, gastrointestinal tract, liver). Prophylaxis and treatment is with immune suppressants (corticosteroids, azathioprine, cyclosporine, FK506, antithymocyte globulin, OKT3).

Acute GVHD is characterized by:

– onset 7–14 days after transplantation (not later than 100 days)
– rash
– hyperbilirubinemia
– diarrhea, protein-losing enteropathy
– decreased activity
– fever, toxicity, edema
– eosinophilia, lymphocytosis, pancytopenia (bone marrow aplasia)
– secondary infections

Chronic GVHD is characterized by:
- onset more than 100 days after transplant
- resembles multisystem autoimmune process
- recurrent infections

BONE MARROW TRANSPLANTATION

Transplant may be autologous (reinfusion of patient's previously stored marrow), syngeneic (from identical twin), or allogeneic (from sibling or unrelated donor). Donor tissue contains lymphocytes able to react to host antigens, resulting in GVHD. Conditioning, myeloablative chemotherapy, and immunosuppression are required.

Complications include opportunistic infections, toxicity from conditioning agents, malignancies, hemolytic uremic syndrome, thrombotic thrombocytopenia, immunoglobulin E (IgE)-mediated hypersensitivity, avascular necrosis of bone, alveolar hemorrhage, and obstructive lung disease.

LIVER TRANSPLANTATION

Common pediatric *indications* include bilary atresia, acute fulminant hepatitis, α-antitrypsin deficiency, intrahepatic cholestasis, and inborn errors of metabolism. Preoperative ABO but not HLA matching and postoperative immunosuppression are necessary.

Complications include coagulopathy, graft failure and rejection, bleeding, vascular thrombosis, ischemic injury and peritonitis, infections, hypertension, oliguria, metabolic alkalosis, right lung atelectasis, phrenic nerve palsy, pleural effusion, encephalopathy, cholangitis, hepatitis, and lymphoma.

RENAL TRANSPLANTATION

Renal transplantation is *indicated* primarily for management of end-stage renal disease (ESRD). *Contraindications* include active systemic infection, IV drug abuse, systemic malignancy, and irreversible brain or other vital organ injury.

Preoperative donor–recipient crossmatch of donor's lymphocytes against recipient is indicated to identify preformed cytotoxic antibodies that cause humoral vasculitis-like rejection directed against ABO or HLA antigens. ABO and HLA matching correlates with graft survival, and mismatch requires immunosuppression.

The procedure is not technically difficult, and the recipient's kidney is left in place. Infants given adult kidneys may have massive fluid and electrolyte losses.

Rejection is manifested by fever, anorexia, malaise, hypertension, oliguria, abdominal pain, allograft swelling and tenderness, increase in blood urea nitrogen and creatinine, and biopsy findings.

HEART TRANSPLANTATION

In infants, heart transplantation may be *indicated* for complex congenital heart lesions such as hypoplastic left heart syndrome. In older children, transplantation may be indicated for irreversible heart disease, including cardiomyopathies, myocarditis, and myocardial tumors. *Contraindications* include ABO or cytotoxic antibody mismatch, uncontrolled infection, poorly controlled diabetes mellitus, and elevated pulmonary vascular resistance.

Complications include arrhythmias, low output, opportunistic infections, hypertension, lymphoproliferative disease, and graft coronary atherosclerosis.

Rejection despite immunosuppressants is manifested by fever, fatigue, heart failure, arrhythmias, and endomyocardial biopsy findings.

LUNG, HEART–LUNG, AND PANCREAS TRANSPLANTATION

Experience with such transplants is limited in children.

PREANESTHETIC AND POSTANESTHETIC CARE
(*NELSON TEXTBOOK*, SECS. 6.48–6.53)

PREANESTHETIC EVALUATION

This should include the following information:

  child's previous anesthetic and surgical procedures
  family history of major anesthetic complications
  history of apnea, breathing irregularities, or cyanosis (especially in infants under age 6 mo)
  recent upper respiratory tract infection
  exposure to exanthems
  previous laryngotracheitis (croup)
  history of allergies, drug hypersensitivities, asthma, or wheezing during respiratory infections
  abnormal weight loss
  exercise intolerance
  bleeding tendencies
  blood transfusion reactions
  current medications
  prior administration of corticosteroids
  emotional reactions of the child to the proposed operation
  when and what the child last ate (especially in emergency procedures)

Special anesthetic problems also may occur in infants and children receiving cortisone, antiepileptic or sedative drugs, and certain antibiotics; in premature infants (e.g., postoperative apnea); in children with cardiopulmonary abnormalities at physical examination; and in infants less than 6 mo of age.

PREANESTHETIC PREPARATION AND SEDATION

Young children (1–4 yr) are usually frightened, and the pre- and postoperative period may produce subsequent serious psychological disturbances that can be ameliorated by parental and professional explanations and reassurances and sedation.

  oral sedation preferred (atropine, meperidine, diazepam, phenobarbital)
  clear liquids with glucose should usually be given up to 4 hr prior to induction
  dehydration, fever, acidosis, and volume depletion should be corrected before operation

INTRAOPERATIVE MANAGEMENT

Anesthesia should be provided unless it is likely to cause cardiac arrest because of the patient's condition; blocking the stress of pain decreases morbidity and mortality.

  halothane, isoflurane, and nitrous oxide with nondepolarizing muscle relaxants are agents of choice
  tracheal intubation usually indicated
  physiologic monitoring always indicated; volume and temperature regulation especially critical in infants
  Malignant hyperpyrexia with unexplained temperatures above 41° C may occur during or following inhalation anesthesia or succinylcholine administration. It requires immediate treatment, including cessation of anesthesia, hyperventilation with oxygen, rapid temperature reduction, fluid resuscitation, sodium bicarbonate, and dantrolene.

POSTANESTHETIC RECOVERY

The child recovering from anesthesia requires monitoring and maintaining of airway patency, ventilation, and circulatory stability. Postanesthetic excitement, vomiting, and pain are common and may require pharmacotherapy. Patients with upper airway anomalies, operations, or history of obstruction and those who have been intubated should receive more prolonged intensive care.

PAIN MANAGEMENT IN CHILDREN
(*NELSON TEXTBOOK*, SEC. 6.54)

Pain is subjective, involving sensory and emotional components, and its intensity and the capacity to cope with it vary greatly among individuals for any given injury. Neurosensory pathways are anatomically and functionally intact at birth, and infants have a broad repertory of physiologic, biochemical, and behavioral responses to pain.

Clinical manifestation vary with age. Infants may be diagnosed by cry, facial expression, autonomic responses, and behavior or motor activity; preschoolers' response is modified by limited cognitive ability.

Treatment may require medical and psychosocial evaluation. Systemic opioids (e.g., morphine, fentanyl) are a mainstay whose need can be modified or eliminated by other analgesic medications (e.g., acetaminophen or nonsteroidal anti-inflammatory drugs) or local anesthetics (e.g., regional blocks).

Whenever possible, children should be given analgesics orally or through an existing IV line. Postoperative pain is best treated by continuous or intermittent dosages, not prn dosing. The apnea risk of opiates is increased in infants less than 3 mo of age.

Cancer and other pain syndromes require determination of whether pain is caused by disease process, side effects of medications, or diagnostic and therapeutic procedures. Patient-controlled analgesia (PCA) may be helpful in older children, and corticosteroids in those suffering from tumor invasion, nerve compression, or elevated ICP.

Anxiety and pain related to procedures may require psychological (e.g., hypnosis, conditioning) as well as pharmacologic management.

PRINCIPLES OF DRUG THERAPY
(*NELSON TEXTBOOK*, SEC. 6.55)

Most drugs are absorbed from the gastrointestinal tract by passive diffusion, and the rate and extent of *absorption* is determined by physicochemical factors (e.g., molecular weight, ionization) and by many age-dependent patient factors (e.g., gastric pH and emptying time, intestinal motility, pancreatic enzyme activity, bile salt pool size, bacterial colonization, disease process). The apparent *volume of distribution* of drugs is determined by many age-dependent variables, such as composition and size of body water and fat compartments, protein binding characteristics, hemodynamic factors, and membrane permeability.

Drug *metabolism* is dependent primarily on the maturation of biochemical processes in the liver, although the kidney, intestine, lung, adrenal, and skin also play a role in biotransforming certain compounds. Renal *excretion* of drugs is similarly dependent on age-dependent developmental processes of blood flow, filtration, and tubular function.

In general, the amount of drugs in the body is directly proportional to the dose administered. Individual and maturational variability with respect to drug efficiency and toxicity frequently requires adjustment of dosage regimens for specific patients and may be facilitated by monitoring serum concentrations.

IMAGING PROCEDURES FOR CHILDREN
(*NELSON TEXTBOOK*, SEC. 6.56)

Plain films are the dominant technique for examining the extremities for trauma and evaluation of the lungs for pneumonia, atelectasis, and neonatal pulmonary disease and the abdomen for intestinal obstruction or appendicitis.

Fluoroscopy is excellent for detecting a bronchial foreign body by differential ventilation.

Contrast examination by upper gastrointestinal series and barium enema is especially useful to diagnose malrotation, Crohn disease, ulcerative colitis, Hirschsprung disease, and intussusception.

Intravascular injection of contrast material is useful in the heart (angiocardiography) to refine echocardiographic diagnosis and in the cranium (cerebral arteriography) for suspected arteriovenous malformation, arteritis, or stroke, or to characterize arterial blood supply to unusual tumors.

Voiding cystourethrography (VCUG) using fluoroscopy is used to show valves, ureteroceles, diverticula, reflux, and other bladder and urethra abnormalities.

Ultrasonography is frequently used to evaluate lesions throughout the body, including fetal malformations, intracranial hemorrhage, ventricular dilation, soft tissue masses in face and neck, cardiac conditions, changes in abdominal organs and in the urinary tract, and hip dysplasia.

Computerized tomography (CT) usually requires sedation in young children. It is particularly useful in evaluating the brain for ventricular size, acute hemorrhage, and bony abnormalities; the lungs for pulmonary metastasis, bronchectasis, and interstitial disorders; the abdomen for abdominal organ trauma and retroperitoneal malignancies; and the lower extremities for femoral anteversion, dislocated hips, and destruction of cortical bone.

Nuclear medicine imaging (radionuclide scintigraphy, single-photon emission CT, positron emission tomography) relies on external detection of the distribution of radiopharmaceuticals to produce static or dynamic images that provide a wide spectrum of unique information.

Magnetic resonance imaging is predominantly used to evaluate the CNS in children, especially for brain tumors and demyelinating disorders. It is the procedure of choice to evaluate the spinal cord and canal, but may also be indicated for congenital heart disease and great vessel abnormalities; hilar and mediastinal adenopathy; pleural, chest wall, mediastinal, and hepatic masses; musculoskeletal soft tissue masses; and abnormalities of joints, slipped capital femoral epiphysis, aseptic necrosis of hips, vascular anomalies, and growth plate injuries of bone.

5

PRENATAL DISTURBANCES

PRENATAL FACTORS IN DISEASES OF CHILDREN

MOLECULAR GENETICS
(*NELSON TEXTBOOK*, SEC. 7.1)

The *human genome* consists of 3 billion base pairs of DNA with two copies of the double-stranded helix in each cell nucleus and mitochondria distributed in 23 chromosomes encoding about 50,000 genes (10% of total DNA). Genes expressed on mitochondrion are only of maternal origin.

A *gene* is a functional unit of DNA from which RNA is copied (transcribed) and, in the case of most human genetic diseases, translated (messenger or mRNA) by cellular machinery into a family of proteins in the cytoplasm.

Mutations are variations in DNA that affect the functioning of genes and, thereby, the patient; *polymorphisms* are variations in DNA that do not affect the health or functioning of the organism. Mutations in germ, not somatic cells, are heritable.

Advances are greatly influenced by the technology of sequencing (base pairs); cloning (amplifying a sequence or fragment of DNA to yield large amounts of the DNA segment); inserting and deleting sequences; the use of single-stranded DNA or RNA sequences (probe) to find complementary fragments by hybridization; enzymatic amplification of a DNA segment by polymerase chain reaction (PCR); and the like. Thus, a disease can be diagnosed by examination of an individual's DNA once the disease is suspected to be present in the patient or a carrier.

Human gene linkage maps are developed by locating genes or nongene DNA sequences to a precise site on a chromosome and determining the position relative to each other of individual genes or DNA sequences on the chromosome.

A *disease gene* can be found by:

1. The "forward" or "classic" method, by identifying a specific defective protein, determining its sequence of amino acids and comparing it to a normal sequence to identify the abnormality, and then isolation, cloning, and sequencing the mRNA for the abnormal protein, from which the complementary DNA sequence containing the mutation can be identified.

2. The "reverse" genetic approach, in which the mutated gene is first identified, isolated, and sequenced by direct

TABLE 5-1. MAJOR CLINICAL FEATURES OF THE THREE MOST COMMON AUTOSOMAL TRISOMIC SYNDROMES*

Characteristic Features	21-Trisomy	18-Trisomy	13-Trisomy
General	Mental retardation; hypotonia	Mental retardation; hypertonia; failure to thrive; preponderance of females; low birth weight	Mental retardation; failure to thrive; capillary hemangiomas; increased nuclear projections in neutrophils; persistent fetal hemoglobin; seizures; apneic episodes
Craniofacies	Flat occiput; oblique palpebral fissures; epicanthic folds; speckled irides (Brushfield spots); protruding tongue; prominent; malformed ears; flat nasal bridge	Prominent occiput; small features; micrognathia; low-set, malformed ears	Microcephaly; cleft lip ± palate; midline scalp defects; microphthalmia; colobomata; low-set malformed ears; apparent deafness
Thorax	Congenital heart disease, mainly septal defects, especially in the endocardial cushion	Congenital heart disease, mainly VSD† and PDA‡; short sternum; diaphragmatic hernia	Congenital heart disease, mainly septal defects, PDA

Abdomen and pelvis	Decreased acetabular and iliac angles; small penis; cryptorchidism	Horseshoe kidney; small pelvis; cryptorchidism; limited hip abduction; inguinal or umbilical hernia	Polycystic kidneys; bicornuate uterus; cryptorchidism
Hands and feet	Simian crease; short, broad hands; hypoplasia of middle phalanx of 5th finger; gap between 1st and 2nd toes	Flexion deformity of fingers; short, dorsiflexed big toes; rockerbottom feet or equinovarus; phocomelia (rare)	Polydactyly; hyperconvex or hypoplastic fingernails; simian crease
Other features observed with significant frequency	High-arched palate: strabismus; broad, short neck; small teeth; furrowed tongue; intestinal atresia; imperforate anus; Hirschsprung disease	Cleft lip ± palate; ocular anomalies; simian crease; hypoplasia of fingernails; widely spaced nipples; webbed neck; single umbilical artery; tracheoesophageal fistula	Flexion deformity of fingers; single umbilical artery; shallow supraorbital ridges; micrognathia; retroflexible thumb; rockerbottom feet; omphalocele

* From Behrman RE (ed): Nelson Textbook of Pediatrics, 14th ed. Philadelphia, WB Saunders Company, 1992, p. 283.
† VSD = ventricular septal defect.
‡ PDA = patent ductus arteriosus.

DNA analysis and subsequently the abnormal gene product (protein) or its absence is determined and its pathophysiology elucidated.

Genetic disease can be diagnosed by examining DNA from almost any cell of a patient at any time in the life of an individual. Many therapeutic molecular genetic interventions are being developed.

GENETIC ABNORMALITIES
(*NELSON TEXTBOOK*, SECS. 7.2–7.10)

Single mutan genes exhibit one of the following inheritance patterns:

Autosomal recessive: a child of two heterozygous parents has a 25% chance of being homozygous

Autosomal dominant: a child of an affected parent has a 50% chance of inheriting the genetic disorder

X-linked recessive: each daughter of a carrier has a 50% chance of being a carrier and each son a 50% chance of inheriting the disorder

X-linked dominant: males and females may be affected but all daughters and no sons of an affected father will be affected

Multifactorial inheritance refers to a process in which an abnormality is the result of the additive effects of one or more genes and environmental factors.

CHROMOSOMES AND THEIR ABNORMALITIES
(*NELSON TEXTBOOK*, SECS. 7.11–7.31)

About 1 in 150 newborns have an abnormality in the number or structure of the normally 46 chromosomes in a karyotype. *21-Trisomy* (Down syndrome; mongolism) is the most frequent autosomal syndrome. There is a high correlation between increasing maternal age and nondisjunction resulting in an extra chromosome. Major clinical features of the three most common trisomic syndromes are indicated in Table 5–1.

Translocations (transfer of a segment from one chromosome to another) are the most common structural aberrations. Usually the loss or gain of chromatin material is unbalanced or not reciprocal, resulting in an abnormal phenotype. Chromosomes 9, 11, 13, 14, 15, 21, and 22 are frequently involved.

Deletions are most commonly associated with chromosomes 4, 5, 9, and 11. They result in characteristic clinical features that often include mental retardation. *Breakage* of chromosomes is associated with neoplastic diseases, such as leukemias, and with autosomal recessive disease, such as Bloom syndrome.

About half of chromosome abnormalities involve sex chromosomes: Turner syndrome (e.g., 45,X), Klinefelter syndrome (e.g., 47,XXY), 47,XXX female, XYY male, fragile X syndrome, etc.

CONGENITAL MALFORMATIONS
(*NELSON TEXTBOOK*, SECS. 7.32 AND 7.34–7.36)

Two percent of newborns have major malformations, about half of which are genetic. There are correlations with genetic diseases, chromosomal abnormalities, in utero infections, and teratogens, but the causes of over 40% remain unknown.

Dysmorphology may result from *deformation* (altered shape or structure of a part that has differentiated normally) or *disruption* of a developing previously normal structure, in addition to *malformation* (a primary structural defect arising from a localized error in morphogenesis).

GENETIC COUNSELING
(*NELSON TEXTBOOK*, SEC. 7.33)

A correct diagnosis is fundamental. Sensitive, well-informed discussion with parents is essential to appropriate care and a major responsibility of the health professional.

6

METABOLIC DISEASES

INBORN ERRORS OF METABOLISM
(*NELSON TEXTBOOK*, SEC. 8.1)

NEONATAL PRESENTATIONS

Neonatal metabolic errors are often severe and lethal if appropriate therapy is not promptly initiated. Clinical manifestations usually are nonspecific, similar to those occurring in generalized infections:

  infant is normal at birth

  lethargy, poor feeding, vomiting, and convulsions may develop within hours after birth

  history of a previous infant with severe neonatal illness or death or consanguinity may be obtained because most disorders are autosomal recessive traits

  hepatomegaly is common

  elevated serum ammonia, commonly with normal bicarbonate and pH, is usually due to defects in urea cycle enzymes, but also may be associated with certain organic acidemias

  normal ammonia, pH, and bicarbonate may be associated with other aminoacidopathies such as hyperglycinemia

POSTNEONATAL PRESENTATIONS

There are many milder variants of diseases typically occurring in the neonatal period that have an insidious onset and delayed diagnosis. Mental retardation, developmental delay, motor deficits, failure to thrive, and convulsions are common manifestations. The clinical course may be episodic or intermittent, triggered by stress or infection, and characterized by vomiting, acidosis, mental deterioration, and coma. Hepatomegaly and renal stones may occur.

DEFECTS IN AMINO ACID METABOLISM
(*NELSON TEXTBOOK*, SECS. 8.2–8.14)

PHENYLALANINE

Phenylketonuria (PKU) is caused by phenylalanine hydroxylase deficiency with accumulation of excess phenylalanine and related metabolites. There are many clinical variants. Infants usually are normal at birth and gradually develop mental retardation that is often severe. These children often are blond, fair skinned, and blue eyed. Newborn screening by Guthrie test is effective. Benign and transient forms of hyperphenylalaninemia exist.

TYROSINE

Defects in tyrosine metabolism may result in tyrosinemia, hawkinsinuria, albinism, or alcaptanuria. Each have clinical presentations, courses, and biochemical abnormalities distinct from each other. Furthermore, most of these entities have subtypes with widely varying clinical manifestations. Dietary management is indicated for the first two disorders; liver transplantation has also been used in type I tyrosinemia.

METHIONINE

Defects in methionine metabolism may result in homocystinuria, homocystinemia, hypermethioninemia, or cystathioninemia. The classic common form of *homocystinemia*, type I, is due to cystathionine synthase deficiency (1 in 200,000 births), is associated with thromboembolic disease, usually presents after 3 yr of age, and may respond to high doses of vitamin B_6. Type II is manifest in just a few months of life and responds to vitamin B_{12}.

TRYPTOPHAN

Defects in tryptophan metabolism include Hartnup disease, serotonin deficiency, tryptophanemia, and indicanuria. *Hartnup disease* can be detected in asymptomatic newborn infants. Children develop cutaneous photosensitivity and episodic symptoms. Urinary metabolites are diagnostic, and children may respond to a high-protein diet and nicotinic acid therapy.

VALINE, LEUCINE, ISOLEUCINE, AND RELATED ORGANIC ACIDURIAS

These acidurias usually cause severe metabolic acidosis within the first few days of life. Diagnosis depends on measuring specific organic acids in body fluids (urine) and enzyme assays. Treatment of acute manifestations involves aggressive management of acidosis, removal of abnormal metabolites, and institution of appropriate nutrition. Disorders include deficiency of branched-chain aminotransferase, maple syrup urine disease (MSUD), isovaleric acidemia (sweaty feet odor), β-ketothiolase deficiency, 3-hydroxy-3-methylglutaric acidemia, propionic acidemia, methylmalonic acidemia, and combined methylmalonic aciduria and homocystinuria.

The several *forms of MSUD* often are suspected because of the peculiar odor of body fluids. Clinical manifestations vary from vomiting, lethargy, and coma within the 1st wk of life, with subsequent death if untreated, to mild retardation later in childhood. Treatment is directed at quick removal of branched-chain amino acids and their metabolites by peritoneal dialysis, fluid management, and subsequent nutritional therapy.

Biotin therapy also may be helpful in treating multiple carboxylase deficiency and *vitamin B₁₂* in treating methylmalonic acidemia.

GLYCINE

Abnormalities in glycine metabolism include hyperglycinemia, nonketotic hyperglycinemia, sarcosinemia, D-glyceric acidemia, trimethylaminuria, and hyperoxaluria and oxalosis. Elevated levels of glycine occur in a number of other inborn errors of metabolism, including propronic acidemia, methylmalonic acidemia, isovaleric acidemia, and β-ketothiolase deficiency, collectively referred to as *ketotic hyperglycinemia*.

Nonketotic Hyperglycinemia usually is a rapidly progressive, often fatal disease presenting in the 1st wk of life with lethargy, coma, and seizures; survivors have severe mental retardation. Milder forms also are characterized by seizures and mental retardation. There is no effective treatment.

Hyperoxaluria is characterized by manifestations related to renal stones and nephrocalcinosis.

PROLINE AND HYDROXYPROLINE

Abnormalities in proline and hydroxyproline metabolism result in rare primary disorders, several of which do not require treatment.

GLUTAMIC ACID

Abnormalities in glutamic acid metabolism include deficiencies of a variety of enzymes in the pathway to glutathione, the major product of glutamic acid. *Glutathione synthetase deficiency* may manifest as severe disease with chronic metabolic acidosis and hemolytic anemia in the first days of life, exacerbated by certain drugs, or milder disease, with only a red cell enzyme deficiency. Decreased production of γ-aminobutyric acid (GABA) may result in seizures and psychomotor retardation that are responsive to vitamin B₆ (vitamin B₆ or pyridoxine dependency).

UREA CYCLE AND HYPERAMMONEMIA ABNORMALITIES

These may be due to primary deficiencies of any of six enzymes involved in the Krebs-Henseleit (urea) cycle. Ammonia also may be elevated secondary to several other inborn errors.

Clinical manifestations in the neonatal period mostly are related to brain dysfunction and are similar regardless of the cause after a few days of protein feeding: refusal to feed, vomiting, tachypnea, lethargy, convulsions, and coma. In infants and older children, ataxia, mental confusion, agitation, irritability, and combativeness are common and alternate with periods of lethargy and somnolence.

Diagnosis usually is established by blood ammonia levels above 200 μmol/L (normal <35 μmol/L).

Treatment should be prompt and include removal of ammonia from the body by renal excretion, arginine administration, dialysis, and intravenous provision of calories and essential amino acids to halt further breakdown of endogenous proteins.

HISTIDINE

Histidine metabolism disorders include histidinemia and urocanic aciduria, characterized by mental and growth retardation, and asymptomatic histidinuria.

ASPARTIC ACID

Abnormal aspartic acid metabolism may lead to Canavan disease, characterized by spongy degeneration of the white matter of the brain.

LYSINE

Disorders of lysine metabolism include hyperlysinermia, α-aminoadipic acidemia, ketoadipic acidemia, glutaric aciduria type I, pipecolatemia, and lysinuric protein intolerance. Children with glutaric aciduria type I may develop normally for 2 yr and then develop progressive dystonia and dyskinesia, siezures, and hypotonia. Acute episodes associated with infection may resemble Reye syndrome and lead to coma.

DEFECTS IN METABOLISM OF LIPIDS
(*NELSON TEXTBOOK*, SECS. 8.15–8.35)

DISORDERS OF FATTY ACID OXIDATION

The most common clinical manifestations are fasting-induced episodes of coma and hypoglycemia or chronic progressive muscle weakness and cardiomyopathy. Clinical recognition is difficult because manifestations may not occur until after a prolonged fast, but some defects may present with severe neonatal disease.

These disorders have an autosomal-recessive inheritance and may result from:

defects in the intramitochondrial oxidation pathway that may present with "hypoketotic hypoglycemia," elevated organic aciduria, and secondary carnitine deficiency (e.g., short-, medium-, and long-chain acyl-CoA dehydrogenase deficiencies; long-chain 3-hydroxyacyl-CoA dehydrogenase deficiency; electron-transfer flavoprotein enzyme deficiencies; glutaric aciduria type II)
defects in transportation of fatty acids into mitochondria that do not have organic aciduria (e.g., various deficiencies in the transport and metabolism of carnitine)
defects in ketone synthesis and utilization

DISORDERS OF VERY-LONG-CHAIN FATTY ACIDS—PEROXISOMAL DISORDERS

These are inherited disorders due to failure to form or maintain the peroxisome or a defect in an enzyme normally located in this organelle (Table 6–1). These serious diseases have a wide range of phenotypes and a great diversity of clinical manifestations.

LIPID STORAGE DISEASES (Lipidoses)

(*NELSON TEXTBOOK,* SEC. 8.18)
Each of these diseases is caused by deficiency of a specific hydrolase, resulting in the storage of lipid material within the lysosomes and leading to characteristic pathophysiology, depending on which tissues are involved. Tay-Sachs, Sandhoff, Niemann-Pick, and Gaucher diseases are more common in Ashkenazi Jews.

G$_{M1}$ Gangliosidoses

These are a group of disorders with variable clinical manifestations caused by a deficiency of the lysosomal enzyme β-galactosidase. The *infantile form* is characterized by hepatosplenomegaly, edema, rashes, psychomotor retardation, macular cherry red spot, seizures, dysostosis multiplex, and cardiomegaly. The *late-onset form* manifests with ataxia, dysarthria, and cerebral palsy–like spasticity.
   Diagnosis is by absent enzyme in white blood cells or cultured skin fibroblasts.

Tay-Sachs Disease (G$_{M2}$ Gangliosidosis Type 1)

This is a devastating disease that primarily involves the central nervous system (CNS), has no peripheral physical signs, and is caused by a deficiency of β-hexosaminidase A. Infants usually develop normally until about 5 mo, when decreased eye contact and focusing, a macular cherry red spot, and hyperacusis are noted. Subsequently, blindness, hypotonia, and developmental retardation occur, culminating in death at 2–4 yr of age. A late-onset variety may also occur.
   Diagnosis is based on demonstrating enzyme deficiency in plasma or cells. *Prevention* depends on genetic counseling, and there is no treatment.

Sandhoff Disease (G$_{M2}$ Gangliosidosis Type 2)

Sandhoff disease results from deficiency of β-hexosaminidase A and B. Its manifestation is similar to Tay-Sachs disease but it also has hepatosplenomegaly in its infantile form.

Niemann-Pick Disease

Classic Niemann-Pick disease (type A) is one of four forms (A, B, C, D) and usually the most severe. Onset is usually at 3–4 mo with failure to thrive, neurologic deterioration, hepatosplenomegaly, and foam cells in bone marrow. There may be a macular cherry red spot.
   Diagnosis is based on demonstrating sphingomyelinase deficiency. There is no treatment.

TABLE 6–1. CLASSIFICATION OF PEROXISOMAL DISORDERS*

Group 1	Group 2	Group 3
Peroxisomes reduced or absent; multiple enzyme defects	Peroxisome normal; single enzyme defect	Peroxisomes present, but structure abnormal; more than one defective enzyme
Zellweger syndrome	X-linked adrenoleukodystrophy	Rhizomelic chondrodysplasia punctata
Neonatal adrenoleukodystrophy	Acatalasemia	Zellweger-like syndrome
Infantile Refsum disease	Hyperoxaluria type 1	
	3-oxoacyl-CoA thiolase deficiency "pseudo-Zellweger syndrome"	
	Acyl-CoA oxidase deficiency	
	Bifunctional enzyme deficiency	

* From Behrman RE (ed): Nelson Textbook of Pediatrics, 14th ed. Philadelphia, WB Saunders Company, 1992, p. 339.

Gaucher Disease

This may present in a variety of forms throughout life as a result of storage of a glucocerebroside in the reticuloendo-thelial system. The classic, chronic or adult form presents with splenomegaly. Hypersplenism and bone marrow failure may occur.

Diagnosis is by demonstrating deficiency of β-glucosidase. *Treatment* includes splenectomy, enzyme replacement, and bone marrow transplantation.

Other Lipidoses

Other rare disorders include Fabry disease (X-linked and often characterized by adolescent extremity pain crisis); Schindler disease (onset at 1–2 yr with developmental regression); metachromatic leukodystrophy (neurologic deterioration in the late infantile form, the most severe and common of many forms); Krabbe disease (seizures, optic atrophy, mental deterioration); Batten disease; Farber disease; Wolman disease; and fucosidosis.

MUCOLIPIDOSES
(*NELSON TEXTBOOK*, SEC. 8.19)

These disorders exhibit features of lipidosis and mucopoly-saccharidosis. They are autosomal recessive with no specific treatment. Types of mucolipidosis (ML) include ML-I or sialidosis type 2, ML-II or I-cell disease, ML-III or pseudo-Hurler polydystrophy, and ML-IV.

DISORDERS OF LIPOPROTEIN METABOLISM AND TRANSPORT
(*NELSON TEXTBOOK*, SECS. 8.20–8.35)

Screening is recommended, selectively, for children and adolescents with family history suggesting coronary heart disease (CHD) or an increased risk for it. *Treatment* is indicated for low-density lipoprotein (LDL) cholesterol of 110 mg/dL or more.

FAMILIAL HYPERCHOLESTEROLEMIA. This disorder is dominantly inherited. *Heterozygous* children have a strong family history of CHD, total cholesterol above 250 mg/dL with LDL cholesterol above 200 mg/dL, and, occasionally, tendon xanthomas and tendonitis. *Homozygous* children have cholesterol of 600 mg/dL or more from birth, usually widespread xanthomas, arcus corneae, coronary atherosclerosis, and early adult myocardial infarction (MI). Treatment may include diet, pharmacotherapy, and, for homozygous children, plasmapheresis and surgery.

FAMILIAL COMBINED HYPERLIPIDEMIA. This is the most frequently inherited multiple hyperlipoproteine-mia. There is a high risk of MI, but children may not manifest elevated triglycerides or cholesterol until the 2nd or 3rd decade, and elevation may be modest. Response to dietary treatment alone is variable.

Hyperapobetalipoproteinemia may be associate with premature CHD.

FAMILIAL DYSBETALIPOPROTEINEMIA. Xanthomas along palmar creases are common, as well as on the trunk, elbows, and knees. Vascular disease is common. Dietary treatment is very effective in this disorder, and usually effective in *sitosterolemia, familial (endogenous) hypertriglyceridemia,* and *endogenous and exogenous hyperlipidemia.*

EXOGENOUS HYPERTRIGLYCERIDEMIA (Hyperchylomicronemia). Lipoprotein lipase (LPL) deficiency results in hypertriglyceridemia shortly after birth. Manifestations include xanthomatosis, mild hepatosplenomegaly, lipemia retinalis, and pancreatitis.

SECONDARY HYPERLIPIDEMIAS. *Hypertriglyceridemia* may be secondary to obesity, diabetes mellitus, renal disease, hypothyroidism, excessive alcohol intake, oral contraceptives, and thiazide diuretics. *Hypercholesterolemia* may be secondary to hypothyroidism, nephrotic syndrome, congenital biliary atresia, anorexia nervosa, systemic lupus erythematosus, and steroids.

HIGH-DENSITY LIPOPROTEIN (HDL) DEFICIENCY STATES. Low levels of HDL or abnormal particles are associated with increased risk of atherosclerosis. There may be enlarged yellow tonsils, hepatosplenomegaly, or neuropathy.

ABETALIPROTEINEMIA AND HYPOBETALIPOPROTEINEMIA. These disorders are characterized by fat malabsorption, diarrhea, cerebellar ataxia, and acanthocytosis.

DEFECTS IN METABOLISM OF CARBOHYDRATES
(NELSON TEXTBOOK, SEC. 8.36–8.42)

GALACTOSE

Galactosemia

The two types of galactosemia result from:

deficiency of galactokinase in red cells and liver

- leads to cataracts without other clinical manifestations
- there is galactosemia and galactosuria
- galactose-free diet prevents cataracts

deficiency of galactose-1-phosphate uridyl transferase ("classic" galactosemia)

- results in substrate accumulation in and injury to kidney, liver, and brain
- clinical manifestations include jaundice, hepatomegaly, hypoglycemia, vomiting, seizures, lethargy, irritability, feeding problems, poor weight gain, liver injury, aminoaciduria, cataracts, splenomegaly, and mental retardation
- early diagnosis is by identifying urinary galactose
- diet restriction ameliorates untoward effects

Deficiency of uridyl diphosphogalactose-4-epimerase

This leads to an asymptomatic disorder or disease manifestations identical to those of classic galactosemia.

FRUCTOSE

Benign *fructosuria* due to fructokinase deficiency is asymptomatic. *Deficiency of 1-phosphofructaldolase* results in chemical manifestations similar to "classic" galactosemia and is treated by a fructose elimination diet.

LACTIC ACIDOSIS–RELATED DISORDERS

These disorders are suggested by Kussmaul respiration and signs of impending shock.

Deficiency of glucose-6-phosphatase (glycogen storage disease type I) may be clinically minor or life threatening.

Deficiency of fructose-1,6-diphosphatase is asymptomatic while infants are taking only human milk, but fructose or sucrose intake leads to hypoglycemia, seizures, and shock.

Deficiencies of pyruvate decarboxylase, dihydrolipoyl transacetylase, dihydrolipoyl dehydrogenase, pyruvate carboxylase, pyruvate dehydrogenase phosphate, and enzymes involved in biotin metabolism have been described and, in general, are characterized by CNS manifestations.

Carnitine deficiency states and *congenital idiopathic lactic acidosis* may present with recurrent attacks of severe acidosis, hypoglycemia, and hepatomegaly.

Leigh subacute necrotizing encephalopathy is characterized by acidosis, seizures, and psychomotor retardation. Transitory improvement with thiamine and tris-hydroxymethylaminomethane (THAM) treatment may occur.

GLYCOGEN STORAGE DISEASES

These disorders result from abnormal concentrations or structures of glycogen and are classified by enzymatic defects and/or distinctive clinical features. *Clinical manifestations* vary with different disorders and may include hypoglycemia, seizures, enlarged liver or kidneys, lactic acidosis, neutropenia, cardiomegaly, hypotonia, hyperlipemia, developmental delays, muscle weakness, neurologic deterioration, and growth retardation. *Diagnosis* is based on postnatal tissue analysis of biopsies and, in some instances, antenatally on analysis of cultured cells.

DISORDERS OF MUCOPOLYSACCHARIDE METABOLISM
(*NELSON TEXTBOOK*, SEC. 8.43)

The mucopolysaccharidoses (MPSs) are inherited disorders (autosomal recessive, except for Hunter syndrome) caused

by incomplete degradation and storage of acid mucopolysac-
charides (glycosaminoglycans).

Clinical manifestations result from accumulation of muco-
polysaccharides in various organs and, because they are
major components of the intracellular substance of connective tissue, from bony changes. Similar features are found
in a variety of nonmucopolysaccharides.

Diagnosis differentiating among these various disorders is
based on clinical and radiologic manifestations, pattern of
urinary mucopolysaccharide excretion, and deficiency of
specific enzymes. The major syndromes are presented
below.

HURLER SYNDROME (MPS IH)

This most severe disorder is due to α-L-iduronidase deficiency, with accumulation of dermatan and heparan sulfates
in almost every tissue and organ of the body.

Clinical manifestations usually progress relentlessly from
normal appearance at birth to death by early teenage years,
and include hepatosplenomegaly, kyphosis, nasal discharge, coarse facial features, enlarged head with frontal
bossing, corneal clouding, developmental and mental retardation, joint abnormalities, and dysostosis multiplex (roentgenographic skeletal deformities).

Diagnosis depends on demonstration of enzyme deficiency
in blood cells, serum, or skin fibroblasts.

SCHEIE SYNDROME (MPS IS)

This is the mildest disorder, and is due to accumulation of
dermatan sulfate in tissues. Intelligence is normal, the cornea usually clouded, and there is onset of milder clinical
features after 5 yr. Life expectancy is normal.

HUNTER SYNDROME (MPS II)

Clinical manifestations in this X-linked disorder are milder but
similar to, and progression slower than in, Hurler syndrome
in terms of skeletal and mental defects, but mental retardation may be severe in type A compared to type B.

SANFILIPPO SYNDROME (MPS III)

Coarse facial appearance and skeletal involvement milder
than in Hunter or Hurler syndrome mark Sanfilippo syndrome. Only heparan sulfate is stored in tissues and excreted
in the urine. Developmental delays and other initially
mild clinical features progress to severe neurologic and
mental deterioration, joint stiffness, hepatosplenomegaly,
dysostosis multiplex, and death in midteens.

MORQUIO SYNDROME (MPS IV)

Keratan sulfate and chondroitin-6-sulfate are stored in tissues and the former is found in urine. Two different enzyme

defects result in identical phenotypes. Clinical manifestations similar to those in Hurler syndrome are severe and appear during the 1st yr, but there is no mental retardation.

DEFECTS IN METABOLISM OF PURINES, PYRIMIDINES, AND OTHER PROTEINS
(*NELSON TEXTBOOK*, SECS. 8.44–8.48)

Purines and pyrimidines combine with other substances to form nucleotides, RNA, and DNA and, thus, are important in genetics and regulation of proteins. Uric acid is the final product of purine metabolism.

Purine disorders include gout, Lesch-Nyhan syndrome (motor delay in first few months of life and rapidly progressive general neurologic deterioration, including compulsive self-destructive behavior); hyperuricemia (usually due to marked increase in cell number and destruction with myeloproliferative disease); xanthinuria (may be associated with urinary calculi); and adenosine deaminase deficiency (severe combined immunodeficiency). Orotic aciduria is seen with several rare *disorders of pyrimidine metabolism*.

A variety of inborn errors of metabolism of enzymes and proteins cannot be assigned naturally to specific metabolic systems (e.g., analbuminemia, haptoglobin deficiency, hypophosphatasia, intestinal enterokinase deficiency, pancreatic enzyme deficiencies).

DEFECTS IN HEME PIGMENT METABOLISM
(*NELSON TEXTBOOK*, SECS. 8.49–8.51)

THE PORPHYRIAS

These syndromes are characterized biochemically by various errors in pyrrole metabolism and clinically by photodermatitis and visceral and neuropsychiatric manifestations. These usually dominantly inherited disorders are classified as erythopoietic (two types) or hepatic (six types) depending on locus of metabolic error. The onset may be from infancy through adulthood. Acquired or toxic porphyrias also may occur.

Clinical manifestations have an insidious onset and then run an undulating acute exacerbating course throughout life.

Skin lesions (erythema, edema, vesiculations, pain, heat) occur with exposure to sunlight and trauma and may become urticarial, eczematoid, and disfiguring.

Colicky abdominal pain and neuropsychiatric features (personality changes, weakness, paresthesias, paralysis) usually occur together and may be precipitated by infection, menstruation, pregnancy, alcohol, and other drugs. Leukocytosis and fever are common, and there may be vomiting, constipation, tachycardia, and hypertension.

Urine is initially colorless but contains porphobilinogen. Later it may become red, especially if barbiturates are given.

Severe fluid and electrolyte disturbances may occur.

Diagnosis depends on recognizing the clinically intermittent exacerbating course and the sequence of manifestations, and demonstrating pyrroles in excreta.

Treatment includes correction of homeostatic disturbances, support of vital functions, increased carbohydrate intake, management of pain, hematin, and avoidance of inducing agents.

HEREDITARY METHEMOGLOBINEMIAS

These disorders are characterized by abnormal amounts of hemoglobin iron in the ferric state (nonfunctioning) as a result of a deficiency of NADH cytochrome b5 reductase or the presence of abnormal methemoglobins (hemoglobin M diseases). Cyanosis without cardiorespiratory distress is the usual presentation. Blood may have a chocolate hue.

Diagnosis is based on elevation of methemoglobin and identification of M hemoglobins.

Treatment includes methylene blue and ascorbic acid.

HEMOCHROMATOSIS

The structure and function of organs is deranged because of idiopathic or acquired excessive iron storage (e.g., hepatitis, bronze skin, diabetes mellitus, cardiac arrthymias). Treatment is by chelation.

DIABETES MELLITUS
(*NELSON TEXTBOOK*, SECS. 8.52–8.58)

Type I, or insulin-dependent diabetis mellitus (IDDM), the most common metabolic–endocrine disorder of childhood, is caused by a progressive deficiency of insulin secretion resulting in abnormal carbohydrate, protein, and fat metabolism. Autoimmunity, genetic susceptibility, and triggering factors such as infections play important roles in the etiology and pathogenesis.

The pathophysiology results from derangements in the regulation of glucose metabolism caused by insulin deficiency and increased concentration and action of counterregulatory hormones (epinephrine, cortisol, growth hormone, and glucagon).

Increased production and decreased utilization of glucose leads to hyperglycemia and glucosuria, resulting in osmotic diuresis with loss of electrolytes and water and hyperosmolarity.

Lipolysis and lipid synthesis increase, leading to the formation and accumulation of ketoacids (β-hydroxybutyrate and acetoacetate) and acetone, resulting in metabolic acidosis.

CLINICAL MANIFESTATIONS

There is usually a history of polyuria, polydipsia, polyphagia, and weight loss for less than 1 mo. Onset may be insidious, with lethargy and weakness. Ketoacidosis may manifest as vomiting, dehydration, Kussmaul respirations, and acetone breath. There may be abdominal pain.

Laboratory findings include glucosuria, ketonuria, hyperglycemia, ketonemia, metabolic acidosis, electrolyte abnormalities, leukocytosis, and hyperlipidemia.

DIAGNOSIS

Hyperglycemia (plasma glucose >200 mg/dL) and associated glucosuria with or without ketonuria is diagnostic. A glucose tolerance test is not needed if polyuria and polydipsia are associated with hyperglycemia and glucosuria.

Diabetic ketoacidosis (DKA) is diagnosed by glucose >300 mg/dL, positive ketones at greater than 1:2 serum dilution, pH <7.3 and bicarbonate <15 mEq/L, glucosuria, ketonuria, and clinical manifestations. Nonketotic hyperosmolar coma (glucose >600 mg/dL, acidosis, dehydration) must be distinguished from DKA.

TREATMENT

Ketoacidosis (DKA) Phase

1. Monitor vital signs, input and output, glucose, fluid and electrolytes, and acid–base status.
2. Correct intravascular volume deficit with isotonic saline (0.9%) gradually (50–60% in first 12 hr) and administer IV glucose when blood glucose is about 300 mg/dL to avoid rapid fall in serum osmolality and onset of cerebral edema.
3. Administer potassium phosphate after urine flow is established to avoid hypokalemia secondary to depletion, correction of acidosis, and insulin therapy.

Severe acidosis (pH of 7.2 or less) not corrected by provision of fluids, electrolytes, glucose, and insulin may require slow infusion (over 2 hr) of bicarbonate. *Cerebral edema* with elevated intracranial pressure, the major life-threatening complication of DKA, requires prompt therapy with mannitol and hyperventilation.

Continuous low-dose regular insulin infusion is indicated (0.1 U/kg priming dose and then 0.1 U/kg/hr) and should be adjusted to response, with subsequent transition to IM or SC bolus injections.

Postacidotic/Transition Phase or IDDM without Ketoacidosis and Dehydration

Adequate oral fluid and nutrition should be provided. SC regular insulin (0.1–0.25 U/kg every 6–8 hr before meals) should be given. Patient and parent education is directed at facilitating their understanding and management of the disease (including insulin injection).

CONTINUING (CHRONIC) MANAGEMENT

The goals of chronic management include adequate nutrition for normal growth and development and an active life, exogenous insulin sufficient to avoid acute clinical manifestations, and metabolic control sufficient to minimize long-term complications (e.g., ocular, cardiovascular, renal). Usually, two daily combined doses of short- (regular) and intermediate-acting insulin are recommended. Initially the dose is based on two thirds of the total daily dose required during the transition phase. Adjustments are made in 10–15% increments or decrements to achieve control. There are no special nutritional requirements other than those necessary for optimal growth, development, and activity, but regular eating patterns are important for optimal insulin administration. Blood and urine glucose and glycosylated hemoglobin (HbA$_{1c}$) monitoring are essential.

A *"honeymoon"* *period* of progressive reduction in insulin requirements secondary to residual beta cell function is common after initial stabilization.

Hypoglycemic reactions (insulin shock) may develop suddenly and may manifest as pallor, sweating, apprehension, trembling, tachycardia, hunger, drowsiness, confusion, and coma or other CNS changes. Insulin shock is due to too much insulin relative to food intake and energy expenditure and is primarily treated by immediately increasing carbohydrate intake or, if oral intake is not feasible, by administration of glucagon.

Intercurrent illnesses require additional insulin. Cystic fibrosis, various autoimmune diseases, and rare genetic syndromes are also associated with diabetes mellitus.

HYPOGLYCEMIA
(*NELSON TEXTBOOK*, SEC. 8.59)

DEFINITIONS

Neonate: blood glucose <40 mg/dL (2.2 mmol/L) should be treated as presumptive hypoglycemia, especially after 2–3 hr of life (nadir); blood glucose is usually 50 mg/dL (2.8 mmol/L) or more after 12–24 hr

Older infants and children: blood glucose <40 mg/dL is significant hypoglycemia necessitating treatment

SIGNIFICANCE AND SEQUELAE

Glucose is a major source of fuel and energy storage, and the developing brain is critically dependent on glucose. Prolonged hypoglycemia may lead to severe neurologic damage.

CLINICAL MANIFESTATIONS IN CHILDHOOD

Features associated with activation of autonomic nervous system and epinephrine release include anxiety, perspiration, palpitation, pallor, weakness, and hunger. Features associated with cerebral glucopenia include headache, mental confusion, visual disturbances, personality changes, inability to concentrate, seizures, coma, and dizziness.

MAJOR CAUSES

- Neonatal

    prematurity
    small-for-gestational-age birth
    low birth weight
    severe illness
    maternal toxemia
    infants of diabetic mothers
    erythroblastosis fetalis

- Neonatal/Infantile/Childhood

    hyperinsulinemic states (e.g., nesidioblastosis, leucine sensitivity, Beckwith-Wiedemann syndrome)
    hormone deficiency (e.g., panhypopituitarism, adrenal insufficiency, isolated growth hormone deficiency)
    limited substrate disorders (e.g., ketotic hypoglycemia, MSUD)
    glycogen storage disease
    disorders of gluconeogenesis (e.g., acute alcohol intoxication, salicylate poisoning, IDDM)
    other enzyme deficiencies (e.g., galactosemia, fructose intolerance)
    disorders of fat metabolism (e.g., carnitine deficiency)
    drugs (e.g., insulin, propranolol)
    liver disease (e.g., Reye syndrome, hepatitis)
    amino acid and organic acid disorders
    systemic disorders (e.g., sepsis, heart failure, malnutrition, shock, diarrhea)

TREATMENT

Prevention is especially important during the neonatal period and early childhood, when CNS development is rapid. Hypoglycemia in a neonate or infant should be treated with 2mL/kg of $D_{10}W$, followed by continuous glucose infusion of 6–8 mg/kg/min, adjusting the rate to maintain normal blood levels. Persistent hypoglycemia during infancy or childhood may require high rates of glucose infusion, hydrocortisone, growth hormone, diazoxide, octreotide, pancreatic surgery, dietary management, or other therapy, depending on the specific diagnosis of the underlying disorder.

7

THE FETUS AND NEONATAL INFANT

DEFINITIONS

Neonatal mortality refers to death within the first 4 wk of life; the highest rate is in first 24 hr.

Perinatal mortality refers to deaths of fetuses and neonates from 20 wk gestation to 28 days after birth.

Infant mortality refers to deaths from birth through 12 mo/ 1,000 live births.

Low birth weight (LBW) refers to infants weighing 2,500 g or less at birth.

Very low birth weight (VLBW) refers to infants weighing 1,500 g or less at birth.

NEWBORN INFANT
(*NELSON TEXTBOOK*, SECS. 9.1–9.6)

The neonatal period is a time of high mortality and morbidity because of increased vulnerability secondary to the transition from intrauterine to extrauterine life and the immature developmental stage. Family and pregnancy history and physical examination are important to anticipation and early detection of problems. Infants born after high-risk pregnancies or deliveries, those with family histories of heritable disorders, or infants with abnormal physical findings should be placed under special observation.

ORDINARY CARE

- Basic requirements

    assistance at birth, primarily to establish respiration
    provision of adequate nutrition
    support to maintain normal body temperature
    avoiding contact with infection
    constant care, alert to signs of illness
    minimum separation from mother

- Delivery room care

    clearing and maintaining airway
    Apgar assessment (heart rate, respiratory effort, muscle tone, response to nostril catheter, color)
    limiting heat loss

asceptic skin and cord care
eye drop protection against gonorrhea
neonatal disorder screening

Breast-feeding should be encouraged.

HIGH-RISK PREGNANCIES AND THE FETUS
(NELSON TEXTBOOK, SECS. 9.7–9.14)

Many clinical problems of the newborn infant are related to intrauterine and/or maternal factors. About half of perinatal morbidity and mortality can be identified with high-risk pregnancies or deliveries.

Major *risk factors* of pregnancy are economic (e.g., poverty, poor access to prenatal care); cultural–behavioral (e.g., cigarette, alcohol, and drug abuse; unmarried status; black race; short interpregnancy interval); biologic–genetic (e.g., previous LBW infant, hereditary diseases, poor maternal nutrition); reproductive (e.g., prolonged gestation or labor, breech lie, infection, uterine bleeding, polyhydramnios and oligohydramnios, prior infertility, premature rupture of membranes, fetal disorders); and medical (e.g., maternal diabetes mellitus, hypertension, cardiopulmonary disease, or ingestion of legal or illegal drugs).

Fetal growth and maturity are assessed by history of last menstrual periods, ultrasonic measurements, and determination of amniotic fluid surfactant content. *Fetal distress* and various *fetal diseases* are diagnosed by a variety of antepartum and intrapartum imaging (e.g., ultrasound), biochemical (e.g., fetal tissue and fluid analysis), and biophysical (electronic monitoring) methods, which may provide the basis for various maternal (e.g., maternal steroids for idiopathic thrombocytopenic purpura), fetal (e.g., RhoGAM, fetal blood transfusion for Rh disease), or neonatal (e.g., acid–base resuscitation for fetal hypoxic encephalopathy) preventive or treatment regimens.

HIGH-RISK INFANTS
(NELSON TEXTBOOK, SECS. 9.15–9.19)

Infants at particular risk during the neonatal period should be identified as soon as possible before or after birth and closely observed in order to decrease morbidity and mortality. *Risk factors* include demographic–social (e.g., illicit drug, alcohol, or cigarette use; poverty; unmarried status); past medical history (e.g., maternal diabetes, hypertension, chronic medication); prior pregnancy (e.g., fetal or neonatal death, premature or LBW birth, congenital malformation); present pregnancy (e.g., vaginal bleeding, multiple gestation, inadequate prenatal care, acute illness); labor and delivery (e.g., premature labor, fetal distress, breech presentation, low Apgar score, prolonged pregnancy, abnormal placenta, immature lecithin–sphyngomyelin ratio); and neonatal (e.g., birth weight <2,500 or >4,000 g, gestation <37 or >42 wk, disproportionate growth for gestational age, tachypnea, cyanosis, pallor, plethora, or congenital malformations).

DISEASE IN LBW INFANTS

Immaturity tends to increase the severity but decrease the distinctiveness of clinical manifestations.

Infants with intrauterine growth retardation (IUGR) and those small for gestational age (SGA) are a heterogeneous population distinguished from infants that are premature (by gestational age) but of appropriate or larger size for their gestational age or developmentally immature at any gestational age. Important disorders in these groups of infants include:

hemorrhage
sepsis
respiratory distress syndrome
major malformations
apnea
hypoglycemia
necrotizing enterocolitis (NEC)
hyperbilirubinemia
retinopathy of prematurity
dysfunctions related to organ system immaturity

Intensive care nurseries have been specially adapted to the needs of these and other high-risk infants. These hospital units provide physiologic and biochemical monitoring.

DISEASES OF THE NEWBORN INFANT: PREMATURE AND FULL TERM
(*NELSON TEXTBOOK*, SECS. 9.20–9.29)

CLINICAL MANIFESTATIONS IN THE NEONATAL PERIOD

Recognizing disease depends on knowledge about the disorder and evaluation of a limited number of signs and symptoms:

central cyanosis—usually indicates respiratory insufficiency, which may be due to pulmonary conditions, central nervous system (CNS) conditions, or shock; however, it may also be due to and difficult to distinguish from congenital heart disease (CHD)
pallor—may be due to hemorrhage, hypoxia, hypoglycemia, sepsis, shock or adrenal failure
convulsions
lethargy
irritability
hyperactivity
failure to feed well
hyperpyrexia or hypopyrexia
jaundice
vomiting, diarrhea, or abdominal distention

CONGENITAL ANOMALIES

Common life-threatening anomalies include choanal atresia, Pierre Robin syndrome, diaphragmatic hernia, tracheoesophageal fistula, intestinal obstruction, gastroschisis, omphalocele, renal agenesis, neural tube defects, and ductal-dependent CHD.

BIRTH INJURIES

Birth injuries are avoidable or unavoidable mechanical or anoxic trauma incurred during labor and delivery, such as:

cranial injury (e.g., caput succedaneum, cephalohematoma, skull fracture)
intracranial (intraventricular) hemorrhage, which is highly associated with LBW
spinal cord traction
peripheral nerve injuries (brachial palsy, phrenic nerve paralysis, facial nerve paralysis)
visceral trauma (to spleen, liver, or adrenals)
fracture of clavical or extremities

Hypoxic–ischemic encephalopathy (asphyxia) may occur before or after birth and is an important cause of subsequent CNS disability.

DELIVERY ROOM EMERGENCIES

Failure to initiate and maintain respiration is the most common and important emergency. This may represent CNS failure (e.g., intraventricular hemorrhage, asphyxia, drug narcosis) or a pulmonary disorder. A chest film is necessary. Resuscitation must be initiated promptly.

Shock requires fluid resuscitation.
Convulsions require anticonvulsants and oxygen.

DISTURBANCES OF ORGAN SYSTEMS

RESPIRATORY TRACT
(*NELSON TEXTBOOK*, SECS. 9.30–9.40)

Transition from placental to pulmonary respiration requires removal of fetal lung fluid, establishing and maintaining gas-containing functional residual capacity, and developing a ventilation (alveoli)–perfusion (blood) relationship for optimal O_2–CO_2 exchange. Prolonged apneic pauses associated with illness must be distinguished from a periodic breathing pattern. Monitoring and treatment (e.g., stimulation, ventilation, airway pressure, drugs) may be required.

Hyaline Membrane Disease (Respiratory Distress Syndrome)

This major cause of death in LBW infants is due to surfactant deficiency in the lungs with progressive atelectasis and hypoventilation. Rapid, shallow respirations are usually noted shortly after birth. Grunting retractions, nasal flaring, and cyanosis are common. Secondary circulatory insufficiency

jaundice hue is primarily due to accumulation of unconjugated indirect-reacting, lipid-soluble bilirubin pigment derived from hemoglobin breakdown. It can be neurotoxic at certain concentrations and under certain circumstances. Normally its principle route of elimination is via conjugation and excretion by hepatic cells into the biliary system and gastrointestinal tract.

ETIOLOGY. Unconjugated hyperbilirubinemia may be caused or increased by factors that: (1) increase the load to be metabolized in liver (e.g., hemolytic anemia); (2) damage or reduce the activity of conjugating transferase enzymes; (3) compete for or block transferase enzymes (e.g., drugs); and (4) lead to an absence of or decreased amounts of enzyme or reduction in bilirubin liver uptake (e.g., genetic disease, prematurity).

Toxic effects are due to factors that reduce retention of bilirubin in the circulation, (e.g., hypoproteinemia, displacement of bilirubin from albumin binding sites) or increase the permeability of the blood–brain barrier or nerve cell membranes to unconjugated bilirubin, such as occurs with asphyxia and prematurity.

CLINICAL MANIFESTATIONS. Jaundice, a bright yellow or orange color, may be present at birth (e.g., Rh disease) or appear at any time during the neonatal period. Infants are often asymptomatic but may be lethargic or feed poorly.

DIFFERENTIAL DIAGNOSIS. Time of onset may be helpful:

at birth or within 1st 24 hr suggests erythroblastosis, concealed hemorrhage, sepsis, or congenital infection

on 2nd or 3rd day suggests "physiologic" jaundice or Crigler-Najjar syndrome

after 3rd day suggests septicemia

after 1st wk suggest breast milk jaundice, septicemia, bile duct atresia (direct-reacting or conjugated bilirubin also present), or spherocytosis

Significant levels of hyperbilirubinemia require a diagnostic evaluation.

PHYSIOLOGIC JAUNDICE (Icterus Neonatorum). Under normal circumstances the following levels of indirect-reacting bilirubin occur in *full-term infants:*

1–3 mg/dL (17.1–51 μmol/L) in umbilical cord serum

rate of increase is <5 mg/dL/24 hr, resulting in 5–6 mg/dL peak at 2nd–4th day of life (6–7% have 12.9 mg/dL)

Premature or LBW infants' serum bilirubin levels tend to rise at a similar rate or a little slower than term infants, but the rise is of longer duration, resulting in higher levels.

Peak levels of 8–12 mg/dL (136–205 μmol/L) tend to occur at 5th–7th day

levels are very dependent on weight, maturity, and clinical status of these infants

PATHOLOGIC HYPERBILIRUBINEMIA. This is defined as a time of appearance, duration, or pattern of serially determined serum bilirubin concentrations that varies significantly from that of physiologic jaundice or, if the concentrations do not vary, as a circumstance in which other reasons exist to consider that the infant is at special risk of neurotoxicity (kernicterus).

JAUNDICE ASSOCIATED WITH BREAST-FEEDING. This may occur as a consequence of decreased fluid and nutritional intake or a benign condition in which a substance in breast milk inhibits hepatic bilirubin conjugation.

KERNICTERUS. This is a neurologic syndrome resulting from the deposition of unconjugated bilirubin in brain cells. The risk is probably crudely related to the serum bilirubin level of whatever cause. A number of factors (e.g., prematurity, anoxia, meningitis, acidosis) increase the risk of kernicterus. *Clinical manifestations* usually appear 2–7 days after birth, but they can occur at any time during the neonatal period and include lethargy, poor feeding, loss of Moro reflex, respiratory distress, seizures, opisthotonos, high-pitched cry, and rigidity. *Prognosis* is usually poor. Survivors have severe motor abnormalities and hearing loss.

TREATMENT OF HYPERBILIRUBINEMIA. Therapy is directed at preventing blood indirect-reacting unconjugated bilirubin from reaching neurotoxic levels (Table 7–1). The risk of CNS injury should be balanced against risks of the treatment modality. Underlying causes such as sepsis must be treated.

Exchange transfusion is usually indicated in full-term infants to keep bilirubin under 20 mg/dL (342 μmol/L) (see above).

Phototherapy should be started below toxic levels because 12–24 hr of treatment may be necessary before a measurable effect occurs.

TABLE 7–1. GUIDELINES FOR MAXIMAL PERMISSIBLE TOTAL SERUM BILIRUBIN CONCENTRATIONS (mg/dL)*†

Birthweight Category (g)‡	Uncomplicated Course	Complicated Course§
Less than 1,250	13‖	10
1,250–1,499	15	13
1,500–1,999	17	15
2,000–2,499	18	17
2,500 and up	20	18

* From Gartner LM: *In* Behrman RE (ed): Neonatal-Perinatal Medicine. St. Louis, CV Mosby, 1977.

† Direct-reacting bilirubin concentrations are not subtracted unless they amount to more than 50% of the total serum bilirubin concentration. This table is applicable during the first 28 days of life.

‡ Equivalent gestational age categories may be used in lieu of birth weight for small for gestational age (SGA) infants.

§ Complications include perinatal asphyxia and acidosis, postnatal hypoxia and acidosis, significant and persistent hypothermia, hypoalbuminemia, meningitis, and other significant infections, hemolysis, hypoglycemia, and signs of clinical or CNS deterioration.

‖ To convert mg/dL to μmol/L, multiply by 17.1.

potentially neurotoxic bilirubin in the skin absorbs light energy, which converts it to a nontoxic configurational photoisomer that is excreted in bile (4Z,15E bilirubin) and a structural isomer (lumirubin) excreted in the urine

peak levels may be reduced by 3–6 mg/dL

eyes need to be covered and temperature and bilirubin monitored

complications include loose stools and rashes

BLOOD
(*NELSON TEXTBOOK*, SECS. 9.46–9.49)

Newborn Anemia

At birth, anemia may manifest as pallor, congestive heart failure, or shock. It is usually caused by hemolytic disease of the newborn, but may be due to acute blood loss, transplacental hemorrhage, internal hemorrhage, intrauterine infection, or twin–twin transfusion.

Anemia appearing in *first few days after birth* usually also is due to hemolytic disease, but may result from umbilical cord hemorrhage, cephalohematoma, intracranial hemorrhage, and subcapsular bleeding from the liver, spleen, adrenals, or kidneys.

Anemia of prematurity may occur in LBW infants 1–3 mo of age, manifesting as failure to thrive or tachypnea and tachycardia. It may be a consequence of earlier disease, phlebotomy, or decreased hematopoiesis.

Treatment depends on severity and the presence of comorbid disease. It may include iron, blood transfusion, or erythropoietin administration.

Hemolytic Disease of the Newborn
(Erythroblastosis Fetalis)

An increased red cell destruction results from transplacental passage of maternal antibody active against red blood cell antigens of the infant.

DUE TO Rh INCOMPATIBILITY. Ninety percent of cases are due to D antigen inherited from an Rh-positive father and antibody production by a previously sensitized (from blood transfusion or transplantal passage of fetal cells containing antigen) Rh-negative (D−) mother.

Clinical Manifestations. These range from mild laboratory evidence of hemolysis (anemia, jaundice) to severe symptomatic anemia and hydrops fetalis.

Hydrops fetalis includes severe anemia, hyperbilirubinemia, signs of cardiac decompensation (cardiomegaly, respiratory distress, anasarca, edema, circulatory collapse), and massive enlargement of the liver and spleen (as a result of hyperplasia of erythropoietic tissue). It may also occur from nonimmune disorders such as intrauterine infections, congenital anomalies of the cardiac, pulmonary, or renal systems, or tumors.

Intrauterine therapeutic transfusion or compensatory extramedullary hematopoiesis may mask anemia.

Diagnosis. Diagnosis requires demonstration of blood group incompatibility and antibody bound to the infant's red blood cells.

Antenatal diagnosis is based on a history of sensitization (previous transfusion, abortion, or pregnancy), paternal–maternal blood type incompatibility, elevated maternal blood immunoglobulin G (IgG) antibodies to D antigen, ultrasound diagnosis of hydrops fetalis, percutaneous umbilical blood sampling, and amniocentesis (amniotic fluid bilirubin levels).

Postnatal diagnosis is based on positive direct Coombs test, demonstration of anemia, hyperbilirubinemia, and blood type incompatibility between infant and mother.

Treatment. Goals are (1) to prevent morbidity and death from severe anemia and hypoxia and (2) to avoid neurotoxicity from hyperbilirubinemia. *Intrauterine transfusion* of packed red cells is indicated for hydrops or anemia in a fetus that is too immature to survive without significant morbidity if delivered. Life support, including airway and fluid resuscitation, and stabilization and monitoring may be needed at birth for severely affected infants.

Transfusion or partial or full exchange transfusion should use fresh, low-titer, group O, Rh-negative blood cross-matched against maternal serum. Exchange transfusion of an infant is indicated if there is a high risk of rapid development of a dangerous degree of anemia or hyperbilirubinemia. Severe hemolysis is manifested by a hemoglobin of 10 g/dL or less, a bilirubin of 5 mg/dL (85 μmol/L) or more, and reticulocyte counts greater than 15% at birth.

Bilirubin should be monitored and kept below levels indicated in Table 7–1 by exchange transfusion and/or phototherapy.

Prevention of Rh Sensitization. This is accomplished by IM injection of 300 mg of human anti-D globulin (RhoGAM) within 72 hr of delivery or abortion.

DUE TO A-B AND OTHER BLOOD GROUP INCOMPATIBILITIES. Most cases are mild, with jaundice as the only clinical manifestation, but may require management of anemia and hyperbilirubinemia. *Diagnosis* is based on demonstrating blood group incompatibility, positive direct Coombs test, spherocytosis, and reticulocytosis. *Treatment* with phototherapy is usually sufficient for mild disease.

Plethora of the Newborn Infant

A ruddy, deep purple appearance associated with a high hematocrit (central of 65% or higher) is often due to polycythemia.

Clinical manifestations are varied and include cyanosis, respiratory distress, seizures, and hyperbilirubinemia. Many infants are asymptomatic.

Treatment includes phlebotomy and saline or albumin replacement.

Hemorrhagic Disease in the Newborn

Rare episodes of spontaneous and prolonged bleeding are due to accentuation and prolongation of deficiency of vitamin K–dependent blood coagulation factors (II, VII, IX, and X) that are normally transiently depressed after birth. Hemorrhagic disease is more common in premature than term infants and in breast-fed infants between the 2nd and 5th days of life.

Treatment with IV vitamin K_1 (1–5 mg) is usually effective within a few hours. *Prevention* is often effective in full-term infants with administration of 1 mg of natural oil–soluble vitamin K IM at birth.

MASTITIS NEONATORUM
(*NELSON TEXTBOOK*, SEC. 9.52)

Engorgement of the breasts is physiologic in newborn infants. Infection may occur as a result of manipulation and is manifested by redness, heat, swelling, and pain. *Treatment* includes systemic antibiotics and local compresses.

UMBILICUS
(*NELSON TEXTBOOK*, SEC. 9.53)

A *single umbilical artery* is associated with congenital anomalies.

Omphalocele, herniation or protrusion of the abdominal contents into the base of the cord, requires surgical treatment.

Hemorrhage may be due to inadequate ligation of the cord, failure of normal thrombus formation, hemorrhagic disease of the newborn, or infection.

Granuloma with discharge may result from mild infection and is usually responsive to local treatment with cleansing alcohol. More exuberant local granulation requires silver nitrate cauterization.

Inflammation of the umbilical region requires prompt systemic antibiotic administration and local management.

Umbilical hernias of 1–5 cm are common and do not require treatment.

SUBSTANCE ABUSE
(*NELSON TEXTBOOK*, SEC. 9.54)

Substance abuse during pregnancy may have untoward effects on the fetus and infant. Usually multiple substances are abused, including tobacco, and there are many other socioeconomic and medical risk factors present.

Heroin addiction is associated with LBW births and stillbirths. Infants may be depressed at birth. Infant withdrawal symptoms usually occur within 48 hr but may occur as late as 4–6 wk after birth. Tremors and hyperirritability are most often prominent manifestations but there may also be tachypnea, vomiting, and diarrhea.

Methadone addiction results in a pattern of infant clinical manifestation similar to that of heroin addiction, but seizures and late withdrawal signs and symptoms are more common.

Alcohol addiction is more common than heroin and methadone addiction, but withdrawal manifestations are uncommon. Hypoglycemia and acidosis occur. *Fetal alcohol syndrome* results from high levels of alcohol ingestion during pregnancy and consists of retarded body and head growth, facial dysmorphology, cardiac anomalies, delayed development, and various degrees of mental retardation.

Cocaine addiction is associated with premature labor, abruptio placentae, LBW, microcephaly, and neurodevelopmental abnormalities, many of which are transient. There are no withdrawal manifestations.

INFANTS OF DIABETIC MOTHERS
(*NELSON TEXTBOOK*, SEC. 9.56)

Infants of diabetic women and those who later develop diabetes may share certain morphologic characteristics and morbidity risks. Diabetic mothers also have a high incidence of polyhydramnios, their fetal mortality rate is greater than that of nondiabetic mothers, and when vascular disease is present their LBW rate is high.

The *pathophysiology* probably primarily relates to maternal hyperglycemia with resultant fetal hyperglycemia and hyperinsulinemia.

Clinical manifestations include large size for gestational age, plump plethoric puffy cushingoid appearance, macrosomia (esp. heart, liver, spleen), and hyperexcitability or tremulousness, although hypotonia and lethargy also may occur. Hypoglycemia is common and often asymptomatic. Hypocalcemia and hypomagnesemia may also occur. Respiratory distress, cardiac failure, congenital anomalies, polycythemia, hyperbilirubinemia, asphyxia, and renal vein thrombosis are associated morbidities.

Treatment is supportive, depending on morbidity, and includes glucose administration for asymptomatic hypoglycemic infants.

HYPOGLYCEMIA
(*NELSON TEXTBOOK*, SECS. 8.59 and 9.57)

Diagnosis is based on serum glucose levels significantly lower than the range among postnatal age–matched normal infants: term infants are rarely less than 35 mg/dL at 1–3 hr of life, 40 mg/dL at 3–24 hr, and 45 mg/dL after 24 hr. Diagnosis in older infants and children requires a careful history and may necessitate provocative testing with glucagon. Low serum glucose levels are associated with increased risks of neurodevelopmental deficits. Those at increased risk include:

1. Infants with hyperinsulinism due to maternal diabetes mellitus or gestational diabetes, severe erythroblastosis fetalis, insulinomas, beta cell nesidioblastosis or hyperplasia, or **Beckwith syndrome** (macroglossia, large size, visceromegaly, omphalocele).
2. Infants who are premature or have intrauterine growth failure.
3. Severely ill infants, especially those having associated hypoxia and hypothermia.
4. Infants with various inborn errors of metabolism.

Clinical manifestations, when present, include jitteriness or tremors, apathy, cyanosis, seizures, intermittent apnea or tachypnea, weak or high-pitched cry, lethargy, difficulty feeding, sweating, pallor, hypothermia, and cardiac failure.

Treatment initially consists of an intravenous bolus of 2–4 mL/kg of 10% glucose followed by infusion of 8 mg/kg/min. Additional pharmacologic or surgical therapy depends on the underlying etiology.

INFECTIONS OF THE NEWBORN
(*NELSON TEXTBOOK,* SECS. 9.58–9.75)

GENERAL CONSIDERATIONS

Infections are a frequent cause of neonatal mortality and morbidity due to varying modes of transmission in the perinatal period, the immune status of the infant, coexisting diseases, and the extreme variability of the manifestations of infection in the neonate. Infections may be acquired at any time during pregnancy, just before or during delivery (perinatal), or postnatally (during the first 28 days of life). Prematurity or LBW is the most important factor predisposing to infection.

Clinical manifestations are highly variable, ranging from asymptomatic to severe fulminant presentations, acute to chronic, and involving single or multiple organs. Infections with different microorganisms usually cannot be distinguished by clinical features alone and are often indistinguishable from noninfectious processes. Nonspecific signs and symptoms are presented in Table 7–2.

Diagnosis is often suggested by maternal history, and a variety of screening test are available to detect intrauterine and perinatally acquired newborn infection.

Treatment is usually required before definitive diagnosis because of the high morbidity and mortality and the difficulty of assessing nonspecific signs of neonatal infection. Antibiotics are selected on the basis of expected sensitivity patterns of anticipated pathogens. Dosages must be specifically tailored to this age group.

NOSOCOMIAL NURSERY INFECTION

Neonatal infections developing later than 48–72 hr after birth usually are considered to have been acquired in the hospital (nosocomial), although some late-onset perinatal infections and delivery room–acquired infections are exceptions. These infections are uncommon in normal full-term infants and, when they occur, usually involve the skin (*Staphylococcus aureus* and *Candida*). They are common among LBW infants and among infants requiring neonatal intensive care. The use of equipment, antibiotics, and invasive procedures are special risk factors.

NEONATAL SEPSIS (Septicemia)

This usually consists of bacteremia plus a constellation of signs and symptoms caused by microorganisms or their toxic

TABLE 7–2. NONSPECIFIC CLINICAL MANIFESTATIONS OF INFECTION IN THE NEWBORN INFANT*

General
  Fever, hypothermia
  "Not doing well"
  Poor feeding
  Sclerema

Gastrointestinal System
  Abdominal distention
  Anorexia, vomiting
  Diarrhea
  Hepatomegaly

Respiratory System
  Apnea, dyspnea
  Tachypnea, retraction
  Flaring, grunting
  Cyanosis

Cardiovascular System
  Pallor, mottling, cold, clammy skin
  Tachycardia
  Hypotension
  Bradycardia

Central Nervous System
  Irritability, lethargy
  Tremors, seizures
  Hyporeflexia, hypotonia
  Abnormal Moro reflex
  Irregular respirations
  Full fontanel
  High-pitched cry

Hematologic System
  Jaundice
  Splenomegaly
  Pallor
  Petechiae, purpura
  Bleeding

* From Behrman RE (ed): Nelson Textbook of Pediatrics, 14th ed. Philadelphia, WB Saunders Company, 1992, p. 497.

products in the circulation during the first month of life. The *incidence* varies from 1 to 8/1,000 live births. The *etiology* varies with time and geographic area, but group B streptococci and *Escherichia coli* cause about 75% of early-onset sepsis.

Clinical manifestations initially are usually nonspecific (Table 7–2) or minimal and occur in many noninfectious disorders. Temperature instability and poor feeding are common. Late manifestations include apnea, cyanosis, and shock. An *early-onset pattern* (<7 days) often is characterized by respiratory distress, pneumonia, and shock, in contrast to a *late-onset pattern,* characterized by fever and CNS or focal signs.

Diagnosis is based on organism culture or demonstration of endotoxin or bacterial antigen. A "sepsis work-up" usually includes blood culture, a lumbar puncture and cerebrospinal fluid (CSF) examination and culture, urine examination and culture, and a chest roentgenogram.

Treatment should be started once the diagnosis is suspected and appropriate cultures have been obtained. Usually this consists of ampicillin and an aminoglycoside (often gentamicin) because of the pattern of disease and organisms common during the neonatal period (group B streptococcus and *E. coli*). Nosocomial infections usually are due to staphylococci, Enterobacteriaceae, *Pseudomonas,* or *Candida.* An antistaphylococcal drug thus often is substituted for ampicillin. Once the pathogen is known, the most appropriate antibiotic should be used. Supportive therapy also is essential.

CONJUNCTIVITIS

Conjunctivitis in the newborn infant usually is due to inflammation from silver nitrate or infection with *Neisseria gonorrhoeae*, *Chlamydia trachomatis*, or *S. aureus*.

Clinical manifestations from silver nitrate drops usually occur 6–12 hr after birth and clear by 24–48 hr. Gonococcal conjunctivitis begins with mild inflammation and serosanguineous discharge that becomes thick and purulent within 24 hr, with tense eyelid edema and marked chemosis. Chlamydial disease may vary from mild to severe inflammation and usually is manifest 5–18 days after birth.

Treatment of suspected gonococcal ophthalmia should be promptly initiated with 25–50 mg/kg/day of ceftriaxone for 7 days on the basis of a positive Gram stain.

For *prevention*, at birth all infants should receive 0.5% erythromycin or 1% silver nitrate instilled directly into open eyes. This will not be effective against active infection with gonococcus or for prophylaxis of chlamydia conjunctivitis or pneumonia.

HEPATITIS

The *etiology* of neonatal hepatitis frequently cannot be identified, but infections may occur from hepatitis virus A, B, C, and E, enterovirus, cytomegalovirus, rubella, herpes simplex, and human immunodeficiency virus.

Clinical manifestations include anorexia, vomiting, jaundice, and elevated hepatic enzyme levels. Fulminant disease is characterized by very high enzyme levels and decreased production of coagulation proteins, often with bleeding, shock, and death. Infants with hepatitis B virus usually become HB$_s$Ag positive and remain asymptomatic, developing either persistent antigenemia with evidence of chronic liver involvement or mild anicteric hepatitis.

For *prevention and treatment*, infants of HB$_s$Ag-positive mothers should be given hepatitis B immunoglobulin (HBIG), 0.5 mL, as soon after birth as possible, and all infants should receive hepatitis B virus vaccine at birth, 1 mo, and 6 mo of age.

MENINGITIS

Meningitis in the neonate often is associated with sepsis and causes significant morbidity and mortality. *Etiologic* agents usually are similar to those causing sepsis, but a great variety of bacterial, fungal, parasitic, and viral organisms may cause neonatal meningitis.

Clinical manifestations may initially be indistinguishable from those of sepsis and noninfectious neonatal disorders (Table 7–2). Temperature instability, apnea, brachycardia, poor feeding, high-pitched cry, cyanosis, tachycardia, tachypnea, lethargy, seizures, and shock are prominent.

Diagnosis is confirmed by CSF examination, culture, and antigen detection. Bacterial culture is diagnostic in 70–85%

of neonates. Lumbar puncture is contraindicated in the presence of raised intracranial pressure.

Treatment is similar to that of neonatal sepsis.

PNEUMONIA

Pneumonia is an important cause of morbidity and mortality in the neonate. Infection may be acquired transplacentally, perinatally, or postnatally. Pneumonia acquired transplacentally or perinatally often is termed congenital pneumonia, is associated with bacteremia, and is frequently associated with prolonged rupture of the membranes, prematurity, and fetal distress.

Clinical manifestations are frequently nonspecific (Table 7–2) and include poor feeding, lethargy or irritability, poor color, temperature instability, abdominal distention, and signs of respiratory distress such as grunting, flaring of alae nasi, tachypnea, tachycardia, retractions, and apnea. Group B streptococci may cause a fulminant sepsis and pneumonia.

Diagnosis is based on chest roentgenogram, Gram stain of tracheal aspirate, and culture.

Treatment is similar to that of neonatal sepsis because the bacterial organisms usually are the same. Because it is often difficult to distinguish pneumonia from hyaline membrane disease in LBW infants, these infants are often treated with broad-spectrum parenteral antibiotics when severely ill.

GROUP B STREPTOCOCCAL INFECTION

Group B streptococcal (GBS) infection is a major cause of severe systemic and local newborn disease.

Epidemiology

The organism commonly colonizes the maternal genitourinary and gastrointestinal tracts, and newborns usually acquire the disease by vertical transmission from an asymptomatic mother. Horizontal nursing transmission also occurs and has been responsible for late-onset disease, which is most often of type III.

Pathogenesis

Early-onset disease is associated with an immature host defense mechanism, especially among LBW infants, and prolonged exposure to heavy maternal colonization. Late-onset GBS additionally may be associated with elaboration of large amounts of GBS type III capsular polysaccharide and reduced amounts of maternal antibody.

Clinical Manifestations

Early-onset infections range from asymptomatic bacteremia to pneumonia to overwhelming infection characterized by shock, asphyxia, and persistent pulmonary hypertension. There may be acute meningitis and onset may begin at birth. *Late-onset infections* commonly manifest as meningitis, usually indistinguishable from other forms of neonatal meningitis, and may occur at any time during the neonatal period as an acute or more indolent infection.

Diagnosis

Diagnosis is established by isolation of the organism from normally sterile sites or antigen detection of GBS. CSF examination usually reveals an elevated neutrophil cell count.

Treatment

Empiric systemic administration of ampicillin and an aminoglycoside are indicated until GBS is identified. GBS is uniformly sensitive to penicillin G, which may be substituted after several days of a good response to initial therapy. Intensive supportive management is often necessary because of life-threatening presentations.

URINARY TRACT INFECTIONS

Clinical manifestations are varied and nonspecific (Table 7–2) but may be insidious in onset during the neonatal period, consisting of low-grade fever, vomiting, diarrhea, irritability, jaundice, and failure to gain weight. Some infants may be asymptomatic; others, especially LBW infants, may present with a sepsis syndrome.

Diagnosis is confirmed by urine culture. *Treatment* initially is the same as for sepsis and then is specific for the cultured organism. Renal ultrasound is indicated.

Genital mycoplasma potentially may be responsible for neonatal meningitis or pneumonia or may be markers for premature labor with subsequent neonatal colonization.

CYTOMEGALOVIRUS

Humans are the only known source of maternal (usually asymptomatic) congenital or perinatal infection. Risk of symptomatic congenital cytomegalovirus (CMV) infection may be increased with maternal infection during the first half of pregnancy.

Symptomatic congenital CMV infection may be a multiorgan systemic illness characterized by IUGR, hepatosplenomegaly, jaundice, hepatitis, rash, choreoretinitis, periventricular cerebral calcifications, and macrocephaly. This severe form occurs in less than 10% of congenitally infected infants, the majority of whom are asymptomatic.

CNS infection is highly associated with psychomotor retardation, and hearing loss is common.

Postnatal CMV infection, associated with blood transfusion, is characterized by septic appearance, hepatitis, pallor, deteriorating respiratory status, hemolytic anemia, thrombocytopenia, and neutropenia.

Diagnosis is based on viral cultures and the pattern of IgG antibody titers. *Treatment* is nonspecific. *Prognosis* of congenital infection is poor, especially among symptomatic patients with CNS manifestations.

ENTEROVIRUS (ECHOVIRUSES, COXSACKIEVIRUSES, POLIOVIRUSES)

These common pathogens may produce diverse, serious neonatal disease. A *sepsis-like illness* may occur characterized by fever, irritability, poor feeding, lethargy, hepatitis, apnea, hypotonia, vomiting, diarrhea, and rash. Patterns range from subclinical to overwhelming fatal infection. Mild *febrile illness* with viremia or aseptic meningitis occurs most commonly in full-term infants. *Myocarditis* manifesting as cyanosis, lethargy, tachycardia, tachypnea, arrhythmias, or heart failure particularly is associated with coxsackievirus B1–B4 infection. Upper respiratory infection and rashes are common.

Diagnosis depends on virus isolation. *Treatment* is supportive and may be lifesaving but is not specific for the virus infection.

HERPES SIMPLEX

Etiology

Herpes simplex virus (HSV) type 2 and occasionally type 1 produce significant neonatal and sometimes fetal disease. Type 2 is usually acquired from a maternal genitourinary tract infection during pregnancy or parturition and type 1 from a mucocutaneous infection about the mouth or the skin above the waist. However, both types can cause oral or genital infections and are neurotropic.

Clinical Manifestations

Intrauterine infection due to HSV 2 is evident at birth and characterized by cutaneous scars or vesicles, choreoretinitis, microphthalmia, keratoconjunctivitis, microcephaly, hydranencephaly, intracranial calcifications, and hepatosplenomegaly.

Intrapartum or postpartum infant infection may result in disseminated illness, disease limited to the skin, eye, and mouth, or encephalitis.

Disseminated disease manifestations are similar to bacterial sepsis. It is characterized by lesions in the skin, lungs, adrenals, CNS, trachea, esophagus, kidney, spleen, and heart.

Skin, eye, or mouth disease lesions are typically 1–3 mm diameter, erythematous-based vesicles that may progress to bullous-sized lesions. They may be discrete or grouped and linear. These lesions may disseminate if therapy is delayed or not provided, and they may recur during the first 6–12 mo of life. Ocular lesions include keratoconjunctivitis or late choreoretinitis.

Encephalitis occurs in most patients with disseminated disease but also may occur as an isolated infection, usually of later onset. Manifestations include fever, irritability, lethargy, coma, seizures, and a high-pitched cry.

Diagnosis

Diagnosis can be made in 1–3 days by viral culture.

Treatment

Early diagnosis and prompt administration of vidarabine or acyclovir is critical for decreasing morbidity and mortality. Despite effective antiviral therapy, disseminated HSV infections and localized encephalitis have considerable morbidity and mortality.

PARVOVIRUS B19

This virus may cause erythema infectiosum, aplastic crisis in patients with hereditary hemolytic anemia, chronic red cell aplasia in immunocompromised patients, and fetal anemia and death in seronegative mothers who acquire the infection during pregnancy. There is no specific treatment.

CONGENITAL RUBELLA SYNDROME (German Measles)

This viral infection during pregnancy is associated with variable rates and degrees of fetal infection and rates of teratogenesis before 20 wk gestation that are gestational age dependent. Fetal infection and dissemination may produce permanent organ malformations and tissue injury, transient neonatal manifestations, or a delayed, late-onset illness due to chronic infection or autoimmune phenomena. *Congenital anomalies* frequently noted include congenital heart disease (esp. patient ductus arteriosus, peripheral pulmonic stenosis, and pulmonary valve stenosis), microphthalmia, microcephaly, and deafness.

Clinical manifestations in the newborn period include hepatosplenomegaly, "blueberry muffin" rash, purpura, jaundice, intrauterine and postnatal growth retardation, cataracts, retinopathy, sensorineural hearing loss, thrombocytopenia, adenopathy, bony radiolucencies, panencephalitis, myocarditis, hepatitis, and pneumonia. Many infants are asymptomatic in the newborn period and then later develop evidence of congenital rubella. The most significant *delayed manifestations* include hearing loss, congenital heart disease, mental retardation, and cataract or glaucoma, but many of the inflammatory manifestations that usually occur in the newborn also may occur later in infancy.

Diagnosis is based on viral isolation coupled with typical manifestations.

Treatment is nonspecific and directed at the particular injury (e.g., cardiac surgery for a correctable heart anomaly).

Prevention can be accomplished by vaccine administration in infancy and during adolescence and young adulthood.

VARICELLA (Chickenpox)

The risk of fetal infection following maternal infection is about 25%, and congenital malformations occur in about 5% of those infected before the 3rd trimester. About 25% of newborns delivered to mothers having varicella during the last 3 wk of pregnancy develop a clinical infection. If maternal varicella occurs 5–21 days prior to delivery, neonatal disease occurs in the first 4 days of life and the prognosis is good because of the passage of maternal varicella IgG antibody. If maternal varicella occurs between 5 days before and 2 days after delivery, neonatal varicella appears at 5–10 days of age. Illness may be mild or severe, with 30% mortality.

Clinical manifestations include congenital anomalies such as cicatricial dermatomal scarring, unilateral limb hypoplasia and paresis, rudimentary digits, microcephaly, cortical and cerebellar atropy, psychomotor retardation, seizures, cataracts, chorioretinitis, and microphthalmia. *Neonatal illness* may be mild or severe and includes fever, rash, pneumonia, and generalized necrotic visceral lesions.

Diagnosis is usually made clinically from history and the characteristic pustular rash. The virus can be isolated and antigens detected.

For *treatment and prevention*, acyclovir may be effective in moderate to severe cases but may rarely produce renal or neurotoxicity. Varicella-zoster immune globulin (VZIG) is recommended for infants born to mothers who develop varicella within 5 days before to 2 days after delivery and for infants less than 1,000 g or 28 wk gestation. Infants and mothers should be isolated. Special precautions are needed for family and health care workers.

CANDIDA

Candida albicans is the most common species causing infection in the newborn.

Clinical Manifestations

Thrush consists of white curd-like plaques on the tongue, gums, or oral mucosa that, when removed, reveal an erythematous base. The skin manifestations are erythematous maculopapular or vesicular scaling lesions.

Congenital candidiasis presents as a generalized erythematous eruption in the first 12 hr of life. It may desquamate and become pustular. Systemic disease is characterized by pneumonia, shock, meningitis, bone infection, and a high mortality.

Nosocomial or delayed congenital invasive candidiasis manifests similar to acute neonatal sepsis coupled with skin manifestations characteristic of congenital infection. However, the sepsis often is indolent. This disseminated disease, which involves one or more organ systems and has positive cultures from normally sterile body fluids or tissues, must be distinguished from catheter-associated transient candidemia, which usually responds to catheter removal.

Diagnosis

Diagnosis is confirmed by organism identification from scraped mucosal or skin lesions. Blood cultures must be incubated for prolonged time periods in special media.

Treatment

Thrush should be treated with oral nystatin and skin infections with topical nystatin. *Systemic candidiasis* should be treated with IV amphotericin alone or in combination with oral flucytosine.

8

SPECIAL HEALTH PROBLEMS DURING ADOLESCENCE

This period of development is characterized by a low utilization of health services; a low rate of insurance coverage; a high incidence of undiagnosed disorders in presumably healthy 12–17-yr-olds; high morbidity and mortality from accidents (esp. automobile and motorcycle), homicides, and suicides; and a high incidence of sexually transmitted disease and health-destructive behaviors (cigarette, alcohol, and other drug abuse) (see *Nelson Textbook*, Secs. 10.1–10.22).

DEPRESSION

Adolescence is a time of mood swings, which may be difficult to distinguish from true clinical depression.

Diagnosis may be based on persistence of depressed mood (lasts for at least 3 consecutive hr for three or more periods each week), absence of corresponding periods of elation, inability to function, and expression of hopelessness and helplessness. Disturbances of eating and sleeping are not as pervasive in adolescents as in adults but may be severe. A family history of depression and suicide are particularly important associations. Inquiries should be made about suicidal feelings, ideation, and planning for self-destruction. Any affirmative response or increase in risk-taking behavior requires immediate psychiatric consultation. Acting-out behavior may mask depression.

Treatment will vary depending on the severity of depression, from close observation to psychiatric interventions.

SUICIDE

Higher adolescent suicide rates occur in females, Native and Asian–Americans, and the chronically ill. Ingestion is the most common method of adolescent suicide. Males tend to use more violent methods such as hanging or shooting. The medical lethality correlates poorly with seriousness of intent, but the patient's expectation of lethality, extent of premeditation, and likelihood of rescue correlate well with seriousness of intent. Suicidal attempts require short-term hospitalization and psychiatric consultation.

SUBSTANCE ABUSE

Drug use, alcohol ingestion, and marijuana smoking is experienced at some time by more than 90% of teenagers. Twenty percent of adolescents smoke cigarettes and 40% use some illicit drug other than marijuana. Therefore, the clinician needs to assess the role of drug use in each adolescent's life and the effects of specific drugs on their physical and functional parameters. Multiple variables are associated with adolescent drug use that is likely to result in a significant health or psychosocial problem, such as family history of drug abuse, setting of drug use, school performance, use before driving, and type of drug.

PATHOPHYSIOLOGY

Pubertal physical growth and development may be adversely affected by drug use (e.g., menstrual abnormalities from heroin, impaired sleep and gonadotrophin secretion from amphetamines). Metabolism of prescribed drugs may be affected by coincident abuse of illicit drugs or alcohol (e.g. alcohol acceleration of metabolism of estrogen-containing contraceptives increases vulnerability to pregnancy).

HEROIN

Pharmacology

Route of administration influences timing of onset (e.g., IV immediate, 30 min for inhalation).

Clinical Manifestations

Major effect is euphoria and analgesia. Other features include neuropathies, vasodilation, respiratory depression, pulmonary granulomatosis, fibrosis or edema, hypertrophic linear scars following course of veins, fat necrosis, loss of libido, constipation, and infections.

Overdose syndrome is a reaction often resulting in death. Clinical signs include stupor, coma, seizures, respiratory depression, pulmonary edema, cyanosis, and miotic pupils. *Treatment* consists of naloxone for ventilation and life support.

Withdrawal (abstinence syndrome) usually occurs after 8 hr in an addict and over 24–36 hr consists of yawning, tearing, mydriasis, insomnia, "gooseflesh," cramping of voluntary muscles, diarrhea, tachycardia, hypertension, and, rarely, siezures. Diazepam and methadone may be used for *detoxification*.

HALLUCINOGENS

Hallucinogens include lyseric acid diethylamide (LSD), phencyclidine (PCP), certain mushrooms, and jimsonweed. They may cause serious toxicity, terrifying flashbacks (LSD), and death.

PCP can be taken orally or smoked, resulting in euphoria,

nystagmus, ataxia, emotional lability, hallucination with bizarre distortions of body image, and panic reactions. High doses may result in toxic psychosis with disorientation, hypersalivation, and abusive language; alternating coma and wakefulness with dystonic posturing, muscular rigidity, hyperreflexia, and myoclonic jerks; and hypotension, generalized siezures, cardiac arrhythmias, hypothermia, and shock. Death may occur. *Treatment* may include decreased external stimuli, life support, diazepam, and urine acidification to promote excretion.

Mushrooms have cholinergic and anticholinergic effects in addition to euphoria and hallucinations. Usually these are self-limited and do not require therapy. Some cause LSD-like reactions and agitation, requiring *treatment* with diazepam. Fatal poisoning also may result from some toxic mushrooms.

Jimsonweed contains atropine as well as a hallucinogenic chemical and may produce restlessness, disorientation, lethargy, coma, hypertension, siezures, and delirium as well as dry mouth, hot skin, fever, mydriasis, urinary retention, and sinus tachycardia. *Treatment* with supportive care and an anticholinesterase may be indicated.

VOLATILE SUBSTANCES

Volatile substances of many varieties may cause euphoria and enjoy varying popularity among adolescents. Most are toxic, and many may result in death.

Airplane glue can result in cerebral and pulmonary edema and acute myocardial dysfunction in addition to chronic central nervous system (CNS) and renal disorders.

Gasoline sniffing may result in excitement, ataxia, nausea, coma, and encephalopathy.

Aerosol products, such as hair spray and deodorants, which contain fluorocarbon propellants (freons), may result in arrhythmias and death.

MARIJUANA

In addition to elation and euphoria, marijuana may cause impairment of short-term memory, poor performance of tasks requiring divided attention (e.g., driving), loss of critical judgment, distortion of time perception, visual hallucinations, transient hypertension, and tachycardia.

COCAINE AND CRACK COCAINE

Effects of cocaine include euphoria, increased motor activity, decreased fatigability, paranoid ideation, tachycardia, hypertension, and hyperthermia. Binge patterns of use are common. Psychological dependence may occur. *Treatment* is similar to that for other opiates, such as heroin.

ALCOHOL

Alcohol has become a major threat to the normal functions of teenagers and to the lives of others jeopardized by drunken drivers. It is a CNS depressant that, dependent on dose, produces euphoria, grogginess, talkativeness, impaired short-term memory, increase in pain threshold and the time needed to brake a car, vasodilation, hypothermia, and, at very high doses, respiratory depression.

Physiologic dependence may develop over weeks with daily ingestion, and *withdrawal* manifestations include anxiety, tremors, insomnia, and irritability. *Treatment* with librium is usually effective.

Overdose syndrome includes disorientation, lethargy, coma, and respiratory depression. *Treatment* is life support.

SMOKING

Smoking duration correlates with cardiovascular and respiratory disease incidence. Therefore, adolescents who continue to smoke as adults are at increased risk from these disorders. In addition, during adolescence they are at increased risk of low-birth-weight pregnancies, cough, and wheezing.

ANABOLIC STEROIDS

Anabolic steroid ingestion by adolescent athletes is associated with hepatocarcinoma and cholestasis. In males, endocrine effects include gynecomastia and testicular atrophy; in females, these include hirsutism, baldness, deepening voice, breast atrophy, acne, menstrual abnormalities, and clitoral enlargement. Additional adverse effects include untoward serum lipid profile, advanced epiphyseal closure, and serious psychological affects with high doses.

SLEEP DISORDERS

Sleep disorders may be related to depression. In addition, narcolepsy and sleep apnea–hypersomnia syndrome first become symptomatic during this period. Insomnia affects 10–20% of teenagers.

ANOREXIA NERVOSA AND BULIMIA

The incidence of these disorders has increased; about 1 in 100 females 16–18 yr old has anorexia nervosa, and the ratio of females to males is 10:1.

DIAGNOSIS

Diagnosis is based on clinical criteria. *Anorexia* includes:

intense fear of becoming obese that does not decrease with weight loss

disturbance in the way the patient perceives his or her body image

refusal to maintain body weight over a minimal age-for-height ratio

absence of at least 3 consecutive menstrual cycles

Other characteristics of anorexia include excess physical activity, denial of hunger, and preoccupation with food preparation.

Bulimia includes:

recurrent episodes of binge eating, at least 2 episodes/wk for 3 mo

fear of not being able to stop eating

regularly engaging in self-induced vomiting, use of laxatives, or fasting/dieting to counter effects of binge eating

CLINICAL MANIFESTATIONS

Anorexia and bulimia result in disturbances in many organ systems either directly or as a consequence of severe malnutrition:

10% death rate is due to severe electrolyte abnormalities, arrhythmias, or congestive heart failure

bradycardia, amenorrhea, hypotension, and hypothermia are common

bone marrow hypoplasia occurs

constipation, vomiting, and esophagitis are common

TREATMENT

Treatment includes psychotherapy, behavior modification techniques, and nutritional rehabilitation.

PROBLEMS RELATED TO ADOLESCENT SEXUALITY

PREGNANCY

The U.S. adolescent pregnancy rate is the highest among developed countries. An increasing number are unintended pregnancies to unmarried mothers.

Diagnosis is usually based on history of sexual intercourse, nausea, and breast tenderness and physical findings of increased nipple pigmentation, linea alba, cyanosis and softening of the cervix, and an enlarged uterus. The serum β-subunit human chorionic gonadotropin is positive.

Primary *prevention* includes counseling about abstinence and contraception, including use of condoms, diaphragms, cervical caps, spermicides, various systemically administered hormones, and intrauterine devices (IUDs).

SEXUALLY TRANSMITTED DISEASES

Adolescents have the highest rate of sexually transmitted diseases (STDs).

Gonorrhea infection occurs via the urethral, cervical, anal, pharyngeal, or conjunctival route. Ceftriaxone is the treatment drug of choice.

Syphilis incidence is rising, and screening with the sensitive VDRL test is advisable. Penicillin benzathine treatment is effective and ceftriaxone also is effective against incubating disease.

Chlamydia infections have increased dramatically in the past decade and often resemble or are coexistent with gonococcal disease. Treatment with cefoxitin and doxycycline is indicated.

Chancroid usually presents as a painful purulent ulcer requiring biopsy for definitive diagnosis. Ceftriaxone treatment is indicated.

Herpes progenitalis may present with sharp pain radiating from the perineum and/or a characteristic skin/mucosal lesion. Symptomatic relief in primary infections may be achieved with oral acyclovir.

Human Papillomavirus (HPV) causes significant morbidity, and some types are associated with cervical cancer.

Trichomonas usually causes a frothy discharge and can be effectively treated with metronidazole.

Haemophilus (Gardnerella) vaginalis causes a foul-smelling discharge and responds to metronidazole treatment.

Human immunodeficiency virus (HIV) infection rate is increasing significantly among adolescents.

MENSTRUAL PROBLEMS

Amenorrhea

Primary amenorrhea indicates menarche has not occurred after the age at which it normally occurs (10–16 yr). *Secondary amenorrhea* refers to the cessation of menses for more than 3 mo after a regular menstrual cycling has been established.

Primary amenorrhea may be due to chromosomal or congenital abnormalities, such as gonadal dysgenesis or the triplex syndrome, or to pregnancy. Secondary amenorrhea is usually due to pregnancy. Either may be caused by chronic illness, especially that associated with malnutrition or hypoxia, CNS or adrenal tumors, hyperthyroidism, anomaly of the müllerian duct system (e.g., imperforate hymen), ovarian pathology, anabolic steroid or other drug abuse, and psychogenic factors.

Menometrorrhagia

Menometrorrhagia (excessive menstrual bleeding) may constitute a gynecologic emergency because of associated shock and anemia. Most often dysfunctional uterine bleeding is secondary to anovulatory cycles that normally occur in the 1st yr after menarche. Hormonal treatment is indicated only if bleeding is significant. Rarely, endometrial currettage is necessary.

Bleeding may also be due to congenital coagulopathies (e.g., von Willebrand disease), aspirin, thrombocytopenia, improper use of oral contraceptives, hypothyroidism, and other rare disorders. Bleeding due to trauma, infection, or pregnancy is usually accompanied by pain.

Dysmenorrhea

Dysmenorrhea, or painful menstrual cramps, is experienced by two thirds of postmenarcheal teenagers.

Primary dysmenorrhea is frequent and due to myometrial contractions caused by prostaglandins $F_{2\alpha}$ and E_2. Prostaglandin synthetase inhibitors (e.g., naproxin sodium) administered before a menstrual period or shortly after it begins are usually effective. Oral contraceptives may be required in severe cases.

Secondary dysmenorrhea should be ruled out by gynecologic examinations before treating as a primary disorder. Causes include structural abnormalities of the cervix or uterus, a foreign body, endometritis, and endometriosis.

PREMENSTRUAL SYNDROME

This is a complex of physical signs and behavioral symptoms occurring during the second half of the menstrual cycle that may resolve with the onset of menses. It is uncommon among adolescents.

Clinical manifestations include breast fullness and tenderness, bloating, fatigue, headache, mood swings, and irritability.

THE BREAST

Cysts should be monitored and, if they persist or enlarge over 3 menstrual cycles, surgical consultation is indicated. Carcinomas are rare in adolescence and mammography is not indicated.

Fibrocystic disease suggested by multiple small lumps should be monitored regularly by examinations. Combination oral contraceptives of low progesterone potency may be beneficial.

Gynecomastia in males usually is transient and only requires reassurance.

Nipple discharge usually is due to local stimulation, drugs (oral contraception), or pregnancy, and rarely to infection (purulent) or neoplasm (bloody).

DELIVERY OF HEALTH CARE

Examination, education, anticipatory guidance, immunization (reimmunization against measles, mumps, and rubella), and screening should be provided on a regular schedule.

The right of a minor to consent to treatment without parental knowledge is governed by state law; usually self-consent is granted when there is suspicion of STDs and for provision of contraceptives. Parental consent is not needed for (1) *emancipated* minors (live away from home, economically self-supporting, married, member of the military, or not subject to parental control); (2) medical emergencies if delay would jeopardize life or health, and (3) minors of sufficient maturity to understand their illness and the risks and benefits of treatment (this *Mature Minor Rule* is increasingly recognized).

Screening tests include urinalysis and culture, hematocrit, tuberculosis skin test, VDRL, gonococcal culture, HIV test, pap smear, audiometry, vision tests, blood pressure determination, scoliosis examination, breast or scrotum examination and self-examination instruction, and psychosocial assessment.

9

IMMUNITY, ALLERGY, AND DISEASES OF INFLAMMATION

THE IMMUNOLOGIC SYSTEM
(*NELSON TEXTBOOK*, SECS. 11.1–11.3)

This system is that part of host defenses that includes macrophages, leukocytes, lymphocytes, cytokines, immunoglobulins, and the complement system. Its primary function, together with physical barriers such as the skin and motile cilia, is to protect against invasion of infectious agents. The cost of this protection is allergy, autoimmunity, and rejection of organ transplants.

Lymphoid stem cells differentiate into *T cells* (in thymus) and *B cells* (in bone marrow), which each further differentiate into various subpopulations. These include T-helper, suppression, and killer cells and various B-cell subpopulations each responsible for the production of various major classes of immunoglobulins (IgM, IgG, IgA, IgD, and IgE).

IgM, the first immunoglobin formed in response to antigen, is found intravascularly and efficiently enhances various immune processes of complement fixation and agglutination. *IgG* supports passive immunization and recall immunity. *IgA* protects mainly secretory surfaces (gastrointestinal tract, eyes). *IgE* effects release of pharmacologically active agents from mast cells that are major factors in eliminating parasites and causing asthma, hay fever, and anaphylaxis.

The production of immune cell lines following exposure to antigen requires cellular interaction involving T and B cells and macrophages. T cells are assessed by peripheral blood lymphocyte count, roentgenograms of the chest to evaluate the thymus, skin tests for hypersensitivity, and various studies to identify surface markers and observe in vitro responses. B cells can be enumerated in blood by various markers, commonly IgM molecules on the surface of B lymphocytes, and their function can be assessed by measurement of serum immunoglobulin levels.

PRIMARY IMMUNODEFICIENCY
(*NELSON TEXTBOOK*, SEC. 11.4)

Generally disorders of the T cell system have graver prognoses than those of the B cell system (hypogammaglobulinemic syndromes). Disorders involving both systems carry the worst prognosis.

Clinical differentiation among primary deficiencies is uncertain, but some manifestations are suggestive (Table 9–1).

PRIMARY B CELL DISEASES
(*NELSON TEXTBOOK*, SECS. 11.5–11.11)

Panhypogammaglobulinemia (Congenital Agammaglobulinemia, Bruton Disease)

This disease involves all three major classes of immunoglobulins and has various modes of inheritance. Many patients are asymptomatic until later in life.

Clinical manifestations characteristically relate to repeated bacterial infections. There may be growth failure, but usually there is no lymphadenopathy or splenomegaly. Skin disorders and later pulmonary dysfunction are frequent.

Diagnosis is based on the levels of gamma globulin.

Treatment includes administration of gamma globulin and antibiotics.

Common Variable Immunodeficiency

This term encompasses most deficiency states with prominent B cell and minimum T cell defects. There is a later onset of clinical manifestations, especially sinopulmonary infections and malabsorption (similar to panhypogammaglobulinemia).

Selective Deficiencies

These may involve IgA, secretory component, IgM, and IgG subclass deficiencies.

IgA deficiency is characterized by recurrent respiratory infections and diarrhea. Autoimmune disorders are associated, but many children are asymptomatic. Serum and secretory IgA disorders maybe distinguished, but they are usually not isolated defects.

IgM deficiency patients are at high risk of rapid hematogenous spread of bacterial infections, requiring prompt treatment.

IgG subclass deficiency patients show increased susceptibility to infections, normal total IgG, and variable response to IgG administration.

PRIMARY T CELL DISEASES
(*NELSON TEXTBOOK*, SECS. 11.12–11.15)

These are characterized primarily by fungal or viral infections, interstitial pneumonia, nasal discharge, and neutropenia.

DiGeorge anomaly (DGA) is probably caused by an embryologic field defect that often results in conotruncal heart malformations, facial anomalies, urinary tract abnormalities, parathyroid deficiency, and immune defects resulting from thymic abnormalities.

Nezelof syndrome usually does not have the cardiac or parathyroid involvement of DGA, and *cartilage–hair hypoplasia*, a bone dysplasia, is associated with short-limbed dwarfism and immune deficiencies similar to DGA.

TABLE 9–1. CLINICAL SYMPTOMS OF IMMUNODEFICIENCY*

Suggestive of T cell defect
  Systemic illness following vaccination with any live virus or BCG†; unusual life-threatening complication following infection with ordinarily benign viruses (e.g., giant cell pneumonia with rubeola; varicella pneumonia)
  Chronic oral candidiasis after 6 mo of age
  Chronic mucocutaneous candidiasis
  Features (fine, thin hair; short-limbed dwarfism with characteristic roentgenographic features of cartilage–hair hypoplasia [CHH])
  Intrauterine graft-verus-host disease—most characteristic feature is scaling erythroderma and total alopecia (absence of eyebrows quite striking)
  Graft-versus-host disease after blood transfusion
  Hypocalcemia in newborn (DiGeorge anomaly, especially with characteristic facies, ears, and cardiac lesion)
  Small (less than 10 μm diameter) lymphocytes count persistently less than 1,500/mm³; must rule out gastrointestinal loss or loss from lymphatics

Suggestive of B cell defect
  Recurrent proved bacterial pneumonia, sepsis, or meningitis
  Nodular lymphoid hyperplasia

Suggestive of B and T cell defect (combined immunodeficiency disease [CID])
  Features of all above except chronic mucocutaneous candidiasis and nodular lymphoid hyperplasia
  Features of Wiskott-Aldrich syndrome (draining ears, thrombocytopenia, and eczema)
  Features of ataxia–telangiectasia

Suggestive of immunodeficiency without clearly implicating T or B cell defect
  Pneumocystis carinii pneumonia
  Intractable eczema
  Ulcerative colitis in infants less than 1 yr of age
  Intractable diarrhea
  Unexplained hematologic deficiency (RBC†, WBC†, platelet)
  Severe generalized seborrheic dermatitis (Leiner disease) suggests C5 deficiency; seborrhea common in combined immunodeficiency disease
  Recurrent pyogenic infections seen in C3 deficiency

Suggestive of biochemical defect
  Features of combined immunodeficiency with characteristic bony lesions (adenosine deaminase deficiency)
  Features of Diamond-Blackfan aplastic anemia (nucleoside phosphorylase deficiency)

Suggestive of abnormality of polymorphonuclear leukocytes
  Primarily skin infections (if associated with asthma, eczema, and coarse facies, think of Buckley syndrome‡)
  Chronic osteomyelitis with Klebsiella or Serratia species, draining lymph nodes (chronic granulomatous disease)

Suggestive of secondary deficiency
  Concomitant or preceding viral infection
  Lymphoid malignancy (chronic lymphatic leukemia, Hodgkin disease, myeloma)

---

* From Behrman RE (ed): Nelson Textbook of Pediatrics, 14th ed. Philadelphia, WB Saunders Company, 1992, p. 551. (Modified from Hong R: Immunodeficiency. In Rose NR, Friedman H [eds]: Manual of Clinical Immunology. Washington, DC, American Society for Microbiology, 1976.)
† BCG = bacille Calmette-Guérin; RBC = red blood cell; WBC = white blood cell.
‡ From Buckley RH, et al: Extreme hyperimmunoglobulinemia E and undue susceptibility to infection. Pediatrics 49:59, 1972.

COMBINED T AND B CELL DISORDERS
(*NELSON TEXTBOOK*, SECS. 11.16–11.21)

Combined immunodeficiency disease (CID) may be a mild or severe (SCID) disorder leading to death within several years of birth.

the type of infections that occur depend on the combination and degree of T or B cell defect

wasting, skin manifestations, gastroenteritis, and hepatitis are common

bone marrow transplantation may be successful

Combined immunodeficiency disease and Letterer–Siwe syndrome (Omenn disease) is characterized by skin eruptions, hepatosplenomegaly, and eosinophilia.

Wiskott–Aldrich syndrome, an X-linked recessive disorder, is characterized by thrombocytopenia, draining ears (otitis), pneumonia, and eczema during the first 6 mo of life. Hepatosplenomegaly and lymphadenopathy are common. Serum IgG and IgE levels are markedly elevated.

Ataxia–telangiectasia is characterized by ataxia, ocular and cutaneous telangiectasias, chronic sinopulmonary disease, and endocrine abnormalities. The neurologic signs progress to severe disability.

Chronic mucocutaneous candidosis of the mucous membranes and skin rarely may become systemic. Endocrine deficiencies are associated. IV amphotericin is effective treatment.

SECONDARY IMMUNODEFICIENCY DISEASES
(*NELSON TEXTBOOK*, SEC. 11.22)

Secondary immunodeficiency diseases due to causes outside the lymphoid system include adenosine deaminase and nucleoside phosphorylase deficiencies, hypoproteinemia from protein loss, nutritional deficiency, immune suppression, and various viral infections (see Chap. 10 for acquired immunodeficiency syndrome and human immunodeficiency virus infection).

COMPLEMENT AND ASSOCIATED DISEASES
(*NELSON TEXTBOOK*, SECS. 11.23–11.28)

Complement is a complex system of interacting proteins that play a number of important roles in the host's defenses against infection.

Primary deficiencies of complement components have been described for all 11 component proteins of the classic pathway and factor D of the alternative pathway. Infections and collagen vascular disease (esp. vasculitis) are the major clinical manifestations.

Primary deficiencies of complement control proteins (factor I, properdin, complement receptor 1, C1 inhibitor) result in a variety of diverse clinical syndromes presenting with infection, systemic lupus erythematosus (SLE), and angioedema.

Secondary complement deficiencies occur in a great variety of disorders, including SCID, nephritis, SLE, malnutrition, hemoglobinopathies, renal disease, shock, and burns.

Diagnosis depend on measurement of specific components. Total hemolytic complement activity (CH_{50}) is useful for screening.

Treatment consists of supportive management and is not based on complement component replacement.

THE PHAGOCYTIC SYSTEMS AND ASSOCIATED DISEASES
(NELSON TEXTBOOK, SECS. 11.29–11.33)

LEUKOCYTE ADHESION DEFICIENCY

The *etiology* is an inherited defect in three leukocyte membrane glycoproteins that confer adhesiveness on lymphocyte, monocyte, and granulocyte surfaces, facilitating protection of epithelium against microbial invasion and promoting wound repair.

Clinical manifestations include delayed umbilical cord separation; progressive skin, mucous membrane, and subcutaneous infections characterized by decreased pus formation; ear, nose, and throat infections; poor wound healing; and persistent granulocytosis. Life-threatening systemic infections are common.

Diagnosis is based on laboratory identification of abnormal adhesiveness of the affected cells and decreased adherence of monoclonal antibodies to adhesive glycoproteins on all surfaces. Neutrophilia is common.

Treatment of infections with antibiotics is indicated.

NEUTROPHIL GRANULE DEFECTS

Etiology

There are three phenotypic genetic disorders:

  hereditary myeloperoxidase (MPO) deficiency of azurophilic granules
  congenital specific granule deficiency (SGD)
  Chédiak–Higashi syndrome (CHS)—giant granules formed by fusion

Clinical Manifestations

MPO deficiency is usually asymptomatic but may be associated with severe candidiasis, diabetes mellitus, or other severe infections.

SGD is a rare disorder characterized by recurrent bacterial and fungal infections of the skin and lungs, adenitis, and otitis. Onset is usually during the first few years of life.

CHS presents during early childhood with photophobia, rotary nystagmus, partial albinism, gingivitis, and recurrent infections of the skin, mucous membrane, and respiratory tract. Progressive motor and sensory abnormalities occur subsequently in surviving patients.

Diagnosis

Blood count and differential may suggest a neutrophil granule defect: with SGD, there are bilobed nuclei and decreased intracytoplasmic granularity in neutrophils; with CHS, there are giant granules. Cytochemical stains of blood cells and phagocytic cell function studies usually are the basis for definitive diagnosis.

Treatment

Appropriate antibiotics should be used against infections. Bone marrow transplantation for CHS has been successful.

CHRONIC GRANULOMATOUS DISEASE

Chronic granulomatous disease (CGD) is the most common inherited disorder of phagocyte function.

Etiology

The X-linked and autosomal dominant forms are associated with missing components or subunits of the phagocyte NADPH oxidase complex, which plays a pivotal role in the respiratory burst after phagocyte activation, leading to subsequent killing of catalase-positive microbes.

Clinical Manifestations

These usually include chronic and recurrent pyogenic infections during the first 2 yr of life, lymphadenopathy, hepatosplenomegaly, pneumonia with unusual microbes, abscesses, osteomyelitis, and dermatitis. Granuloma formation may lead to various obstructions.

Diagnosis

Neutrophils demonstrate normal chemotaxis, phagocytosis, and degranulation but do not generate superoxide anion. The presence of the latter is measured by reduction of nitroblue tetrazolium (NBT screening test).

Treatment

Treatment consists of a combination of long-term prophylaxis with trimethoprim–sulfamethoxazole, other antimicrobials for active infections, selective short-term granulocyte infusions for persistent infections, and administration of γ-interferon. Bone marrow transplantation has had limited success.

ALLERGIC DISORDERS
(NELSON TEXTBOOK, SECS. 11.34–11.39)

These are specific, acquired changes in host reactivity mediated by immune mechanisms, causing untoward reactions. Some of these may be characterized.

Type I hypersensitivity, mediated by IgE, is characterized by circulatory basophils and tissue mast cells around blood vessels becoming sensitized through binding of IgE antibodies to their cell surfaces. Injury relates to allergic interaction with cell bound IgE antibody molecules and a variety of subsequent immune events.

Type II hypersensitivity (cytotoxic) interactions occur between antigen and antibody at cell surfaces; IgG or IgM immunoglobulins react with antigenic determinants that either are integral parts of the cell membrane or have become adsorbed to or incorporated into the membrane. Complement is activated and the cell is destroyed.

Type III immunopathologic (Arthus or immune-complex) mechanism of tissue injury involves antigen–antibody complexes formed in extravascular spaces that are toxic to the tissues in which they are deposited.

Type IV, cell-mediated or delayed hypersensitivity results in pathologic changes due to interaction of antigen with specifically sensitized, thymus-derived T lymphocytes.

RESPIRATORY ALLERGY
(*NELSON TEXTBOOK*, SECS. 11.40 AND 11.41)

The respiratory tract is the system most commonly involved in childhood allergies.

ALLERGIC RHINITIS

Pathophysiology

Inhaled pollens, mold spores, and animal or mite antigens deposited on nasal mucus initiate production of local IgE. IgE-stimulated synthesis and release of mast cell mediators and subsequent recruitment of other cells results in early- and late-phase reactions.

Clinical Manifestations

These include sneezing (often paroxysmal); rhinorrhea (watery and profuse); nasal obstruction caused by boggy pale blue edeminous mucosa; itching of the eyes, nose, palate, pharynx, and ears; and tearing and redness of eyes.

Diagnosis

Smear of nasal secretions shows eosinophils.

Treatment

Treatment is based on the following principles:

   the patient should avoid exposure to allergens and irritants
   antihistamines and cromolyn nasal spray provide symptomatic relief
   topical corticosteroids (inhalant) for refractory reactions may be indicated

ASTHMA

This leading cause of chronic illness in childhood consists of a diffuse, predominantly reversible obstructive lung disease with hyperreactivity of airways to a variety of stimuli.

Pathophysiology

Airway obstruction is due to bronchoconstriction, hypersecretion of mucus, mucosal edema, cellular infiltration, and desquamation of epithelial and inflammatory cells. These processes are initiated by various allergic and nonspecific stimuli. Various newly synthesized and stored mediators released from mast cells and other cells also play an important role. Obstruction may lead to acidosis and hypoxia.

Etiology

The etiology of this complex disorder involves autonomic, immunologic, infectious, endocrine, and psychological factors.

Clinical Manifestations

These include cough, wheezing, tachypnea, and dyspnea with prolonged expiration and use of accessory respiratory muscles. Hyperinflation, tachycardia, and pulsus paradoxus may be present to various degrees. Wheezing in infancy is a special problem because of the unique vulnerability of young children to obstructive airway disease and infection.

Diagnosis

Diagnosis is based on history and physical findings. Differential diagnosis includes congenital malformations, foreign bodies in the airway or esophagus, infectious bronchiolitis, cystic fibrosis, and rare conditions.

Treatment

Treatment involves avoiding allergens, improving bronchodilation, and reducing mediator-induced inflammation.

   oxygen should be administered to most children during an acute attack
   epinephrine, 0.01 mL/kg of 1:1,000 concentration of an injectable aqueous preparation, is a common initial therapy
   bronchodilator aerosols such as albuterol are usually effective; IV aminophylline may be necessary
   a short course of steroids may hasten resolution

STATUS ASTHMATICUS

Status asthmaticus is a clinical diagnosis characterized by increasingly severe asthma not responsive to usually effective drugs. It may be life threatening. Management consists of:

   admission to hospital, preferably intensive care
   monitoring of vital signs, arterial blood gases, oxygenation, and serum theophylline levels
   appropriate respiratory and fluid support and treatment of acidosis
   pharmacotherapy consisting of sympathomimetic bronchodilator aerosols, intravenous aminophylline, and systemic corticosteroids

DAILY MANAGEMENT OF THE ASTHMATIC CHILD

Daily chronic management of the asthmatic child must be adjusted to different degrees of illness. Mild disease requires only bronchodilator medication when symptomatic and usually responds to aerosol adrenergic agents. In contrast, severe disease may require a variety of daily bronchodilators, including systemic or aerosolized corticosteroids.

ATOPIC DERMATITIS (Infantile or Atopic Eczema)
(*NELSON TEXTBOOK*, SEC. 11.42)

This inflammatory, hyperactive skin disorder characterized by erythema, edema, pruritus, exudation, crusting, and scaling is frequently associated with a marked elevation of serum IgE.

Clinical manifestations typically occur in three stages:

1. In *infancy* (usually begins within first 2–3 mo) features include erythematous weepy patches on the cheeks with subsequent extension to the face, neck, wrists, hands, abdomen, exterior aspects of extremities, and popliteal and antecubital fossae. Pruritus is marked, and scratching leads to weeping, crusting, and secondary infection.
2. At *3–5 years* disease is characterized by a tendency to remission; usually the disease is quiescent by 5 years. Mild to moderate ezema occurs in the antecubital and popliteal fossae, on the wrists, behind the ears, and on the face and neck.
3. *Childhood* disease is commonly manifested by antecubital and popliteal lesions and involvement of the extensor surfaces of extremities. The skin drys and thickens with age, especially in the involved areas on the neck, forehead, and eyelids. The face takes on a whitish hue.

Diagnosis is based on a family history of allergy, clinical features, elevated serum IgE, antibodies to a variety of foods and inhalants, and eosinophilia.

Treatment includes:

avoidance of environmental precipitants (including foods) and the itch–scratch–itch (often with infection) cycle
use of soaps and detergents that do not defat skin (minimize bathing)
local therapy: wet Burow solution dressings and topical steroids between dressings during acute flare-ups
treatment of infection with systemic antibiotics
corticosteroid creams and ointments for longer term use

URTICARIA-ANGIOEDEMA (Hives)
(*NELSON TEXTBOOK*, SEC. 11.43)

Urticaria consist of well-circumscribed, sometimes coalescent, localized or generalized erythematous raised skin lesions (wheals or welts) of various sizes. Lesions appear singly or in crops and usually resolve in 48 hr. *Angioedema* involves deeper tissues and commonly the upper respiratory and gastrointestinal tracts.

The *pathophysiology* involves interaction of antigen with mast cell– or basophil-bound IgE antibody, the complement system, and the plasma kinin-forming coagulation scheme.

The *etiology* involves a broad array of allergies, physical stimuli, and genetic and other diseases.

Treatment may not be needed since the disorder is usually self-limited, but epinephrine provides acute relief and hydroxyzine and combined H_1 and H_2 antihistamines may be helpful in chronic urticaria.

ANAPHYLAXIS
(*NELSON TEXTBOOK*, SEC. 11.44)

This is a sudden life-threatening immunologic reaction; it may result from IgE-mediated sensitivity to foreign substances. These reactions are uncommon in childhood.

ETIOLOGY

Etiologies include drugs, foods, insect stings, food additives, biologic agents, and exercise.

PATHOPHYSIOLOGY

Subsequent exposure to sensitizing antigen results in an explosive antigen–antibody reaction with massive release of chemical mediators such as histamine. Agents also may directly cause mediator release.

CLINICAL MANIFESTATIONS

These include feelings of impending doom, tingling sensation around face and mouth, itching, difficulty swallowing, tightness in the throat or chest, flushing, urticaria, angioedema, inspiratory stridor and respiratory distress, dysphagia, hypotension, bradycardia, and diarrhea.

TREATMENT

This depends on anticipation of and preparation for such reactions.

  a generalized reaction requires administration of epinephrine and a tourniquet if an allergen has been injected into an extremity.
  aminophylline IV may be needed for bronchoconstriction.
  volume expansion may be needed for hypotension.
  airway maintenance is a priority.

SERUM SICKNESS
(*NELSON TEXTBOOK*, SEC. 11.45)

Serum sickness usually is caused by the administration of therapeutic agents.

PATHOPHYSIOLOGY

Antigen–antibody complexes of IgE, IgG, or IgM classes, complement components, and release of mediator from inflammatory cells lead to tissue injury.

CLINICAL MANIFESTATIONS

Symptoms usually begin 7–12 days after an allergic stimulus, but the onset may be as late as 3 wk or as early as 1–3 days if there was previous exposure or reaction.

> fever, malaise, and rash almost always are present
> generalized urticaria is common
> other prominent findings are edema, myalgias, lymphadenopathy, arthralgia, arthritis, nausea, diarrhea, and erythema marginatum
> thrombocytopenia, increased sedimentation rate, and decreased C3 and C4 are common

TREATMENT

Treatment usually consists of aspirin and antihistamines; rarely, corticosteroids are needed.

PROGNOSIS

The course is usually self-limited, with recovery in 7–10 days.

ADVERSE REACTIONS TO DRUGS
(*NELSON TEXTBOOK*, SEC. 11.46)

Untoward drug reactions include toxicity, intolerance, side effects, idiosyncratic responses, drug interactions, and allergic reactions. Many diverse mechanisms are involved in the pathophysiology of these reactions.

Cutaneous eruptions are the most common *clinical manifestation* in children and may be accompanied by fever. Urticaria and exanthematous and eczematoid reactions predominate, but almost any morphology may occur. Renal and pulmonary disease is rare.

Diagnosis is usually dependent on history.

Treatment depends on the mechanism of drug reaction and the manifestations.

INSECT ALLERGY
(*NELSON TEXTBOOK*, SEC. 11.47)

Etiologies include:

> inhalation of particulate matter of insect origin, leading to respiratory allergy (often IgE mediated)
> insect bites, resulting in cutaneous reactions (often wheal and flare lesions)

insect stings, which may cause anaphylaxis (many venoms
result in IgE-mediated sensitivity)

Clinical manifestations include:

asthma, rhinitis, and conjunctivitis in reaction to inhaled
insect allergens

papular, vascular, and erythematous rashes in reaction to
bites (occasionally delayed hypersensitivity)

sting reactions ranging from local pain and erythema to
severe anaphylactic episodes

Treatment depends on the type of reaction. Venom immunotherapy may be needed for stings.

OCULAR ALLERGIES
(*NELSON TEXTBOOK*, SEC. 11.48)

Ocular allergies may be IgE or cell mediated.

CLINICAL MANIFESTATIONS

Eyelid swelling (common) often is due to contact dermatitis,
cosmetics, or topical ophthalmic medications.

Conjunctivitis frequently occurs with allergic rhinitis
caused by pollens (hay fever). It is characterized by red,
edematous, itching eyes with discharge.

TREATMENT

Treatment includes the following components:

sensitizers must be identified and eliminated

topical steroids may be needed for acute allergic reactions
of the eyelids

lid hygiene should be instituted

topical sympathomimetics, cromolyn solution, or corticosteroid drops or ointments may be needed

ADVERSE REACTIONS TO FOOD
(*NELSON TEXTBOOK*, SEC. 11.49)

Etiologies include allergy; enzyme deficiencies; adverse reactions to tyramine, nitrites, monosodium glutamate, and food
additives; food poisoning; infections; drug reactions; and
gastrointestinal disorders.

Treatment is directed at clinical manifestations and is related to etiology.

RHEUMATIC DISEASES OF CHILDHOOD
(*NELSON TEXTBOOK*, SECS. 11.50–11.75)

DEFINITION

This group of disorders is associated with inflammatory
changes in connective tissues throughout the body. They

have similar pathologies and overlapping clinical manifestations. The causes are unknown, and the different entities usually may be distinguished from each other on the basis of the clinical course of their signs and symptoms and laboratory findings.

LABORATORY STUDIES

The following tests may be helpful.

Acute-phase phenomena—these plasma constituents appear or increase during the inflammatory state and include erythrocyte sedimentation rate (ESR), C-reactive protein (CRP), serum mucoproteins, various α-globulins, gamma globulins, some complement components, and transferrin.

Rheumatoid factors—these are antibodies that react with the Fc portion of immunoglobulin G from the host, other individuals, or other species. They are produced by protracted immune stimulation, chronic infection, or inflammation.

Antinuclear antibodies (ANAs)—these are antibodies against various nuclear constituents, including deoxyribonucleoprotein (DNP), ribonucleoprotein (RNP), and ribonucleic acid (RNA).

Complement—these proteins mediate certain aspects of inflammation and cell injury.

Immune complex determinations—these antigen complexes may cause tissue damage.

Serum proteins and immunoglobulins—increased levels of α-globulin and gamma globulin frequently occur with active inflammation. Albumin levels may be low.

The histocompatibility (human leukocyte antigen; [HLA]) system—various HLA antigens on the surfaces of human cells are statistically associated with different rheumatoid disorders.

JUVENILE RHEUMATOID ARTHRITIS
(*NELSON TEXTBOOK*, SEC. 11.51)

This group of diseases is characterized by chronic synovitis and a variety of extra-articular inflammatory manifestations. Diagnosis of the various subgroups is important in determining appropriate follow-up, treatment, and prognosis.

Etiology

The etiology of juvenile rheumatoid arthritis (JRA) is unknown but is hypothesized to represent either hypersensitivity or autoimmune reaction to unknown stimuli or infection. Genetic vulnerability also is thought to play a role in some disorders.

Pathology

The arthritis is characterized by chronic nonsuppurative inflammation of the synovium.

Clinical Manifestations

POLYARTICULAR-ONSET DISEASE. This is characterized by involvement of multiple joints, typically including the small joints of the hands, and is unassociated with prominent systemic manifestation. It occurs in about 35% of JRA patients. The course of arthritis may be insidious or fulminant and usually starts in the large joints. It consists of two subtypes that occur predominantly in girls and may involve any joint. Malaise, mild anemia, irritability, and low-grade fever are common.

Rheumatoid factor–negative (about two thirds of polyarticular patients) disorder occurs throughout childhood, rarely involves the eyes, and does not involve the spine. Some 10–15% of patients have severe arthritic morbidity. The ANA test is positive in about 25% of children.

Rheumatoid factor–positive disorder occurs late in childhood, does not involve the eyes, and sacroiliitis occurs rarely. More than 50% of children have severe joint morbidity. The ANA test is positive in about 75%.

PAUCIARTICULAR-ONSET DISEASE. This is characterized by arthritis in four or fewer joints, typically large joints for the first 6 mo, and is rheumatoid factor negative. The two subtypes constitute over 50% of JRA patients. Extra-articular manifestations are usually mild, consisting of low-grade fever, malaise, modest hepatomegaly, and lymphadenopathy.

Type I (35–40% of JRA patients) usually begins before age 4, primarily in girls. It often involves the knee, ankle, or elbow but does not include sacroiliitis; 90% are ANA positive. About a third develop chronic iridocyclitis; approximately 10% going on to ocular damage and 20% to severe polyarthritis.

Type II (10–15% of JRA patients) usually begins in late childhood, occurs predominantly in boys, and often involves the hip girdle and lower extremity joints. There may be sacroiliitis, the ANA test is negative, and 10–20% develop acute iridocyclitis. There is an association with HLA-B27 and subsequent spondyloarthropathy.

SYSTEMIC-ONSET JRA. This subtype (20% of JRA patients) is characterized by prominent extra-articular manifestations. It occurs about equally in boys and girls. High, intermittent fever, often with chills, and an evanescent, recurrent red–pink macular rash are usually the presenting signs. Other major manifestation include hepatosplenomegaly, lymphadenopathy, pleuritis, pericarditis, abdominal pain, leukocytosis, severe anemia, arthralgia, myalgia, and arthritis. Severe arthritis occurs in about 25%, but the onset may be late. Rheumatoid factor and ANA tests are negative, and sacroiliitis and iridocyclitis do not occur.

Course and Prognosis

The various courses of the different JRA entities are highly variable. Chronic joint disease and chronic iridocyclitis are the major morbidities.

Laboratory Findings

There are no specific diagnostic tests. ESR and CRP are usually elevated in chronic disease. Anemia and elevated white blood cell counts are common.

Diagnosis and Differential Diagnosis

The diagnosis is clinical, and depends on the persistence of arthritis or typical systemic manifestations for 3 consecutive mo or more and the exclusion of other diseases.

Other diseases that may present with similar clinical manifestations include septic arthritis, Lyme disease, osteomyelitis, viral arthritis, malignancy, growing pains, rheumatic fever, SLE, Kawasaki disease, and dermatomyositis.

Treatment

This is directed at (1) preserving joint function, (2) providing adequate care for extra-articular manifestations without doing harm, and (3) supporting the family and child in achieving optimal psychosocial adjustment.

Drugs that may be used to suppress the inflammatory process include aspirin and nonsteroidal anti-inflammatory agents such as tolmetin and Naprosyn. There are a few indications for corticosteroids, such as severe systemic disease unresponsive to an adequate trial of salicylates, iridocyclitis uncontrolled by topical steroids, and heart failure due to pericarditis or myocarditis. Steroids are rarely indicated for relief of joint manifestations. Other anti-inflammatory therapies for disease unresponsive to nonsteroidal agents include oral gold treatment, hydroxychloroquine, and methotrexate.

Physical and occupational therapy are important complementary treatments.

Iridocyclitis requires prompt diagnosis and therapy (topical steroids and dilating agents, systemic and locally injected steroids) to preserve vision.

SPONDYLARTHROPATHIES IN CHILDREN
(*NELSON TEXTBOOK*, SECS. 11.52–11.53)

All spondylarthropathies in children are associated with HLA-B27 and are rheumatoid factor and ANA negative.

Ankylosing Spondylitis

Ankylosing spondylitis is a familial disease of young and middle-aged adults that may begin in late childhood. There is a predilection for males.

Clinical manifestations include characteristic ascending involvement of sacroiliac joints and lumbodorsal and cervical spinal, with associated back, hip, and thigh pain; early involvement of large lower extremity joints and, occasionally, varied peripheral arthritis; painful, swollen, warm joints with limited motion; heel pain and inflammation at sites of attachment of tendons and ligaments; associated iridocyclitis and aortitis; and low-grade fever, anemia, and fatigability.

Treatment is directed at relief of pain and maintenance of good posture and function and includes aspirin and nonsteroidal anti-inflammatory agents and physical therapy.

Reiter Disease

Reiter disease classically consists of sterile urethritis, arthritis, and ocular inflammation but often includes gastroenteritis and skin rashes. It may follow infections such as *Shigella*, *Yersinia*, and sexually transmitted diseases. It is usually pauciarticular, involving large joints. Anti-inflammatory agents and antibiotic treatment of infections are indicated.

Arthritis of Inflammatory Bowel Disease

This occurs in about 10% of children with inflammatory bowel disease. It usually waxes and wanes with the activity of the bowel disease and does not result in permanent joint deformity. However, rarely, the latter may occur, especially in association with ankylosing spondylitis.

SYSTEMIC LUPUS ERYTHEMATOSUS (SLE)
(*NELSON TEXTBOOK*, SEC. 11.54 AND 11.55)

This multisystem disease often is progressive but may remit spontaneously or smolder for years. SLE is generally more acute and severe in children than adults.

The *etiology* is unknown, but altered immune regulation or virus infection is hypothesized. Exacerbations may be related to intercurrent infection, and there may be a familial propensity. Lupus-like disease also may occur in reaction to drugs.

The most frequent early *clinical manifestations* are fever, malaise, arthritis, arthralgia, and rash. Anorexia, weight loss, and debility are common. The malar butterfly rash extending over the bridge of the nose is characteristic, but rashes, often photosensitive, may be varied and widespread. Raynaud phenomenon, polyserositis, hepatosplenomegaly, lymphadenopathy, and renal disease also are frequent.

Laboratory findings include ANA in all patients with active disease (antibodies to Sm are relatively specific for SLE), antibodies to double-stranded DNA, decreased C3 in active disease (esp. nephritis), elevated gamma globulin and α-globulin, decreased albumin and hemoglobin, thrombocytopenia, leukopenia, and abnormal urinary sediment.

This disorder may mimic many rheumatoid and nonrheumatoid diseases and, therefore, *diagnosis* depends on the clinical and laboratory findings that become manifest over time.

Treatment is based on the extent and severity of disease, particularly renal involvement. There is no specific therapy. Drugs are used to suppress inflammation and the formation of immune complexes. Salicylates and nonsteroidal anti-inflammatory drugs are used for mild disease without nephritis. Corticosteroids are required for more severe or widespread organ involvement, and for renal disease. The latter also often requires the use of immunosuppressive agents such as cyclophosphamide and azathioprine. Dialysis and renal transplant eventually may be needed. Central nervous system (CNS) manifestations and coagulopathies require other specific therapies.

Neonatal lupus phenomenon occur in infants of mothers with SLE or other rheumatoid disorders and are associated with maternal antibodies to Ro/SSA or La/SSB. An erythematous, circinate rash and fetal and neonatal heart block are common, usually transient, manifestations.

VASCULITIS SYNDROMES
(*NELSON TEXTBOOK*, SECS. 11.56–11.61)

These are syndromes of blood vessel inflammation that may be primary or secondary to another connective tissue disorder, infection, or other process. The patterns of disease may overlap and depend on the size and location of the vessels.

Henoch–Schönlein Purpura (Vasculitis)
(Anaphylactoid Purpura)

ETIOLOGY AND EPIDEMIOLOGY.　The cause is unknown, although allergy, drug sensitivity, and upper respiratory infection sometimes are associated. Most cases occur in boys 2–8 yr of age.

PATHOLOGY.　Capillaries, small arterioles, and venules are usually involved in an inflammatory hemorrhagic reaction.

CLINICAL MANIFESTATIONS.　Henoch–Schönlein purpura is characterized by nonthrombocytopenic, usually dependent, palpable purpuras, arthritis, abdominal pain, and nephritis. The onset may be acute, with simultaneous appearance of several manifestations, or gradual, with sequential appearance of features over weeks. There may be malaise and low-grade fever. The prognosis is good in the absence of significant renal disease.

> *Skin lesions* occur in all patients and usually begin as small wheals or erythematous maculopapules that then become petechial or purpuric.
> *Swollen, tender large joints* occur in two thirds of children.
> *Gastrointestinal symptoms* occur in over half of affected children.
> *Renal involvement* occurs in 25–50%; most recover, but a few develop chronic disease.

TREATMENT.　There is no specific therapy. Life-threatening hemorrhage, intestinal obstruction (intussuception) or perforation, or CNS manifestations may be managed by early use of 1–2 mg/kg/24 hr of prednisone. Acute renal failure is managed similarly to acute glomerulonephritis.

Kawasaki Disease (Mucocutaneous Lymph Node Syndrome, Infantile Polyarteritis)

This febrile disease involves vasculitis of large coronary vessels, with potential for aneurysm, thrombosis, rupture, and myocardial infarction.

CLINICAL MANIFESTATIONS.　Diagnosis is based on clinical features, including fever lasting at least 5 days; bilateral nonpurulent conjunctival injection; changes in mucosa of the oral pharynx (infection, dry fissured lips, strawberry tongue); peripheral extremity findings such as edema, erythema of hands or feet, and desquamations (usually beginning periungually); primarily truncal, nonvesicular polymorphous rash; and cervical lymphadenopathy.

Onset is usually abrupt.

Transient arthritis, iridocyclitis, and a large variety of multisystem manifestations may also occur.

Cardiac involvement occurs in 10–40% of children within the first 2 wk of illness, and its seriousness requires vigilance in detection and prompt management. Prognosis is primarily related to this complication.

Laboratory findings include leukocytosis, thrombocytosis, anemia, and elevated ESR and CRP.

TREATMENT. Treatment includes IV gamma globulin, 400 mg/kg/24 hr, given during the period of acute febrile illness, and salicylates to achieve serum concentration of 20–30 mg/dL during the febrile phase, followed by lower doses (5 mg/kg/24 hr) for subsequent antithrombotic effects.

Polyarteritis Nodosa

This inflammation of small and medium-sized arteries is rare and presents diverse manifestations typically involving the heart, kidney, skin, and peripheral nervous system. Systemic illness (fever, lethargy, weight loss), arthralgias, and arthritis are common. The prognosis is poor, and systemic steroids are indicated.

Wegener Granulomatosis

This rare syndrome is characterized by destructive granulomatous lesions of the upper respiratory tract and lungs and systemic necrotizing vasculitis of the lungs and kidneys. Corticosteroids may suppress the process.

Takayasu Arteritis (Pulseless Disease)

This rare inflammatory process involves the aorta and its major branches. Absent pulses, hypertension, and fever are common.

DERMATOMYOSITIS
(NELSON TEXTBOOK, SEC. 11.62)

This multisystem disease involves a nonsuppurative inflammation of striated muscle and characteristic skin lesions.

Etiology and Epidemiology

The cause is unknown but it is probably mediated by cellular immune mechanisms. The onset usually is at 8–9 yr, and girls are more affected than boys.

Clinical Manifestations

The *onset* is insidious with slowly developing muscle weakness usually first apparent in proximal muscles of the extremities and trunk, stiffness, and tenderness. Calcium deposition may occur.

Skin lesions often have a distinctive violaceous (heliotrope) erythema; the upper eyelids often are involved. Periorbital and facial edema and a butterfly rash may occur. Many nonspecific and atrophic changes in the skin occur and often involve the extensor surfaces over joints.

Gastrointestinal involvement may occur at any level and includes difficulty swallowing, abdominal pain, perforation, and constipation.

There may be *arthritis* and other systemic manifestations.

Elevation of serum levels of enzymes such as serum glutamic oxaloacetic transaminase, creatine phosphokinase, and lactic dehydrogenase reflect muscle inflammation.

Treatment

Treatment includes acute-phase support of palatorespiratory function, corticosteroids to suppress inflammation, and physical therapy. Untreated patients have a high mortality.

SCLERODERMA
(*NELSON TEXTBOOK*, SEC., 11.63)

This chronic fibrotic disturbance of unknown etiology involves the skin but also may affect the gastrointestinal tract, heart, lungs, kidney, and synovium. It may be remitting or progressive.

Clinical Manifestations

Cutaneous lesions may be focal in patches (morphea) or in a linear distribution or, more rarely, systemic.

Focal scleroderma lesions initially are slightly erythematous and edematous, with an atrophic, shiny appearance, and may be painful. They progress, becoming indurated, violaceous, and elevated. Extensive scarring and fibrosis can occur and be severe enough to limit growth and produce contractions.

Systemic scleroderma usually is associated with Raynaud phenomenon. It is widespread, with diffuse cutaneous fibrosis and serious gastrointestinal, heart, lung, and renal involvement that may be life threatening.

Treatment

There is no specific therapy and, although corticosteroids may be beneficial in the acute edematous phase, a wide variety of immunosuppressive and other agents have not had a clear-cut benefit. Physical therapy is important to maximize function.

RHEUMATIC SYNDROME OF UNCERTAIN CLASSIFICATION
(*NELSON TEXTBOOK*, SECS. 11.64–11.74)

These constitute a large variety of rare disorders, including mixed connective tissue disease, fasciitis, benign rheumatoid nodules, erythema nodosum, Stevens-Johnson syndrome, and a variety of diseases mimicking rheumatoid disorders.

RHEUMATIC FEVER
(*NELSON TEXTBOOK*, SEC. 11.75)

Etiology

Group A β-hemolytic streptococcus is the inciting agent resulting in acute rheumatic fever (ARF), although the exact pathogenic mechanisms are unknown. Some serotypes probably have a greater propensity to initiate this process.

Epidemiology

ARF most frequently occurs in children 5–15 yr of age, who are usually the group most susceptible to upper respiratory tract streptococcal infections. The incidence is increased in socially and economically disadvantaged groups and in closed or crowded populations. Impetigo is not associated with an increased incidence. A recent resurgence of ARF has been associated with several subtypes, especially the virulent mucoid strains.

Pathogenesis

An abnormal immune response by the human host to an undefined component of the organism is the most popular current hypothesis.

Clinical Manifestations and Diagnosis

The clinical and laboratory features that characterize this disorder (Jones criteria) include:

Major: carditis, migratory polyarthritis, erythema marginatum, chorea, and subcutaneous nodules

Minor: fever, arthralgia, previous rheumatic fever, elevated acute-phase reactants (ESR, CRP), prolonged P-R interval in electrocardiogram

Plus: evidence of preceding streptococcal infection (culture, antigen, antibody, scarlet fever)

Pancarditis, mild to very severe, occurs in ARF; insufficiency of the mitral valve with or without aortic valve involvement is common. Stenosis usually occurs later.

The *migratory arthritis* (elbows, knees, ankles, wrists) is exquisitely tender; joints are red, warm, and swollen. However, the arthritis usually is gone after 24 hr of anti-inflammatory treatment, and chronic joint disease does not occur.

Sydenham chorea occurs much later than other manifestations, often occurs alone, and may be very subtle at onset.

Preceding streptococcal infection may result in elevation of antibodies such as antistreptolysin O (ASO), which peaks 3–6 wk after infection; antideoxyribonuclease B (anti-DNase B), which peaks 6–8 wk after infection; or antihyaluronidase (AH). Culture of group A streptococcus is the gold standard evidence of previous infection.

Differential diagnosis includes JRA, other connective tissue disorders, infective arthritis or endocarditis, and Lyme disease.

Treatment

Treatment involves three approaches:

1. Antibiotic therapy (usually penicillin) for group A streptococcus infection.
2. Anti-inflammatory drugs (usually salicylates):
   - Prompt, dramatic relief of arthritis usually occurs; therefore, salicylates should not be given until diagnosis is established.
   - Mild carditis without heart failure usually responds to salicylates alone. Corticosteroids are indicated if there is congestive heart failure or significant carditis, although there is no objective evidence that salicylates or corticosteroids prevent subsequent valvular disease.
3. Supportive therapy
   - Congestive heart failure should be treated conventionally, including diuretics and cardiac glycosides.
   - Chorea may require sedatives, diazepam, or haloperidol.

Prevention

Prevention and treatment of group A streptococcal infection can prevent ARF.

Primary prophylaxis by antibiotic treatment of streptococcal infection within 1 wk of an upper respiratory tract infection almost completely eliminates the risk of ARF.

Secondary prophylaxis by continuous antibiotic administration should prevent colonization or infection of the upper respiratory tract of those who already have had an attack of ARF and avoid recurrences of rheumatic fever. This can be accomplished by oral therapy or regular monthly injections of penicillin for at least 5 yr after the most recent attack or when the 18th birthday is reached; many recommend a longer duration of treatment.

10

INFECTIOUS DISEASES

GENERAL CONSIDERATIONS
(*NELSON TEXTBOOK*, SECS. 12.1–12.5)

FEVER

Fever is an elevation of body temperature mediated by an increase of the hypothalamic heat regulatory set-point. Normal homeostatic regulation of temperature may be altered by various disease states, the most common of which are the infectious diseases. Other causes of fever include:

malignancy
tissue injury (e.g., crush injuries)
collagen vascular (autoimmune) diseases (e.g., juvenile rheumatoid arthritis [JRA], systemic lupus erythematosus [SLE])
endocrine disorders (e.g., hyperthyroidism)
metabolic disorders (e.g., uremia)
reaction to vaccines (e.g., diphtheria–tetanus–pertussis)
reactions to biologic agents (e.g., interferon)
reactions to drugs (e.g., antibiotics)

Body temperature also may be elevated by mechanisms not primarily related to the hypothalamus. These include increased endogenous heat production (vigorous exercise, malignant hyperthermia), decreased heat loss (bundling, atropine intoxication), or prolonged exposure to high environmental temperatures (heat stroke).

FEVER AS A MANIFESTATION OF SERIOUS BACTERIAL DISEASE

Fever is a common manifestation of many infectious diseases, some benign and some potentially life threatening. The severity of the situation is dictated by both the infectious agent and the host. Some situations are known to be high risk, warranting a thorough evaluation (Table 10–1). Evaluation consists of:

thorough history (being attentive to potential ill contacts and baseline medical state)
use of an Acute Illness Observation Scale in an effort to assess the global toxic appearance of the child (see Table 4–1)
thorough physical examination (remembering that infections of the ears, pharynx, lungs, intestines, urinary tract, skin, bones, joints, and meninges are common in children)

TABLE 10–1. HIGH-RISK FEBRILE PATIENTS

Condition	Comment
Previously Normal Patients	
Neonate (<28 days)	Group B streptococcus, *Escherichia coli, Listeria monocytogenes,* herpes simplex
Infants <3 mo	Serious bacterial disease 10–15%, bacteremia 5%: seasonal viral illness—respiratory syncytial virus winter, enterovirus summer
Infants 3–24 mo	Risk of occult bacteremia increased if fever is >40°C, WBC[†] <5,000 or >15,000, positive exposure history
Hyperpyrexia (>41°C)	Meningitis, bacteremia, pneumonia. Heat stroke, hemorrhagic shock–encephalopathy syndrome
Fever with petechiae	Bacteremia, meningitis. Meningococcus, *Haemophilus influenzae* type b, pneumococcus
Immunocompromised Patients	
Sickle cell anemia	Pneumococcal sepsis, meningitis
Asplenia	Encapsulated bacteria
Complement/properdin deficiency	Meningococcal sepsis
Agammaglobulinemia	Bacteremia, sinopulmonary infection
AIDS[‡]	Pneumococcus, *H. influenzae* type b, *Salmonella*
Congenital heart disease	Risk of endocarditis
Central venous line	*Staphylococcus aureus, S. epidermidis, Corynebacteria, Candida*
Malignancy	*Pseudomonas aeruginosa, S. aureus, S. epidermidis, Candida*

* From Behrman RE (ed): Nelson Textbook of Pediatrics, 14th ed. Philadelphia, WB Saunders Company, 1992, p. 649.
† WBC = white blood cell count.
‡ AIDS = acquired immunodeficiency syndrome.

if no source is found, the following lab tests should be considered:

– complete blood count with differential
– chest roentgenogram (if lower respiratory symptoms are present)
– cultures of blood, urine, cerebrospinal fluid (CSF) (if meningitis is considered), and stool (if gastrointestinal symptoms are prominent)

If the patient is in a high-risk situation or any of the above tests are abnormal, hospitalization and intravenous antibiotics should be considered. In contrast, if the patient (1) is not in a high-risk situation, (2) is nontoxic appearing, and (3) has a normal physical examination and lab tests, and (4) if good follow-up is assured, the patient may be discharged to home on no therapy. At some centers, the outpatient use of intramuscular antibiotics, such as ceftriaxone, is advocated.

FEVER OF UNKNOWN ORIGIN

Although definitions vary as to what precisely constitutes a fever of unknown origin (FUO), it is widely agreed that this term should be reserved for (1) fever of greater than 14 days' duration without a source and (2) fever for which all of the usual lab work-up is unremarkable.

The differential diagnosis of a FUO is extensive. Common causes include (1) infectious diseases not diagnosed by a typical laboratory work-up (e.g., tuberculosis, malaria, abscesses); (2) collagen vascular diseases (JRA, SLE, inflammatory bowel disease); and (3) neoplasm (esp. leukemias).

History should include questions about exposures to animals, pica, exposures to medicines and drugs, travel history, and family history. Physical examination should be especially attentive when searching for deep abscesses and possible bone infections. Although no formal laboratory work-up is universally agreed on, a staged work-up might include:

- Level I: history and physical examination

  complete blood count, erythrocyte sedimentation rate, chemistry panel
  urine analysis and culture
  stool guaiac
  chest roentgenogram
  blood cultures
  VDRL, antinuclear antibodies, rheumatoid factor, C3, and total complement
  purified protein derivative (PPD) and anergy panel
  1 extra tube of serum for acute serologic titers

- Level II: bone marrow aspirate and culture

  ultrasound and echocardiography
  computerized tomography (CT) and/or magnetic resonance imaging (MRI)

- Level III: nuclear medicine scans (biopsies, angiography, etc.)

CLINICAL USE OF THE MICROBIOLOGY LABORATORY

Although culture remains the "gold standard" in the diagnosis of infectious diseases, culturing various pathogens can be expensive, labor intensive, and time consuming. Fortunately, there are a growing number of tools that may aid in the diagnosis of infectious disease. These tools include techniques in which the microbe is visualized, such as Gram stain, microscopy with fluorescent antibodies, and electron microscopy. Immunologic techniques may be used, such as latex agglutination, fluorescent antibody stains, enzyme-linked immunosorbent assay (ELISA), and radioimmunoassay. Additionally, through use of polymerase chain reactions, in which the DNA of the microbe is amplified, a growing number of infectious diseases can be diagnosed.

DISORDERS CAUSED BY A VARIETY OF INFECTIOUS AGENTS
(*NELSON TEXTBOOK*, SECS. 12.10–12.13)

DIARRHEA

Diarrhea is one of the symptoms most frequently encountered by pediatricians. It may be due to causes extrinsic or intrinsic to the gastrointestinal tract. Common extrinsic causes include urinary tract infections and otitis media, both of which frequently have diarrhea as one of their manifestations. The most common intrinsic cause of acute diarrhea is infection, and in the United States, a *viral etiology* most often is to blame. Of the viruses that cause diarrhea, rotavirus is the most commonly isolated virus during the winter months and may be proven by culture or ELISA techniques. During summer months, the enteroviruses are prominent. Epidemic spread of diarrhea has been noted with enteric adenovirus and the Norwalk agent.

A *bacterial cause* of diarrhea should be sought in patients who have traveled abroad, patients who have had contact with others with known bacterial diarrhea, patients who have been exposed to tainted or ill-cooked foods, and hospitalized patients. A bacterial cause should be sought in all patients who have either blood or leukocytes in their stool because bacterial pathogens are associated with these findings. Bacterial causes of diarrhea include *Salmonella, Shigella, Campylobacter, Yersinia,* and pathogenic *Escherichia coli.*

Parasitic causes of diarrhea are endemic in other parts of the world, but are less of a public health problem in the United States. Parasitic infections include those due to *Giardia lamblia,* which is very common in day-care centers and residential facilities, and cryptosporidium, which, although still uncommon, has been associated with acquired immunodeficiency syndrome (AIDS).

ACUTE ASEPTIC MENINGITIS

Acute aseptic meningitis is a relatively common illness caused by a variety of factors. Diagnosis rests on finding CSF pleocytosis without micro-organisms on Gram stain or routine culture.

Etiology

Eighty-five percent of aseptic meningitis is caused by the enteroviruses, especially coxsackievirus B5 and echoviruses 4, 6, 9, and 11. Arboviruses account for another 5%. The most common nonviral cause of aseptic meningitis is partially and improperly treated bacterial infection. Other infectious agents, such as tuberculosis, mycoplasm, and leptospirosis, and malignancy are uncommon causes of aseptic meningitis.

Clinical Manifestations

In infants, irritability and resentment while being handled are the most common signs. A full fontanel and fever may be the only signs. In children, headache, fever, nausea, and vomiting are common presenting complaints. Nuchal rigidity and photophobia are commonly found on physical examination.

Laboratory Manifestations

CSF contains few to several thousand white blood cells/mm³. Early in the disease, these cells are often polymorphonuclear; later they are chiefly mononuclear. No organisms are seen on Gram stain. Protein levels are normal to slightly elevated, whereas the glucose level is typically normal.

Treatment and Prognosis

Patients with aseptic meningitis are typically hospitalized because of the possibility of nonviral etiology, which warrants immediate treatment with antibiotics and steroids. Once viral etiology is certain, the patient may be treated at home with supportive therapy, including rest and pain control with non–aspirin-containing analgesics.

ENCEPHALITIS

Encephalitis refers to inflammation of the brain, whereas encephalopathy refers to neurologic symptoms suggestive of encephalitis but without the inflammation (e.g., Reye syndrome). Encephalitis may be global or may involve specific areas of the central nervous system (CNS) (e.g., acute cerebellar ataxia, Guillain–Barré syndrome).

Etiology

Although only 25% of the cases of encephalitis reported to the Centers for Disease Control have established causes, the vast majority of cases are due enteroviruses, which are transmitted from person to person, and arboviruses, which are spread via an arthropod vector. All of the herpesviruses have been implicated, with herpes simplex viruses (types 1 and 2) being a fairly common and devastating cause of encephalitis, especially in newborns. There are also known bacterial, parasitic, postinfectious, and allergic causes of encephalitis, as well as those attributable to slow-viral disease (e.g., Creutzfeldt–Jakob disease and kuru).

Pathogenesis and Pathologic Findings

It is likely that neurologic damage is caused both by direct destruction of neurologic tissue by the actively multiplying viruses and by a reaction of the patient's nervous tissue to antigens of the virus. The process may be global, as is typically the case with the arboviruses, or localized (herpes simplex tends to severely affect the temporal lobes, and rabies has a predilection for the basal structures).

Clinical Manifestations

Symptoms may appear suddenly or insidiously, with some cases mild and others catastrophic. Initial symptoms may be nonspecific or flu-like, only to be followed by changes in mental status, bizarre movements, seizures, and changes in the neurologic examination. Such changes may be progressive, static, or fluctuating, and they may be permanent or short lived. Complications include convulsions, cerebral edema, hyperpyrexia, abrupt changes in cardiorespiratory function of a central origin, fluid and electrolyte disturbances (e.g., syndrome of inappropriate antidiuretic hormone secretion [SIADH]), and disseminated intravascular coagulation. Patients should be placed in an intensive care unit where such complications can be adequately monitored and treated.

Diagnosis

Brain biopsy is the gold standard for diagnosis. CT scan or MRI may reveal nonspecific global inflammation or focal lesions, such as those frequently found in the temporal lobe with herpes simplex infections. CSF is typically normal, but lumbar puncture should be performed and cultures done. Serum acute and convalescent titers may be of diagnostic help.

Prognosis

This is guarded with respect to both immediate outcome and sequelae. Young infants usually have severe disease and sequelae. Herpes simplex infections carry a worse overall prognosis than do infections with the enteroviruses.

INFECTIONS IN THE COMPROMISED HOST

The normal patient has several lines of defense against infectious diseases. These defenses include *physical barriers* to infection, such as the skin, cilia, and protective "normal" flora colonizing epithelial and endothelial surfaces; *humoral barriers* to infection; and *cell-mediated barriers* to infection. Primary (congenital) immunodeficiencies are rare and may affect either B cell (humoral) or T cell (cellular) function or both. Far more common are secondary deficiencies caused by disease states (e.g., AIDS, malnutrition).

Most commonly, patients are compromised as an iatrogenic complication of the treatment of disease. Some examples of these iatrogenic complications include interference with mechanical barriers to infection (e.g., ventricular shunts, percutaneous large venous catheters, and urethral catheters) and suppression of cellular and humoral immune barriers with various drugs (e.g., corticosteroids, antineoplastic agents, and drugs used to prevent rejection in transplant recipients).

When treating a patient who is compromised, it must be remembered that infections are a major cause of mortality and morbidity. Attempts should be made to prevent them and aggressively treat them. *Preventive management* strategies include sterile technique when handling indwelling catheters, regular administration of IV immunoglobulin if humoral deficiencies are present, avoidance of live virus vaccines if cellular immunity is compromised, and antibiotic prophylaxis. *Treatment* of infectious disease complications includes educating parents about the signs and symptoms of infectious diseases and aggressive work-up and antibiotic therapy whenever an infection may be present.

BACTERIAL INFECTIONS
(*NELSON TEXTBOOK*, SECS. 12.14–12.63)

BACTEREMIA AND SEPTICEMIA

Bacteremia refers to the recovery of bacteria in a blood culture and may be transient or associated with serious disease. *Septicemia*, or sepsis, is a severe form of bacteremia that may progress to septic shock. A *sepsis syndrome* may be present in the absence of documented bacteremia. Indistinguishable from septic shock, it may be due to endotoxemia, prior antibiotic therapy, severe local infection, fastidious slow-growing organisms, or rickettsial or viral infections.

Signs and symptoms of septic shock include temperature instability, tachycardia, hyperventilation, cutaneous lesions such as petechiae and purpura, and changes in mental status. Early septic shock is characteristically "warm," with increased perfusion to the skin, only to become "cold" as shock progresses and peripheral vascular resistance increases.

Treatment includes close monitoring of cardiopulmonary state in an intensive care unit, supporting blood pressure with fluid resuscitation and cardiotonic support, and empiric antibiotic therapy. Controversial adjuvant therapies include use of intravenous immunoglobulin, granulocyte transfusions, and monoclonal antibodies. Corticosteroids are not beneficial in patients with septic shock.

Prognosis depends on initial site of infection, bacterial pathogen, and degree of multiple organ dysfunction, but mortality can be greater than 50% for patients with gram-negative enteric sepsis.

ACUTE BACTERIAL MENINGITIS BEYOND THE NEONATAL PERIOD

Bacterial meningitis is a common severe infection that carries serious morbidity and mortality. In the newborn period, bacteria implicated reflect maternal vaginal flora: group B streptococcus, *Listeria monocytogenes*, and gram-negative enteric flora (see Chap. 7). In children greater than 2 mo of age, causative agents are those commonly associated with childhood sepsis: *Haemophilus influenzae* type b, *Streptococcus pneumoniae*, and *Neisseria meningitidis*.

Epidemiology and Pathogenesis

Ninety-five percent of cases occur between 1 mo and 5 yr of age, with most cases occurring in children less than 1 yr of age. Transmission is probably through infected nasopharyngeal secretions, with subsequent colonization and infection of the susceptible host. Bacterial meningitis typically occurs from hematogenous dissemination of the causative micro-organism; therefore, a concurrent (and antecedent) bacteremia is commonly found. Infection by direct extension (e.g., periorbital cellulitis, cavernous vein thrombosis) also may occur.

Clinical Manifestations

Meningitis can present suddenly or insidiously. The former is more common with *N. meningitidis*, whereas the latter is more characteristic of *H. influenzae* and *S. pneumoniae*. Signs and symptoms associated with meningitis are most commonly nonspecific: fever, anorexia, lethargy or irritability, shocky appearance, and rash. More specific signs and symptoms of meningeal irritation, such as Kernig and Brudzinski signs, irritability with handling, and nuchal rigidity, may be subtle or absent. Seizures are a presenting sign in 20–30% of patients with meningitis. In the infant less than 6 mo of age, the presentation of fever with seizures should be considered as a sign of meningitis until proven otherwise because febrile seizures are rare in this age group.

Complications

Complications of meningitis include seizures, increased intracranial pressure, cranial nerve palsies, stroke, and subdural effusions. SIADH occurs in 30–50% of cases and may exacerbate cerebral edema or seizures as a result of hyponatremia.

Diagnosis

This rests on immediate lumbar puncture and analysis of the CSF. Typical CSF findings include a neutrophilic pleocytosis, with an elevated protein and reduced glucose content in the CSF. Gram stain reveals organisms in greater than 80–90% of cases of bacterial meningitis. Countercurrent immunoelectrophoresis (CIE) or latex agglutination may detect antigens of group B streptococcus, *H. influenzae*, *N. meningitidis*, and pneumococcus with varying degrees of sensitivity and specificity. If spinal tap must be delayed because of (1) evidence of increased intracranial pressure, (2) septic shock and an unstable cardiorespiratory state, or (3) infection of the skin overlying the lumbar spine, treatment still should be instituted promptly.

Treatment

Several studies have noted decreased morbidity when corticosteroids have been administered prior to institution of antibiotic therapy. The rationale for the use of corticosteroids is that they will moderate the inflammatory response that accompanies bacterial lysis after the administration of antibiotics. Although most of these studies have been done with meningitis due to *H. influenzae*, a growing body of literature supports the use of dexamethasone with the other bacterial meningitides. Treatment consists of using (1) dexamethasone 0.15 mg/kg/dose every 6 hr for 16 doses and (2) a broad-spectrum antibiotic with good CNS penetration, such as ceftriaxone or cefotaxime. Duration of therapy is 7–10 days for *H. influenzae*, 7 days for *N. meningitidis*, and 10–14 days for pneumococcus.

Supportive care consists of fluid restriction to one-half or one-third maintenance until it can be established that increased intracranial pressure or SIADH is not present. Seizures are common during the course of meningitis; phenytoin is preferable to phenobarbital in treating seizures because phenytoin produces less CNS depression and permits better assessment of the patient's level of consciousness.

Prevention

Because these pathogens are spread through respiratory secretions, rifampin is generally prescribed to both patients and their close contacts in an effort to eliminate upper respiratory carriage. With *N. meningitidis*, the dose is 10 mg/kg/dose every 12 hr for four doses. With *H. influenzae*, the dose is 20 mg/kg/dose every day for 4 days. With pneumococcus and other bacterial pathogens, prophylaxis is not necessary.

Prognosis

This varies with the age of the patient and the bacteria responsible. Prognosis is poorest in infants <6 mo old and those infected with either gram-negative organisms or pneumococcus. Long-term sequelae are common and include mental retardation, seizures, hearing loss, and visual impairment.

OSTEOMYELITIS

Etiology and Epidemiology

Osteomyelitis is a relatively common infection of childhood that most commonly occurs in infants less than 1 yr of age and children 2–10 yr old. It is 2–4 times more common in boys and often is associated with antecedent trauma. *Staphylococcus aureus* is the most common causative agent in normal hosts, with *Salmonella* species a frequent causative agent in children with sickle cell disease. *Pseudomonas aeruginosa* may be the cause of osteomyelitis in IV drug users and children who suffer deep puncture wounds through the soles of their sneakers.

Infections may result from traumatic inoculation to the bone or hematogenous dissemination from noncontiguous infected tissues. The femur is the bone most commonly affected. Hematogenous osteomyelitis typically begins as a metaphyseal abscess in tubular bones. In infants, this infection may spread into the joint space via transphyseal bridging vessels, resulting in an associated arthritis. Growth plate development typically inhibits such spread in older children.

Clinical Manifestations

The clinical presentation of osteomyelitis in infancy is typically that of an acute febrile illness and sepsis. Bony involvement may be difficult to localize, so a thorough examination of the extremities is essential, with passive and active range of motion assessed. In older children, presentation is frequently a limp, with localized bone pain and guarding of the affected area.

Diagnosis and Differential Diagnosis

Laboratory diagnosis rests on culture of the blood, periosteal fluid, or affected joint fluid. White blood cell counts are typically elevated, as is the erythrocyte sedimentation rate. Triple-phase technetium-99m diphosphate bone scans show increased uptake of isotope within 24–48 hr of infection and may remain positive for many weeks as a result of persistent bone remodeling and turnover. Roentgenograms of the involved site usually are negative for the first 10–14 days of an acute osteomyelitis. The differential diagnosis includes other infections, trauma, malignancy, and sickle cell crisis.

Treatment

This consists of a prolonged course of antibiotics, typically 4–6 wk in duration. Treatment should start with 7–14 days of IV antistaphylococcal antibiotics, with additional coverage for *H. influenzae* and gram-negative species if suspected. After documentation of a good clinical response (decreased symptoms, fever, and a falling erythrocyte sedimentation rate), the remaining therapy may be given with oral antibiotics as long as compliance and effective mean bacteriocidal concentration can be assured.

Surgery is indicated in the treatment of osteomyelitis when there is poor response to proper antibiotic therapy (for drainage and curettage), associated septic arthritis of the hip, or the need for removal of dead necrotic bone.

SEPTIC ARTHRITIS

Etiology and Epidemiology

Septic arthritis is slightly more common than osteomyelitis. It occurs most commonly in children under 3 yr and adolescent females. Although septic arthritis typically results from hematogenous spread of bacteria, it also can result from contiguous osteomyelitis (esp. in newborns) or in joints in which the joint capsule extends beyond the growth plate (e.g., hip, shoulder, and elbow). The knee is the most commonly affected joint, followed by the hip, elbow, and ankle.

S. aureus is the most common causative organism in neonates and children greater than 5 yr, whereas *H. influenzae* type b is the most common organism found in patients 2 mo to 5 yr of age (*S. aureus* is second in this age group). *Neisseria gonorrhoeae* is the most common causative organism in sexually active adolescents. *S. pneumoniae* is common in patients with sickle cell disease and children less than 2 yr.

Clinical Manifestations

As is true with osteomyelitis, the clinical presentation of septic arthritis is nonspecific in infants: a physical examination that is especially attentive to pain with passive or active motion is very important. In older children, one may find pseudoparalysis of the affected limb, pain on motion, limp, or antalgic positioning of the affected joint (positioning the limb in such a way that intracapsular pressure in the affected joint is reduced to a minimum).

Diagnosis and Differential Diagnosis

Diagnosis rests on culture of the affected synovial fluid, blood culture, and, in the case of *N. gonorrhoeae*, culture from the throat, cervix, and rectum. One also may find an elevated erythrocyte sedimentation rate, C-reactive protein, and white blood cell count. Roentgenograms may show soft tissue swelling, an enlarged joint space, and/or loss of the fat pads. Differential diagnosis is the same as in osteomyelitis, with consideration also given to other nonpyogenic causes of arthritis and toxic synovitis. In this latter condition, the child, typically less than 5 yr old, develops a limp following an upper respiratory infection. Symptoms are generally mild, with low-grade fever, slight limp and decreased range of motion, and normal to slightly elevated erythrocyte sedimentation rate and white blood cell count.

Treatment

Therapy consists of antibiotics appropriate for the suspected causative agent. Therapy for disease due to *S. aureus* should be continued for 4–6 wk, whereas disease due to *H. influenzae*, pneumococcus, and group A streptococcus requires at least 14–21 days of therapy. Septic arthritis caused by *N. gonorrhoeae* should be treated for 7–10 days. Emergency surgical intervention is indicated for septic arthritis of the hip at the time of presentation in an effort to decrease intra-articular pressure in that joint and prevent avascular necrosis of the femoral head. Poor prognostic features include age <6 mo, hip infection, delayed therapy, and infection with *S. aureus*, gram-negative, or fungal pathogens.

STREPTOCOCCAL INFECTIONS

Etiology and Epidemiology

Streptococci are among the most common causes of bacterial infection in infancy and childhood. They are gram-positive cocci that grow in pairs or chains. Lancefield grouped streptococci by differences in the carbohydrate composition of their cell wall (groups A, B, D, etc.). Additionally, they are classified on the basis of their ability to hemolyze red blood cells (α-, β-, and γ-hemolytic). Virulence depends on several outer membrane proteins, of which the M protein is the most important. Streptococci also elaborate several toxins, enzymes, and hemolysins. Antibodies to some of these—antistreptolysin O, antihyaluronidase B, and antideoxyribonuclease B–are useful in the serodiagnosis of group A streptococcal infection.

Group A streptococci are normal inhabitants of the nasopharynx; colonization rate in children is 15–20%. The most common sites of infection involve the respiratory tract, skin, soft tissues, and blood. Skin infections due to group A streptococci are most common in children <6 yr. Pharyngitis is most common in children 5–15 yr of age. As immunity to the various common serotypes of group A streptococci develops, risk of infection diminishes.

Clinical Manifestations

Infections due to group A streptococci have a number of different clinical presentations, depending on both the site of colonization and the toxins and enzymes elaborated by the bacteria.

Scarlet fever is the result of infection by streptococci that elaborate one of three pyogenic (erythrogenic) toxins. The incubation period lasts 1–7 days (mean is 3 days), followed by the sudden onset of fever, vomiting, pharyngitis, abdominal pain that may mimic a surgical abdomen, and headache. On physical examination, there is an exudative pharyngitis with edematous tonsils and tender anterior cervical lymphadenopathy. Additionally, one may find the characteristic "strawberry tongue" and "sandpaper rash." The latter is typified by its fine papular appearance and its initial presentation in the neck, axilla, and groin areas prior to becoming generalized. The rash typical desquamates after about 1 wk.

The most common skin infection due to group A streptococci is superficial pyoderma or *impetigo*. In impetigo, the skin becomes colonized with the offending bacteria about 10 days prior to infection. Infection is introduced by introdermal inoculation after minor trauma, insect bites, or scratching.

Erysipelas is an acute, well-demarcated infection of the skin involving the face and extremities. The skin is erythematous and indurated. The advancing margins of the rash have a raised firm border. Lesions last from days to weeks. Associated lymphadenitis is common.

Streptococcal *pharyngitis* should be suspected in any school-age child with fever, exudative pharyngitis, tender adenopathy, history of exposure, or scarletiniform rash. It must be borne in mind that 50% of proven "strep throats" are nonexudative and only 25% of exudative pharyngitis is due to streptococcus. Laboratory evaluation is therefore essential in the diagnosis. Culture is the gold standard, and it is recommended that all children with pharyngitis and culture-proven strep throat be treated and recultured.

Complications of streptococcus infection include rheumatic fever and glomerulonephritis. The former may follow streptococcal pharyngitis, whereas the latter may follow either pharyngitis or skin infections due to group A streptococci. A more thorough discussion of these two diseases appears elsewhere in this text.

Diagnosis

Diagnosis of group A streptococcal infection depends on culture of the bacteria from the site of infection, typically the throat or skin. There also are a number of rapid strep assays available that are specific but not as sensitive as culture. Evidence of recent streptococcal infection may be ascertained by identification of antibodies to streptolysin O, hyaluronidase B, and deoxyribonuclease B. These tests are essential in the diagnosis of rheumatic fever or glomerulonephritis.

Treatment

Penicillin is the drug of choice for streptococcal infections. Erythromycin, clindamycin, and cephalosporins are effective drugs if penicillin allergy or resistance is present.

STAPHYLOCOCCAL INFECTIONS

Etiology and Epidemiology

Staphylococci are gram-positive cocci that grow in clusters. Pathogenic species include *S. aureus*, *S. epidermidis*, and *S. saprophyticus*. *S. aureus* is the pathogenic species responsible for most disease in children. It may be normal flora in children, growing especially well in the anterior nares and other moist areas of the body. The skin of infants is especially susceptible to infection with *S. aureus*, as is skin in areas where its integrity has been compromised (wounds, burns, catheters, etc.).

Disease is caused by direct tissue invasion, bacteremia, or any of a number of toxins. Exfoliative toxin is the cause of staphylococcal scalded skin syndrome and bullous impetigo. Ingestion of preformed enterotoxin A or D is associated with food poisoning. Enterotoxins A, B, and TSST-1 have been associated with the toxic shock syndrome.

Clinical Manifestations

Clinical manifestations depend on the site of colonization, bacteremia, or toxin involved. Common syndromes include:

Skin—a number of pyogenic skin infections, such as bullous impetigo, cellulitis, folliculitis, furuncles, and carbuncles, may result from infection with *S. aureus;* scalded skin syndrome is the result of exfoliative toxin.

Respiratory tract—staphylococcal infection in the respiratory tract is uncommon, but may occur, and may be associated with high fever, marked local tissue destruction, empyema, and sepsis.

Bones and joints—*S. aureus* is the most common cause of osteomyelitis and arthritis in children and is usually the result of hematogenous dissemination.

Intestinal tract—food poisoning is commonly caused by enterotoxins A and D. Symptoms include profuse emesis in the absence of fever shortly (1–7 hr) after ingestion of preformed toxin.

Infection of CNS, kidneys, and heart may also occur.

Diagnosis

This is based on Gram stain and culture of body fluid or tissue aspirate of the organs affected.

Treatment

Abscesses must be incised and drained. Effective antibiotics include penicillinase-resistant penicillins, first-generation cephalosporins, and vancomycin. Strict handwashing should be used to prevent person-to-person spread.

Prognosis

Disease resulting from *S. aureus* remains cause for significant worry: although antibiotics have lowered the overall mortality of infections due to *S. aureus*, morbidity remains high.

COAGULASE-NEGATIVE STAPHYLOCOCCAL INFECTIONS

Long thought to be innocent commensal bacteria, coagulase-negative staphylococci are important pathogens in patients in the intensive care nursery and in patients with indwelling foreign devices such as urinary catheters, ventriculoperitoneal shunts, and central venous lines. Because most species of coagulase-negative staphylococci are methicillin resistant, vancomycin is the drug of choice.

TOXIC SHOCK SYNDROME

Etiology and Epidemiology

Toxic shock syndrome (TSS) toxin (TSST-1) is responsible for 90% of cases of this syndrome. TSS is most commonly associated with superabsorbent tampon use in menstruating women. It has also been described in children who have a nidus of staphylococcus colonization, such as nasal packs, abscesses, and pneumonia.

Clinical Manifestations

Signs and symptoms associated with TSS include:

high fever
vomiting and diarrhea
aches: head, muscles
exanthem: sunburn-like, desquamating rash
mucositis
shock

Differential Diagnosis

This includes Kawasaki disease, scarlet fever, rickettsial disease, drug rash (erythema multiforme), and measles.

Treatment and Prevention

Therapy for TSS includes antistaphylococcal antibiotics and treatment of shock. Tampon use should be discouraged in women with TSS because there is a 30% recurrence rate.

PNEUMOCOCCAL INFECTIONS

Etiology and Epidemiology

S. pneumoniae, gram-positive diplococci, are normal flora of the upper respiratory tract but have become one of the main causes of bacterial disease in the pediatric age group. They are the leading cause of bacteremia, otitis media, and bacterial pneumonia in children and are a leading cause of bacterial meningitis. There are 83 known serotypes, each classified by type-specific capsular polysaccharide.

Although all children are susceptible to pneumococcal disease, those at greatest risk are patients with asplenia, such as those with sickle cell disease, and patients with deficiencies in the complement cascade or with humoral immunity. Children with nephrotic syndrome and Hodgkin disease also are at risk. Transmission is by aerosolized secretions.

Clinical Manifestations

Clinical symptoms depend on the organ affected. High fever is generally associated with pneumococcal disease.

Diagnosis

The gold standard of diagnosis is Gram stain and culture of sputum, blood, CSF, or other body fluid infected by this pathogen. CIE and latex agglutination tests may be performed on the serum, CSF, and urine of an infected patient for rapid diagnosis. White blood cell count and erythrocyte sedimentation rate are typically elevated with serious disease.

Treatment and Prevention

Penicillin is the treatment of choice for pneumococcal disease. Duration of therapy varies with site of infection. In cases of penicillin allergy or resistance, erythromycin or cephalosporins may be used.

Patients at risk for severe pneumococcal disease should receive pneumococcal vaccine. Antibody response to this capsular protein–derived vaccine is variable, but response is best if vaccine is delivered to patients (1) over age 2 yr and (2) with a functioning spleen. Additionally, children with sickle cell disease should be placed on prophylactic doses of penicillin in an effort to prevent life-threatening infection.

HAEMOPHILUS INFLUENZAE INFECTIONS

Etiology and Epidemiology

H. influenzae are pleomorphic gram-negative coccobacilli. Of the encapsulated strains (types a–f), type b is the major pathogen associated with serious invasive infections. Although nontypable *H. influenzae* are major causes of upper respiratory disease, they are normal oral flora, whereas only 2–5% of children carry type b.

Transmission occurs by aerosolized secretions; therefore, outbreaks of disease are common in families, day-care centers, and institutions in which there is close contact. Patients at most risk for serious *H. influenzae* disease include those under 4 yr of age and those with asplenia, complement deficiencies, or deficiencies in humoral immunity (especially IgG2).

Clinical Manifestations

These depend on the organs affected. Common serious infections are:

Meningitis—*H. influenzae* type b is the most common cause of bacterial meningitis in children between the ages of 1 mo and 4 yr. Because this disease is a result of hematogenous dissemination of this very invasive bacteria, it is frequently associated with other foci of infection, especially in the lungs, bones, sinuses, and joints.

Acute epiglottitis—*H. influenzae* type b is the cause of this potentially lethal infection of the upper airway.

Septic arthritis—*H. influenzae* type b is the main cause of septic arthritis in children less than 3 yr of age. It commonly affects large joints, such as the knees, hips, ankles, and elbows.

Cellulitis—although *S. aureus* is the main cause of cellulitis overall, *H. influenzae* type b is responsible for 85% of facial cellulitis in children less than 2 yr of age. The cellulitis is classically violaceous in hue and is frequently associated with upper respiratory symptoms, high fever, and toxicity.

Other severe infections, including bacteremia, pneumonia, and pericarditis, are commonly caused by *H. influenzae* type b in children less than 4 yr of age.

Diagnosis

Gram stain and culture of tissue or body fluid aspirates are the gold standard for diagnosis of disease caused by *H. influenzae*. CIE and latex agglutination are helpful for rapid diagnosis.

Treatment and Prevention

Cefuroxime, cefotaxime, and ceftriaxone are the agents of choice in treating disease caused by *H. influenzae* type b. Ampicillin was widely used, but regional prevalence of ampicillin-resistant strains has been estimated to be as high as 40%. Because respiratory spread of the pathogen is common, intimate contacts of children with severe disease who are either under age 4 yr or *in intimate contact with children under age 4* should receive prophylaxis with rifampin to eliminate nasal carriage.

Active immunization with conjugate vaccines is currently recommended for children in the first 2 yr of life because they are at greatest risk for severe disease.

MENINGOCOCCAL INFECTIONS

Etiology and Epidemiology

N. meningitidis is a gram-negative intracellular diplococcus that may normally colonize the nasopharyngeal mucosa. It also may lead to invasive disease, including meningitis and life-threatening bacteremia with septic shock. Colonization rates vary from 2–5% of asymptomatic children to greater than 90% of military personnel. Several serotypes of *N. meningitidis* have been identified on the basis of capsular polysaccharides; groups B, C, Y, and W135 are the most prevalent in the United States. Transmission is via aerosolized secretions; thus, intimate contacts of proband cases are at vastly increased risk of acquiring disease. Patients with IgG2 subclass deficiency and terminal complement deficiencies are at risk for recurrent disease.

Clinical Manifestations

Acute meningococcemia presents as a flu-like illness that rapidly progresses to fulminant septic shock. Features include (1) high fever, (2) morbilliform, petechial, or purpuric rash, and (3) symptoms characteristic of septic shock. Meningococcemia also is associated with acute carditis and arthritis.

Meningococcal meningitis frequently is without the symptoms of meningococcemia, and typically is indistinguishable from other causes of bacterial meningitis.

Diagnosis and Differential Diagnosis

Gram stain and culture of blood, CSF, or skin lesions are the gold standards of diagnosis. CIE and latex agglutination of the serum, CSF, or urine may help in rapid diagnosis. Differential diagnosis of a toxic-appearing, febrile patient with rash includes measles, some enteroviral infections, rickettsial diseases, Kawasaki disease, scarlet fever, and bacterial sepsis caused by other organisms.

Treatment and Prevention

Penicillin is the drug of choice for meningococcal infections, with supportive care as necessary. Intimate contacts of any age should receive prophylaxis with rifampin in an effort to eliminate nasal carriage. Meningococcal vaccine against serogroups A, C, Y, and W135 is available but is not routinely given to children. It should be given to patients over 2 yr of age at risk for severe or recurrent infection. These include patients with asplenia, patients with terminal complement deficiencies or IgG2 deficiency, and military recruits.

GONOCOCCAL INFECTIONS

Etiology and Epidemiology

N. gonorrhoeae is a gram-negative intracellular diplococcus that grows optimally at 3–5% CO_2. Infection occurs only in humans; transmission is by sexual contact. Coinfection with other sexually transmitted diseases (STDs), notably chlamydia, is common. Although commonly seen as a primary infection of the genitals, populations at risk for severe disease include asymptomatic carriers, homosexuals, and immunocompromised hosts. Terminal complement deficiencies increase the risk of recurrent infection.

Clinical Manifestations

About 60–80% of patients infected with *N. gonorrhoeae* remain asymptomatic. These patients are an important reservoir of infection and may go on to develop disseminated disease.

Primary uncomplicated gonorrhea is a STD that occurs after an incubation period of 2–5 days in men and 5–10 days in women. It presents with dysuria and purulent discharge from the genitals. Primary infection occurs in the urethra of men, the vulva and vagina of prepubertal girls, and the cervix of postpubertal women. Primary gonorrhea also may affect the pharynx or rectum. Complications include salpingitis and Fitz-Hugh–Curtis syndrome in postpubertal females.

Gonococcal ophthalmitis may occur at any age, but is commonly seen in the newborn period 1–4 days after birth. It presents with an extremely purulent conjunctivitis that is rapidly progressive if not treated emergently.

Disseminated gonococcal infections present as a tenosynovitis–dermatitis syndrome, with symptoms including fever, skin lesions, and polyarthralgias, or as a monoarticular arthritis, typically involving a large joint.

Diagnosis

Culture and Gram stain remain the gold standard of diagnosis, although enzyme immunoassays are available and may be used with high sensitivity and specificity.

Treatment and Prevention

Because penicillin resistance is increasingly seen, ceftriaxone or other cephalosporins are the drugs of choice in treatment of gonococcal infections. Duration of therapy varies from a single injection for primary uncomplicated gonorrhea to 7–10 days for disseminated disease. The possibility of coexistent chlamydial infection should be considered and treatment instituted if it is present. Sexual partners must also be treated.

Gonococcal ophthalmia neonatorum may be prevented through routine application of either erythromycin eye ointment or silver nitrate solution to the eyes shortly after birth.

DIPHTHERIA

Etiology and Epidemiology

Corynebacterium diphtheriae is a gram-positive bacillus that, when infected with a bacteriophage containing the genome for a lysogenic toxin, causes the life-threatening disease diphtheria. Humans are the only known reservoir of *C. diphtheriae*. Transmission is via aerosolized secretions or tainted fomites.

Clinical Manifestations

The oropharynx usually is the primary site of infection with *C. diphtheriae*. After an incubation period of 2–4 days, the patient experiences nonspecific malaise, sore throat, and low-grade fever. These symptoms then progress over 1–2 days to the classic exudative pharyngitis with pseudomembrane formation over the posterior pharynx. There may be marked edema of the neck (bull neck) and airway compromise. Associated symptoms include carditis and neuritis resulting from systemic absorption of the toxin.

Other less common sites of primary infection include the nose and the skin. Laryngeal diphtheria may result from downward extension of the pseudomembrane from the pharynx.

Diagnosis

This is made by culture of *C. diphtheriae* on special selective media using inhibitors to retard the growth of other organisms.

Treatment and Prevention

Treatment consists of antibiotics (penicillin or erythromycin) to eradicate the bacteria and equine antitoxin to neutralize the circulating toxin. Antitoxin must be given early in the course of the disease because it has no effect on tissue-bound toxin. Therapy should continue until the patient has three negative cultures. Use of antitoxin has reduced the mortality of this disease from 50 to 5%.

The incidence of diphtheria has decreased dramatically thanks to worldwide immunization in the 1st yr of life. Close contacts of cases who are unimmunized or who have waning immunity are at special risk for infection. All close contacts should be observed closely for 7 days and have their throats cultured. They should be treated if cultures are positive. Previously immunized contacts who have not received a booster in the past 5 yr should receive a booster injection of diphtheria toxoid. Contacts whose immunization status is poor or unknown should be treated empirically and watched especially closely.

PERTUSSIS (Whooping Cough)

Etiology and Epidemiology

Although the syndrome may be caused by a few pathogens, pertussis is typically caused by *Bordetella pertussis*, a gram-negative, pleomorphic bacillus that requires special media for growth.

Although the incidence of pertussis has decreased dramatically because of widespread vaccination programs, the incidence of disease remains highest in communities where immunization rates are poor. Immunity afforded by vaccine is not lifelong, and because adults are less severely affected than children, they may serve as the reservoir for further infection. Pertussis is very contagious; transmission occurs through respiratory secretions.

Clinical Manifestations

After an incubation period of 6–14 days, a symptomatic illness lasting 6–8 wk begins. Symptomatic illness is generally divided into three clinical stages:

1. The *catarrhal stage* typically lasts 1–2 wk and is marked by upper respiratory symptoms, including rhinorrhea, cough, and conjunctival injection. Wheezing also may be present. It is during this stage that the patient is most contagious.
2. The *paroxysmal stage* lasts 2–4 wk or longer and is marked by coughing jags interrupted by "whoops"—the sound

made as air is inhaled forcefully against the narrowed glottis. The whoop may not be audible in infants less than 6 mo or adults.
3. The *convalescent stage* lasts 1–2 wk or longer and is marked by persistent chronic cough.

Complications of pertussis may include pneumonia, pneumothorax or pneumomediastinum, and encephalopathy resulting from either *B. pertussis* or hypoxia.

Diagnosis

Unfortunately, pertussis is not suspected during the catarrhal stage, when the patient is most contagious. Suspicion typically begins during the paroxysmal stage. Diagnosis depends on isolation and culture of the bacteria from the nasopharynx. Fluorescent antibody tests are widely available, enabling rapid diagnosis. Associated findings include a high white blood cell count with a predominance of lymphocytes. Chest roentgenograms may reveal perihilar infiltrates or evidence of air trapping.

Treatment and Prevention

Erythromycin eliminates nasopharyngeal carriage and may abort or modify the paroxysmal stage if given early (during the catarrhal stage). Once paroxysms begin, erythromycin will eliminate carriage but it will not affect the course of the disease. Ancillary therapy should include oxygen, corticosteroids, and β-agonists. Mortality due to pertussis may be as high as 40% in infants less than 5 mo.

Pertussis is best prevented through widescale immunization programs. Although currently available, whole-cell vaccine has been associated with a wide variety of adverse effects. Acellular pertussis vaccines are currently under investigation. Close contacts of patients with pertussis all should receive 10–14 days of prophylactic erythromycin. Patients under 7 yr of age who have not been fully immunized also should receive booster vaccines.

INFECTIONS CAUSED BY SALMONELLAE

Etiology and Epidemiology

Eggs and chickens have received considerable attention for their role in harboring the gram-negative bacillus *Salmonella*. Three main groups of *Salmonella* have been named—*S. enteritidis*, *S. typhi*, and *S. choleraesuis*—with all but two of the identified serotypes of salmonella belonging to the first group. The diseases caused by salmonella may be divided into nontyphoidal salmonellosis and typhoid fever.

Nontyphoidal Salmonellosis

CLINICAL MANIFESTATIONS. *Salmonella* are spread by the fecal–oral route or through the ingestion of tainted animal products. After an incubation period of 6–72 hr, the patient experiences the abrupt onset of gastrointestinal symptoms, including nausea, vomiting, and abdominal pain. Diarrhea is watery and often contains mucus, blood, and leukocytes. Symptoms last for 2–5 days in healthy individuals, although stool culture may remain positive for weeks to months following acute illness.

In patients whose immune system is compromised (especially infants, patients with sickle cell disease, and those on chronic immunosuppressive therapy), *Salmonella* may cause bacteremia, osteomyelitis, and other more serious infections. Septicemia is common in infants less than 3 mo of age. *S. choleraesuis* is associated with more severe disease.

DIAGNOSIS AND DIFFERENTIAL DIAGNOSIS. Disease caused by *Salmonella* should be suspected in any child presenting with bloody diarrhea. Culture remains the gold standard of diagnosis.

TREATMENT. Antibiotics are indicated only in patients with severe disease caused by *Salmonella,* such as osteomyelitis or septicemia. Patients at risk for developing severe disease, such as infants, also should be treated. Ampicillin, trimethoprim–sulfamethoxazole, and cephalosporins are commonly used in the treatment of infections caused by *Salmonella*. Antibiotics are not indicated for uncomplicated *Salmonella* enteritis because they neither alter the course of the disease nor shorten the carrier state.

Typhoid Fever

CLINICAL MANIFESTATIONS. Although uncommon in the United States, typhoid fever is an important disease in developing countries. *S. typhi* typically infects humans after the ingestion of contaminated water. The bacteria initially localize in the small intestine, causing mild gastrointestinal symptoms. The bacteria then invade the reticuloendothelial system, causing prolonged septicemia and systemic disease. Symptoms vary from mild gastroenteritis to severe septicemia. Classic symptoms of severe disease include fever, malaise, abdominal pain, hepatosplenomegaly, mental status changes, and a macular rash (rose spots). A paradoxical inverse relationship between fever and heart rate is frequently observed. Complications include intestinal perforation or hemorrhage, encephalopathy, cholecystitis, and secondary infections.

DIAGNOSIS. Early in the disease, mononuclear cells are found on stool examination and blood cultures are frequently positive. Urine and stool cultures turn positive only after the secondary septicemia.

TREATMENT AND PREVENTION. Antimicrobial treatment using ampicillin or trimethoprim–sulfamethoxazole is warranted. Typhoid vaccine should be given to patients who (1) have had intimate contact with a carrier or (2) are traveling into a country in which typhoid is endemic. Typhoid vaccine also should be given to members of a closed community in the event of an outbreak.

SHIGELLOSIS

Etiology and Epidemiology

Shigellae are gram-negative bacilli that are non–lactose fermenting. They are classified into four groups, A–D. A member of group A, *S. dysenteriae*, is the major pathogen world-wide but is rarely encountered in the United States. *S. sonnei*, the single serotype of group D, is the major pathogen identified in the United States. Humans are the major reservoir of *Shigellae*; spread is by the fecal–oral route. As is true with most diseases spread in this manner, outbreaks occur in areas of overcrowding and poor sanitary conditions.

Clinical Manifestations

Although *Shigellae* may cause a mild gastroenteritis, disease resulting from *Shigellae* is often severe. Symptoms include high fever, crampy abdominal pain, and diarrhea that contains blood, mucus, and leukocytes. Neurologic symptoms, including seizures and altered mental status, are common and may mimic primary neurologic disease. Complications include arthritis and hemolytic uremic syndrome.

Diagnosis

This is made by culture of the stool. Fecal leukocytes and blood commonly are seen on stool examination.

Treatment

Trimethoprim–sulfamethoxazole or ampicillin should be used in the treatment of shigellosis because they may shorten the course of the disease and shorten the carrier state.

CHOLERA

Etiology and Epidemiology

Vibrio cholerae are gram-negative, flagellated bacilli. The 01 serotype is the cause of cholera, and non-01 serotypes cause milder gastrointestinal disease. Cholera is endemic in parts of the world in which sanitation is poor. Spread is typically via contaminated water.

Clinical Manifestations

The major symptom of cholera is profuse, watery diarrhea. Disease is due to an enterotoxin elaborated by *V. cholerae*. This enterotoxin increases intracellular cyclic adenosine monophosphate (AMP), which then leads to increased chloride secretion by the intestinal mucosal cells. As water follows the anion, profound water loss and electrolyte disturbances may occur. The incubation period is 6 hr to 2 days, with diarrhea continuing for up to 7 days.

Diagnosis

Diagnosis is based on stool culture and isolation of *V. cholerae* 01.

Treatment and Prevention

Because water loss and progression to shock is rapid, primary treatment consists of good fluid and electrolyte management. Antibiotics have been shown to lessen the severity of the diarrhea and shorten the length of carriage; therefore they should be used. Effective antibiotics include tetracycline and trimethoprim–sulfamethoxazole. Preventive measures include avoidance of contaminated food and water. Vaccine is available but provides only limited protection of a short duration. Additionally, although vaccine seems to be effective in the prevention of severe disease, it does not reduce the rate of carriage.

INFECTIONS CAUSED BY PSEUDOMONAS

Pseudomonas species are gram-negative, strictly aerobic bacilli and are a major cause of opportunistic infection in children. Those most commonly infected include chronically hospitalized immunosuppressed patients, such as those with cancer, burn patients, and patients with cystic fibrosis. Disease caused by *Pseudomonas* species depends on the site of infection, although the skin (ecthyma gangrenosum), blood, and lungs are favored sites. *Pseudomonas* also has been shown to be a major cause of osteomyelitis of the foot following puncture wounds. Antibiotics used in the treatment of infections caused by *Pseudomonas* include piperacillin, ticarcillin, and tobramycin. Antibiotic resistance is common.

LISTERIOSIS

L. monocytogenes is a gram-positive rod most commonly associated with disease in newborn infants, pregnant women, and immunocompromised hosts. It typically causes septicemia and/or meningitis that is indistinguishable from that caused by other organisms. Diagnosis may be made by culture or by demonstration of an antibody response. Ampicillin is the drug of choice when treating disease caused by *Listeria*.

CLOSTRIDIAL INFECTIONS

Clostridia are gram-positive, anaerobic bacilli that elaborate a number of potent toxins. These toxins cause a variety of different diseases, the two most common of which in the pediatric population are tetanus and infant botulism. Other diseases caused by *Clostridia* include gas gangrene, food poisoning, and pseudomembranous colitis.

Tetanus

ETIOLOGY AND EPIDEMIOLOGY. The spores of *C. tetani* are hardy and may survive in soil and dust for years. Disease typically follows wound inoculation with the spores of *C. tetani*. After inoculation, the spores become vegetative and elaborate two toxins, tetanospasmin and tetanolysin, the former of which leads to clinical findings. Infection also may occur in the neonatal period as a result of unsterile cord clamping and is a common cause of infant mortality in developing countries.

CLINICAL MANIFESTATIONS. *Generalized tetanus* is the most common form of disease. After a typical incubation period of 3–14 days, the patient develops the gradual stiffening of muscle groups. Trismus is the presenting symptom in over 50% of cases. Facial muscles may contract, leaving the patient with a fixed, sardonic grin (risus sardonicus). Contraction of the muscles of the trunk may lead to opisthotonus. Tetanic seizures are caused by sudden bursts of tonic contraction in various muscle groups. Symptoms increase during the first week, then plateau, and abate after 2–6 wk.

Tetanus neonatorum is common in countries in which neither vaccine nor antitoxin is widely available. It occurs after infection of the umbilical cord and presents as generalized disease with poor sucking and swallowing, irritability, opisthotonus, and rigidity.

C. tetani may also cause localized disease. Pain and spasm may occur in the muscle groups immediately proximal to the site of injury. In the cephalic form of the disease, symptoms are limited to the cranial nerves and typically follow injury to the face. Both of these forms are uncommon in children.

DIAGNOSIS AND DIFFERENTIAL DIAGNOSIS. Diagnosis is made on clinical grounds, although wound cultures may be positive in a minority of cases. Differential diagnosis includes rabies, hypocalcemia, and ingestions, especially phenothiazines or strychnine.

TREATMENT AND PREVENTION. Therapy is aimed at supporting the patient comfortably, eliminating the source of the toxin, and neutralizing the free toxin. Muscle relaxants, analgesics, paralysis, and mechanical ventilation are effective supportive measures. Penicillin and good wound care should be given to eradicate the vegetative C. tetani. Tetanus immune globulin should be given to neutralize the free toxin.

Tetanus may be prevented by regular immunization with tetanus toxoid. Underimmunized children should be given booster vaccines as part of their emergency wound care. Tetanus immune globulin should be given to underimmunized children who sustain wounds contaminated with soil, dirt, feces, or saliva.

Botulism

ETIOLOGY AND EPIDEMIOLOGY. Botulism is the result of the potent neurotoxins produced by C. botulinum. There are seven antigenically distinct toxins (A–G); they are the most potent toxins known to man. They cause disease by irreversibly binding to the presynaptic junctions, inhibiting acetylcholine release and causing flaccid paralysis. There are three variants of disease caused by C. botulinum: food-borne botulism, wound botulism, and infant botulism. The first two result from inoculation with preformed toxin, and the last results from the ingestion of C. botulinum spores, which germinate in the intestines and elaborate toxin over time.

CLINICAL MANIFESTATIONS. *Infant botulism* is the most common variant of botulism in the United States; 95% of cases occur during the first 6 mo of life. It has been associated with ingestion of honey. Symptoms begin with constipation and poor feeding. Over the next 7–14 days, symptoms progress to more frank bulbar palsies and symmetric descending paralysis. Hypoventilation is a common complication and may occur as a result of either poor airway control or paralysis of the diaphragm.

Food-borne botulism most commonly occurs after ingesting home-preserved foods. Symptoms typically begin 12–36 hr after ingestion of toxin and frequently are severe.

Wound botulism has a course similar to that of food-borne, although illness may be milder and more prolonged. Incubation is 4–14 days.

DIAGNOSIS AND DIFFERENTIAL DIAGNOSIS. Diagnosis is made on clinical grounds and is confirmed by the presence of organisms or toxin in the stool. Electromyography may show characteristic BSAPs (brief, small, abundant potentials) suggestive of botulism. Differential diagnosis includes myasthenia gravis, Guillain–Barré syndrome, polio, and other neuromuscular diseases.

TREATMENT AND PREVENTION. Treatment is supportive, with special consideration given to protection of the airway and maintenance of adequate ventilation. Antibiotics do not shorten the course of disease or decrease intestinal colonization; they may in fact exacerbate symptoms by causing rapid lysis of bacteria and elaboration of toxin. Botulism immune globulin is available, and works by binding and neutralizing free toxin. Although it has been helpful in ameliorating symptoms of food-borne and wound-associated cases, it is unclear whether it will help in infant botulism.

Botulism may be prevented by avoidance of honey and proper food canning techniques.

ANAEROBIC INFECTIONS OTHER THAN CLOSTRIDIAL

Anaerobic bacteria are responsible for a wide variety of infections in humans. They are associated with abscess formation and widespread tissue destruction. Some infections associated with anaerobes are listed in Table 10–2.

CAMPYLOBACTER INFECTIONS

Etiology and Epidemiology

Campylobacter are gram-negative, flagellated rods. Of the eight species that cause disease in humans, *C. jejuni* is the cause of 95% of *Campylobacter* enteritis and *C. fetus* is most commonly associated with systemic infection. The bacteria is commonly found in chickens, turkeys, and other fowl; other animals also may harbor the organism. Transmission is through the ingestion of improperly cooked food or via the fecal–oral route.

Clinical Manifestations

After an incubation period of 2–7 days, *C. jejuni* causes an enteritis that is marked by fever, malaise, and crampy abdominal pain that may mimic a surgical abdomen. Diarrhea is profuse and watery, frequently containing blood, mucus, and leukocytes. Most illness lasts less than 1 wk, although asymptomatic carriage may persist for 7 wk in untreated patients.

TABLE 10–2. INFECTIONS ASSOCIATED WITH ANAEROBIC BACTERIA*

Site	Infection	Anaerobic Bacteria†
Central nervous system	Cerebral abscess, subdural empyema, epidural abscess, secondary to adjacent sinusitis, otitis, mastoiditis	Polymicrobial, *B. fragilis*,‡ *Fusobacterium*, *Peptostreptococcus*, *Veillonella*
Upper airway	Dental abscess, Ludwig angina (cellulitis of sublingual–submandibular space), Lemiere syndrome (septic jugular thrombophlebitis), necrotizing gingivitis (Vincent stomatitis), chronic otitis–mastoiditis–sinusitis, peritonsillar abscess, facial space cellulitis	*Peptostreptococcus*, *Fusobacterium*, *B. melaninogenicus*
Pleuropulmonary area	Aspiration pneumonia Necrotizing pneumonitis Lung abscess, bronchopleural fistula, empyema Periodontal disease, bronchial obstruction, altered gag or consciousness predispose to infection	Polymicrobial *B. melaninogenicus* *B. intermedius* *Fusobacterium*, *Peptostreptococcus*, *Eubacterium*, *B. fragilis*, *Veillonella*
Intra-abdominal region	Abscess, secondary peritonitis (appendicitis, penetrating trauma: colon > > > small intestine)	Polymicrobial, *B. fragilis*, other *Bacteroides*, *Clostridium* sp., *Peptostreptococcus*, *Eubacterium*, *Fusobacterium*
Female genital tract	Bartholin abscess, tubo-ovarian abscess, endometritis, pelvic cellulitis or thrombophlebitis, salpingitis, septic abortion	*B. fragilis*, *B. bivius*, *Peptostreptococcus*, *Clostridium* sp.
	Anaerobic (nonspecific bacterial) vaginosis Intrauterine device	*Mobiluncus* sp. Actinomycosis
Soft tissue	Human and animal bites, decubitus ulcers, perirectal cellulitis, abdominal wounds, pilonidal sinus	Varies with site and contamination with mouth or enteric flora
	Synergistic necrotizing cellulitis, myonecrosis	*Clostridium*, other anaerobes

(continued)

**TABLE 10–2. INFECTIONS ASSOCIATED WITH
ANAEROBIC BACTERIA* Continued**

Site	Infection	Anaerobic Bacteria[†]
Bacteremia	Secondary to intra-abdominal or genitourinary source and synergistic cellulitis	B. fragilis, Clostridium, anaerobic streptococci
	Immunosuppressed or neutropenic patients	Clostridium tertium, C. septicum
Bones and joints	Trauma, decubitus ulcers, jaw (secondary to dental pathology)	Actinomycosis, Clostridium, Bacteroides, Fusobacterium

* From Behrman RE (ed): Nelson Textbook of Pediatrics, 14th ed. Philadelphia, WB Saunders Company, 1992, p. 755.
[†] Infections may also be due to or involve aerobic bacteria as the sole or part of a mixed infection: *brain abscess* may contain aerobic streptococci; *intra-abdominal sepsis* may contain coliforms, enterococci; *salpingitis* may contain N. gonorrhoeae, C. trachomatis.
[‡] *Bacteroides fragilis* is usually isolated from infections below the diaphragm except for brain abscesses.

Bacteremia associated with *C. fetus* is more common in immunosuppressed patients. Symptoms are the same as those associated with bacteremia caused by other bacteria.

Diagnosis and Differential Diagnosis

Diagnosis of *Campylobacter* is suspected in any patient with bloody diarrhea and is confirmed by stool culture.

Treatment

Erythromycin is the drug of choice when treating enteritis caused by *C. jejuni*. Erythromycin effectively lessens the severity of the diarrhea and shortens the carrier state to 2 days. Gentamycin is the drug of choice when treating systemic disease caused by *Campylobacter*.

TUBERCULOSIS

Etiology and Epidemiology

Tuberculosis (TB) is caused by *Mycobacterium tuberculosis,* an aerobic acid-fast bacillus. It remains a major cause of morbidity throughout the world because of persistent overcrowding, antimicrobial resistance, and immunodeficiency states such as AIDS. Spread is through aerosolized sputum. Because children usually do not have productive coughs, infections in children typically arise after exposure to an adult with active disease.

Clinical Manifestations

Whereas adults commonly experience a chronic cough, fever, night sweats, and weight loss, children with TB typically are asymptomatic. They are identified by recent conversion of their cutaneous hypersensitivity tests. A newly positive skin test identifies a patient as exposed, with 90% of exposures never progressing to active disease. Primary disease typically affects the lungs and is identified by chest roentgenograms. Disease also may affect other organs, especially the lymph nodes (more typical of other *Mycobacterium* species), the meninges (especially in children less than 3 yr old), the bones, and the urogenital tract. *Miliary TB* describes diffuse, multiorgan disease and is so named because, on pathologic specimens, the tuberculous lesions are scattered like millet seeds.

Diagnosis

This is based on recent skin test conversion. Skin tests involve the placement of tuberculin antigens beneath the skin of the forearm. An exposed patient with an intact immune system will mount a delayed hypersensitivity response 2–10 wk after exposure.

Two types of cutaneous hypersensitivity tests are available: multiple puncture tests and the intradermal Mantoux test. Multiple puncture tests are screening tests, useful in populations with a low incidence of disease. Because the quantity of tuberculin antigen placed is not standardized, false-positive and false-negative tests are common. Positive tests are those in which any induration is found 48–72 hr after the application. A positive multipuncture test should be followed with the more specific and sensitive Mantoux test.

In areas with a higher prevalence of disease, the standardized Mantoux test should be used. This test utilizes 5 units of PPD placed intradermally on the volar surface of the forearm. A positive test is one in which there are greater than 10 mm of induration at the site 48–72 hr after placement. Positive Mantoux tests should be followed with chest roentgenograms, which, if positive, are indicative of disease. False-negative Mantoux tests may be obtained if the patient has severe systemic TB, malnutrition, immunodeficiency or immunosuppression, or some viral illnesses and their vaccines (notably, measles). False-negative tests also may be obtained if the patient is tested too soon following exposure (prior to development of cutaneous hypersensitivity). False-positive Mantoux tests result from infections with atypical *Mycobacterium*, prior administration of bacillus Calmette–Guerin vaccine, and sensitivity to perservatives in PPD.

Treatment and Prevention

All children should be skin tested for TB (1) prior to receiving measles–mumps–rubella vaccine, (2) at school entry, and (3) in adolescence. Children who live in areas with a high prevalence of TB should be skin tested more frequently, perhaps as often as every 1–2 yr. Children who have been exposed to persons with TB should be skin tested soon after the time exposure, with the test repeated 3 mo after exposure in case a delayed cutaneous hypersensitivity response had not yet been mounted. Any newly positive skin test should be followed with a chest roentgenogram. Additionally, an investigation looking for other infectious or exposed contacts should be undertaken.

Treatment relies on long-term use of antituberculous agents. Isoniazid (INH) is typically given as a single agent to exposed patients for a course of 6–9 mo. Primary tuberculosis should be treated with 6–9 mo of INH and rifampin, with a third agent (pyrazinamide or ethambutol) given for the first 2 mo if resistance to either INH or rifampin is suspected. Patients with or at risk for severe disease should receive a longer course (at least 12 mo) of (at least) the three drugs listed above.

SPIROCHETAL DISEASES

Although there are a number of diseases caused by spirochetes, those most commonly seen in children in the United States are syphilis and Lyme disease.

Syphilis

ETIOLOGY AND EPIDEMIOLOGY. Syphilis is caused by the spirochete *Treponema pallidum*. There are two forms of syphilis seen by pediatricians, acquired and congenital. The former is transmitted by sexual contact, and the latter results from maternal spirochetemia at any time during pregnancy, but is most associated with 3rd-trimester acquisition.

CLINICAL MANIFESTATIONS. Acquired syphilis has three discrete phases. The first stage occurs 3–6 wk following sexual contact and is marked by the appearance of a painless ulcerated lesion (chancre). Although the lesion heals spontaneously, if left untreated, secondary syphilis begins as a flu-like illness with an erythematous rash. The rash begins on the trunk and extremities and later becomes prominent on the palms and soles. Wart-like lesions (condyloma latum) may appear in the warm, moist areas of the body. Meningitis, hepatitis, and glomerulonephritis all may complicate the course. If left untreated, the patient may become relatively asymptomatic (latent syphilis) or go on to tertiary syphilis, a slowly progressive disease that may affect any organ system, including the CNS and heart.

Congenital syphilis is usually the result of the passage of spirochetes across the placenta. As is true with most of the congenitally acquired infections, common signs and symptoms include hyperbilirubinemia, thrombocytopenia, anemia, hepatosplenomegaly, jaundice, and rash. Physical examination also may show wart-like lesions of the mucous membranes (analogous to condyloma lata) and copious, blood-tinged nasal secretions (the "snuffles"), both of which contain treponemes. Radiographic evidence of dental anomalies (Hutchinson teeth, Mulberry molars) and diffuse osteochondritis (especially of the long bone metaphyses) may be seen.

DIAGNOSIS. Because *T. pallidum* cannot be grown in vitro, serologic tests are used in diagnosis. Serologic tests fall into two categories: nonspecific, nontreponemal screening tests such as VDRL and RPR, and specific antitreponemal antibody tests, such as TPI, MHA-TP, and FTA-ABS. Antibodies of either category may cross the placenta, making neonatal diagnosis difficult. Congenital infection is diagnosed and treated if the mother is specific serology test positive and (1) the mother was not adequately treated, (2) quantitative VDRL titers in the infant are as high as or higher than in the mother, or (3) the VDRL in the CSF of the infant is reactive. If the mother was adequately treated or the quantitative VDRL titer of the infant is significantly less than that of the mother and the infant has none of the stigmata of congenital syphilis, the child is treated as for primary syphilis.

TREATMENT. Primary, secondary, or early (less than 1 yr) latent syphilis is treated with a single injection of benzathine penicillin. Late latent syphilis is treated with three weekly injections of benzathine penicillin. Tertiary syphilis and congenital syphilis are treated with 10–14 days of intravenous or intramuscular penicillin.

Lyme Disease

ETIOLOGY AND EPIDEMIOLOGY. A tick-borne illness caused by the spirochete *Borrelia burgdorferi*, Lyme disease was first described in the United States in 1975 after an outbreak near Lyme, Connecticut. The tick vectors responsible are members of the genus *Ixodes*, with the most common species being *I. damini* in the Northeast and Midwest and *I. pacificus* in the West.

CLINICAL MANIFESTATIONS. Lyme disease occurs in three stages. *Stage 1* begins with an erythematous papule at the site of the tick bite. This rash then spreads to form the erythematous annular lesion with central clearing characteristic of erythema chronicum migrans. The patient may experience lethargy, fatigue, headache, fever, and myalgias during stage 1 of the disease.

Stage 2 occurs weeks to months after the initial symptoms. Organ systems commonly affected during this stage are the musculoskeletal system (60%), the CNS (10%), and the cardiovascular system (8%). Musculoskeletal symptoms include migratory arthralgias and arthritis. CNS symptoms are varied and include meningitis, palsy, ataxia, encephalopathy, and depression. Cardiac involvement is brief and usually is marked by varying degrees of atrioventricular block.

Stage 3 is persistent infection and is marked by progressive arthritis and joint destruction associated with CNS manifestations, including depression, intellectual impairment, and demyelinating disease.

DIAGNOSIS. Serologic tests using indirect immunofluorescence or ELISA have been used to augment the clinical diagnosis, but these tests have yet to be standardized.

TREATMENT. Disease may be treated with 10–20 days of tetracycline, penicillin, erythromycin, ceftriaxone, or chloramphenicol.

CHLAMYDIAL INFECTIONS

Etiology and Epidemiology

Chlamydia are obligate intracellular parasites that contain both RNA and DNA. They are divided into two subgroups: group A, which includes *C. trachomatis* and the agent causing lymphogranuloma venereum, and group B, which includes *C. psittaci* and other agents causing a wide variety of diseases in animals. *C. trachomatis* infection in children may be acquired through sexual contact, passage through an infected birth canal, or via the eye–hand–eye route in the case of trachoma.

Clinical Manifestations

Sexual transmission is a common cause of nongonococcal urethritis and epididymitis in males and cervicitis, endometritis, and salpingitis in females. Passage through an infected birth canal commonly causes neonatal disease. Conjunctivitis occurs in 25% of infants exposed and typically presents in the 2nd or 3rd wk of life. Pneumonia occurs in 10% of infants exposed and typically presents with wheezing and rales during the 3rd to 16th wk. Trachoma is a disease of overcrowding and is the leading cause of acquired blindness worldwide.

Diagnosis

Tissue culture is the gold standard. Direct fluorescent antibody stains or ELISA may be used for rapid diagnosis.

Treatment

Erythromycin, sulfisoxazole, and tetracycline are all effective in the treatment of chlamydial infections. Conjunctivitis of the newborn should be treated with 14 days of erythromycin because topical therapy does not eliminate nasopharyngeal carriage. Pneumonia should be treated with erythromycin for 2 wk. Genitourinary infections should be treated with 7–10 days of tetracycline.

MYCOPLASMAL INFECTIONS

Mycoplasma are the smallest known free-living organisms. They are smaller than some viruses and have no cell wall. *M. pneumoniae* is a major cause of pneumonia in school-age children. It should be suspected in any child with bronchitis or pneumonia in whom cough is a major feature. Diagnosis is clinical, although a rise in nonspecific cold hemagglutinins may be demonstrated after the 1st wk of disease. Infection is treated with erythromycin or tetracycline.

M. hominis and *Ureaplasma urealyticum* are human urogenital pathogens. They are a major cause of nongonococcal urethritis and may contribute to premature labor, stillbirths, and neonatal pneumonia. Infections are treated with erythromycin or tetracycline.

VIRAL INFECTIONS AND THOSE PRESUMED TO BE CAUSED BY VIRUSES
(*NELSON TEXTBOOK*, SECS. 12.64–12.93)

MEASLES

Etiology and Epidemiology

Measles is a highly contagious disease caused by an RNA virus of the family Paramyxoviridae. It is endemic over most of the world, although its incidence is decreased as a result of worldwide vaccination programs. It is spread by respiratory secretions, with the patient being contagious from 7–10 days after exposure until 5 days after the appearance of the rash.

Clinical Manifestations

Measles infection is characterized by three clinical stages. *Stage 1* is an incubation period of 10–12 days with few, if any, symptoms. *Stage 2* is the prodromal or catarrhal stage, during which the patient experiences 3–5 days of toxic appearance with cough, low-grade fever, conjunctivitis, and the pathognomonic Koplik spots. *Stage 3* is the final stage, during which the patient experiences spiking fevers heralding the onset of a rash that begins on the face and spreads over the trunk and extremities. The rash initially is maculopapular, then becomes confluent as it spreads. It ultimately turns brownish in hue and desquamates as it fades.

Complications include pneumonia, otitis media, and encephalitis. Subacute sclerosing panencephalitis is a rare chronic encephalitis that may occur years to decades following acute measles infection.

Diagnosis and Differential Diagnosis

Diagnosis is based on clinical criteria; laboratory confirmation is rarely needed. Koplik spots, if seen, are diagnostic. They appear as greyish white dots spread irregularly on the buccal mucosa. The differential diagnosis includes other rashes typically associated with conjunctivitis: Kawasaki disease, serum sickness, erythema multiforme, and rickettsial diseases.

Treatment and Prevention

Treatment is symptomatic, providing fluids and antipyretics as necessary. Isolation is mandatory in inpatient settings.

Active immunization with live virus vaccine is recommended at 15 mo, with a booster dose to be given during the preadolescent school years. Vaccine has been associated with a mild measles-like rash 10–14 days after administration and cutaneous anergy, which may last up to 3 mo. Although vaccine is not recommended for use in patients with T cell dysfunction, it is recommended for use in patients with AIDS because disease in these patients may be life threatening.

Passive immunization with measles immune globulin should be given to patients at high risk as soon as possible following exposure. The standard dose is 0.25 mL/kg; this should be doubled for patients with AIDS.

RUBELLA

Etiology and Epidemiology

Also known as "3-day measles," rubella is a common viral disease of childhood. It is caused by an RNA-containing virus of the family Togaviridae, and is transmitted by respiratory secretions. It also may be transmitted from mother to fetus, causing devastating infection and the congenital rubella syndrome (see Chap. 7). Incidence has decreased as a result of widespread vaccination programs, but because vaccination against rubella is not practiced worldwide, it remains a public health concern.

Clinical Manifestations

After an incubation period of 14–21 days, the patient will experience a short, relatively mild, prodromal phase marked by mild catarrhal symptoms and associated painful retroauricular, posterior cervical, and occipital adenopathy. After at least 24 hr of adenopathy, a rash appears on the head and neck that quickly spreads over the body. The exanthem may be variable in appearance and disappears by the 3rd day. Associated symptoms include pharyngitis, conjunctivitis, and splenomegaly.

Complications are uncommon and may include neuritis and arthritis. Progressive rubella panencephalitis is an exceedingly rare chronic encephalitis analogous to subacute sclerosing panencephalitis.

Diagnosis and Differential Diagnosis

Diagnosis is made on clinical grounds. Differential diagnosis includes diseases with rash and adenopathy; infectious mononucleosis and scarlet fever are most common among them.

Treatment and Prevention

Treatment of acute rubella infection is supportive.

Active immunization with a live virus vaccine is usually given at 15 mo. Antibody develops in 98% of those vaccinated and is believed to be lifelong. Although vaccine has never been shown to cause the congenital rubella syndrome, it is not recommended that vaccine be given during pregnancy.

Passive immunization may given to contacts at risk, especially nonimmune pregnant women in the first trimester of pregnancy, with immune serum globulin 0.25–0.50 mL/kg.

ROSEOLA

Exanthem subitum is a classic viral disease of childhood caused by herpesvirus-6. It is characterized by 3–4 days of high fever followed by rapid defervescence and the appearance of a generalized maculopapular exanthem, which first appears on the trunk. The rash spreads quickly to the neck and arms and then fades within 24 hr. Most cases occur in children 6–18 mo of age after an incubation period of 7–17 days. Treatment is symptomatic.

ERYTHEMA INFECTIOSUM

The fifth of five numbered exanthems of childhood, erythema infectiosum ("fifth disease") is caused by parvovirus B19, a single-stranded DNA virus. The virus is spread by aerosolized secretions and, after a week of incubation, leads to a characteristic series of exanthems. They begin with the sudden onset of bright erythema of the cheeks, giving the child a "slapped cheek" appearance. This rash is followed by a maculopapular rash on the trunk and extremities. In the final phase, the rash fades with central clearing, giving it a lacy or reticular appearance.

Associated symptoms are uncommon in children, but adults frequently experience associated headache, upper respiratory symptoms, myalgias, and arthralgias. Parvovirus B19 also has been identified as a cause of hydrops fetalis and aplastic crisis in patients with hemolytic anemias. Treatment is supportive.

HERPES SIMPLEX VIRUS

Etiology and Epidemiology

Herpetic infections are the result of two antigenically distinct, double-stranded DNA viruses, herpes simplex virus (HSV)-1 and HSV-2. Either may cause oral, genital, or disseminated disease, although HSV-1 is the more common cause of oral herpes infection and HSV-2 is the more common cause of genital infection. HSV-1 infection predominates in children; HSV-2 is the more common cause of primary infection in neonates (see Chap. 7) and sexually active adolescents. Spread of infection is determined by two factors: close contact with the pathogen and trauma to the protective skin or mucous membranes.

Clinical Manifestations

Although 85% of primary infections are asymptomatic, both viruses may cause a variety of clinical syndromes, which may recur. Common syndromes include the following.

ACUTE HERPETIC GINGIVOSTOMATITIS. HSV-1 is the most common cause of stomatitis in children 1–3 yr old. Unlike herpangina, an enteroviral-mediated infection in which oral lesions are small and predominantly in the posterior oropharynx, herpes predominantly affects the anterior tongue, gingiva, and buccal mucosa. Vesicles are typically 2–10 mm in diameter. Symptoms include pain, fetor oris, and fever. Recurrence is common. If the child is a thumb sucker, herpetic whitlow also may be present.

ECZEMA HERPETICUM. Also known as "Kaposi varicelliform eruption," this infection typically results from herpetic infection of atopic skin. It may be associated with high fevers and toxic appearance.

OCULAR LESIONS. Although typically associated with neonatal herpes infection, conjunctivitis and keratoconjunctivitis may occur at any age. Herpes should be suspected whenever a vesicular periorbital rash is seen on physical exam. It is associated with poor-prognosis herpes meningo-encephalitis.

GENITAL INFECTIONS. Although these are predominantly caused by HSV-2, 5–10% are caused by HSV-1. Both are sexually transmitted and lead to a vesicular rash in the perineum. Genital infections frequently recur.

Diagnosis

This diagnosis should be suspected whenever there is a localized vesicular rash. Although culture is the gold standard of diagnosis, rapid diagnosis may be aided by specific immunofluorescent staining or the nonspecific Tzanck stain. ELISA and polymerase chain reactions also have been used in diagnosis.

Treatment

Most herpetic infections are self-limited, usually lasting 1–2 wk. Patients treated with oral acyclovir have been found to have less pain, fewer lesions, and shorter duration of viral shedding than control subjects with uncomplicated herpes infections. Patients at risk for severe disease should be treated with IV acyclovir.

VARICELLA AND ZOSTER

Etiology and Epidemiology

These infections are caused by another of the Herpesviridae, *Herpesvirus varicellae*. Varicella, or chickenpox, represents primary infection with this agent, whereas zoster is due to reactivation of this virus from its dormant state in the dorsal root ganglia.

Clinical Manifestations

Primary infection manifests itself after a 10–21-day incubation period. Symptoms begin with a nonspecific viral prodrome followed by the appearance of the diagnostic rash. Individual lesions evolve from maculopapular to maculovesicular before bursting and scabbing over. Diagnosis is usually made when the patient has lesions in all stages of evolution. Pruritis is intense, and scratching frequently leads to secondary bacterial infection.

Complications are common and include pneumonia, hepatitis, Reye syndrome, and postinfectious encephalitis. Newborns, the elderly, and immunosuppressed patients are at risk for more severe systemic disease.

The virus is transmitted by aerosolized respiratory secretions or by direct contact with vesicular fluid. Patients are contagious from the prodrome until all of the lesions have scabbed over, typically a period of 7–10 days.

Diagnosis

This is usually made on clinical grounds. In atypical cases, the diagnosis may be supported by specific immunofluorescent staining of the vesicular fluid.

Treatment

Treatment is supportive, using fluids and non–salicylate-containing antipyretics. Pruritis may be treated with antihistamines or oatmeal baths.

Active immunization of patients at risk for severe infection with the live attenuated virus vaccine is controversial but should be considered. When high-risk patients are inadvertently exposed, they should be passively immunized with varicella–zoster immune globulin (VZIG) within 72 hr of exposure. If a high-risk patient becomes symptomatic, high-dose acyclovir therapy should be instituted as early as possible.

CYTOMEGALOVIRUS INFECTIONS

Etiology and Epidemiology

Cytomegalovirus (CMV), another of the Herpesviridae, is a ubiquitous organism. Although it frequently leads to asymptomatic infection, it is transmitted for months after acute infection in all bodily secretions. Transmission is common in day-care centers and with sexual contact. CMV also may remain latent in the white blood cells of the host, reactivating later and leading to secondary infection.

Clinical Manifestations

CMV is the most common cause of congenital infection. Intrauterine infection is usually associated with primary CMV infection in the mother and occurs after transplacental viremia. See Chap. 7 of this text for discussion of congenital and postnatally acquired infections.

In the immunocompetent host, CMV frequently leads to asymptomatic infection or a mononeucleosis-like syndrome characterized by fever, malaise, weakness, and hepatosplenomegaly. Symptoms typically last 2 wk or longer. Transplant recipients commonly get CMV pneumonitis, and CMV retinitis is common in patients with AIDS.

Diagnosis

CMV usually is diagnosed by isolation of the virus in bodily secretions or diseased tissues.

Treatment

Ganciclovir is effective in the treatment of CMV retinitis, but is only mildly active in the treatment of more widespread disease, which frequently is fatal.

INFECTIOUS MONONUCLEOSIS

Etiology and Epidemiology

Infectious mononucleosis is caused by the Epstein–Barr virus, another member of the Herpesviridae. As is true with all the members of this family, the disease is very contagious and has the capacity for latent infection in the body. Its predominant sites of infection are the epithelial cells of the pharynx and B lymphocytes; it is from the latter that latent infection may arise. It is spread in the saliva, with virus recoverable for months after symptoms resolve. Distribution of the virus is worldwide; its spread is associated with poverty.

Clinical Manifestations

After an incubation period of 30–50 days, symptoms of infectious mononucleosis include a 1–2 wk prodrome in which vague complaints of malaise, fatigue, headache, and abdominal symptoms are experienced. Complaints of fever and sore throat gradually increase until the patient is brought for medical attention. On presentation, physical exam usually reveals moderate fever, tonsillar enlargement with or without exudates, lymphadenopathy, and hepatosplenomegaly. Severe symptoms last for 2–4 wk, followed by a gradual recovery. Complications include splenic rupture, airway compromise, pneumonia, and a myriad of neurologic symptoms and complaints.

Epstein–Barr virus also has been associated with the chronic fatigue syndrome, the African form of Burkitt lymphoma, and nasopharyngeal carcinoma in Chinese populations.

Diagnosis and Differential Diagnosis

Diagnosis may be suspected from clinical presentation, recognition of atypical lymphocytes in the blood, the presence of heterophil antibodies, or specific Epstein–Barr virus serologic tests. Differential diagnosis of a patient with atypical lymphocytes, lymphadenopathy, and hepatosplenomegaly includes CMV infection, toxoplasmosis, acute human immunodeficiency virus (HIV) infection, and infectious hepatitis. If there is an associated leukopenia, anemia, or thrombocytopenia (all of which may be seen in infectious mononucleosis), leukemia must be ruled out.

Treatment

This is symptomatic. Short-course steroids may have some role in the treatment of dangerous edema, such as that of the airway or spleen, or cases in which anemia or thrombocytopenia are pronounced.

MUMPS

Etiology and Epidemiology

Mumps, or epidemic parotitis, is a paramyxoviral infection in which there is painful swelling of the salivary glands, most commonly the parotids. Infection is spread by respiratory secretions, tainted fomites, and possibly the urine. Viral transmission occurs from 1 day prior to the onset of swelling to 3 days after remission.

Clinical Manifestations

After an incubation period of 14–24 days, the patient experiences acute, painful swelling of the salivary glands. Swelling may be unilateral or bilateral and typically subsides in 3–7 days. Although moderate fever is associated with mumps, associated symptoms are uncommon.

Complications include meningoencephalitis, orchitis, and pancreatitis. Meningoencephalitis may be due to either primary infection of the neurons or postinfectious, immune-mediated demyelination. Orchitis and epididymitis are rare in prepubertal boys, but are common in adolescents and have been associated with impaired fertility. Pancreatitis is typically mild.

Diagnosis and Differential Diagnosis

Although virus may be isolated from the saliva, CSF, urine, or blood, diagnosis typically is based on clinical criteria. Amylase typically is elevated. Acute and convalescent titers may be helpful in diagnosis. Differential diagnosis of parotid masses includes calculus, infection caused by agents other than the mumps virus, and tumors.

Treatment and Prevention

Treatment of mumps is supportive. Active immunization with live virus vaccine induces antibody in approximately 96% of those immunized, and immunity is considered to be lifelong. Although hyperimmune mumps gamma globulin has been developed, passive immunization is not effective in preventing mumps or decreasing the rate of complications.

INFLUENZA VIRAL INFECTIONS

Etiology and Epidemiology

Influenza viruses are large RNA orthomyxoviruses, subject to two types of antigenic change, antigenic shift and antigenic drift. In *antigenic shift*, relatively infrequent, major antigenic changes occur. In *antigenic drift*, changes occur more frequently but have less antigenic impact. Influenza A undergoes both antigenic shift and antigenic drift. For this reason, immunity (whether naturally acquired from disease or artificially acquired from vaccine) is short lived. Severe pandemic influenza A (associated with antigenic shift) occurs every 10–40 yr, whereas smaller epidemics (due to antigenic drift) occur every 2–3 yr. Because influenza B undergoes only antigenic drift, outbreaks with this pathogen occur relatively frequently, every 4–7 yr. Immunity to a particular viral subtype is long lasting but, because of antigenic shift and antigenic drift, reinfection is common.

Clinical Manifestations

These viruses are spread in respiratory secretions. They cause disease in the mucous membranes of the respiratory tract after a short incubation period of 2–3 days. Common signs and symptoms of influenza infection are high fever, pharyngitis, conjunctivitis, rhinitis (especially with influenza B), headache, and cough. In uncomplicated influenza, the fever lasts 2–5 days. The cough may persist for 2–3 wk. Complications include pneumonia, carditis, and encephalitis. Bacterial superinfection is common. Reye syndrome is most commonly associated with salicylate use during influenza B infection.

Diagnosis

This is based on clinical symptoms, although fluorescent staining techniques and culture may be used in cases in which identification of the pathogen is necessary.

Treatment and Prevention

Treatment for uncomplicated influenza infection is largely symptomatic. If given early in the course, amantadine and rimantidine are useful in the prophylaxis and treatment of influenza A infections. Ribavirin is active against both influenza A and B viruses.

Active immunization with potent, antigenically up-to-date inactivated viral vaccine is available. It should be used in those patients with chronic disease involving the cardiorespiratory systems and in other groups at risk for severe infection.

PARAINFLUENZA VIRAL INFECTIONS

There are four serologic types of this RNA paramyxovirus, but types 1–3 are the most clinically significant. They affect the respiratory epithelium almost exclusively: type 1 is the most frequent cause of laryngotracheitis and type 3 accounts for most cases of bronchitis, bronchiolitis, and pneumonia. Symptoms most commonly associated with infection include cough, rhinorrhea, and pharyngitis. Complications are rare, and diagnosis may be definitively made using culture or fluorescent antibody techniques. Although ribavirin is active against parainfluenza viruses, treatment is symptomatic.

RESPIRATORY SYNCYTIAL VIRUS

Etiology and Epidemiology

Along with mumps and parainfluenza viruses, respiratory syncytial virus (RSV) is an RNA paramyxovirus. It is the leading cause of respiratory disease in the 1st yr of life and is the causative agent in 45–75% of cases of bronchiolitis. It has a worldwide distribution and appears in yearly winter epidemics lasting 4–5 mo.

Clinical Manifestations

Although RSV infection is most commonly associated with bronchiolitis, it can cause disease anywhere in the upper or lower respiratory tract. Symptoms typically begin about 4 days after exposure with rhinorrhea, pharyngitis, and cough. Shortly after the cough has developed, lower respiratory symptoms may become apparent. Disease may be limited to the bronchioli or extend to the alveoli. Chest roentgenograms of children hospitalized with bronchiolitis most commonly reveal peribronchial cuffing, hyperexpansion, or interstitial pneumonia. Other organ systems are not typically affected.

Diagnosis

This is based on clinical criteria. In cases in which identification of the etiologic agent is important, the virus may be identified by immunofluorescent techniques or culture. Differential diagnosis of lower respiratory tract disease with wheezing in this age group includes foreign body, asthma, and pneumonitis caused by other viruses, bacteria, or chlamydia.

Treatment

This includes oxygen and judicious use of bronchodilators; because the pathogenesis of bronchiolitis is related more to intraluminal obstruction and edema than to bronchiolar smooth muscle contraction, the clinical utility of bronchodilators is limited. Steroids are not indicated.

Ribavirin has been shown to shorten the duration and severity of symptoms in patients with bronchiolitis, but it is cumbersome to administer. Because most cases of bronchiolitis are self-limited, ribavirin is probably only indicated in very sick infants or those at risk for severe disease, such as those with underlying cardiac or pulmonary disease.

ADENOVIRUSES

DNA viruses of intermediate size, adenoviruses cause 5–8% of acute respiratory disease in infants. They also may cause a wide array of other infections: conjunctivitis, gastroenteritis, hemorrhagic cystitis, and pneumonia. Infections caused by adenovirus may be mild or severe: pneumonia caused by some subtypes can have a mortality of as high as 10%. Diagnosis is based on viral culture or demonstration of a rise in antibody titers. Treatment is supportive.

HEPATITIS

Hepatitis is a major public health problem worldwide that may be caused by a number of different viruses. Although there are differences in the severity of disease and associated symptoms produced by each virus, the clinical diagnosis of hepatitis should be suspected in patients experiencing abdominal pain associated with jaundice, dark urine, and clay-colored stools. Additional symptoms may include fever, nausea, vomiting, diarrhea, skin rash, and arthritis. The various viruses causing hepatitis and some of their characteristics are summarized below.

Hepatitis A

Hepatitis A virus (HAV) is an RNA virus that is typically transmitted by the fecal–oral route. There is no known carrier state. The highest attack rates are in children in day-care centers or those institutionalized. The incubation period is 15–50 days, and the patient is contagious (secreting fecal HAV) during the week or two preceding and following the onset of jaundice. The majority of childhood infections are anicteric.

Diagnosis is based on viral isolation or demonstration of anti-HAV IgM, which typically rises with clinical symptoms.

Treatment is symptomatic.

For *prevention*, household contacts should be treated with immune globulin (0.02 mL/kg) as soon as possible following diagnosis. Those traveling to areas in which HAV is endemic should receive immune globulin (0.06 mL/kg) prior to departure.

Hepatitis B

Hepatitis B is a DNA virus whose transmission is primarily via sexual contact or tainted blood. Neonatal/in utero transmission also is possible. The incubation period is 45–160 days, and the majority of childhood infections are asymptomatic. Complications include chronic carrier state, cirrhosis, and hepatocellular carcinoma. Carriers may have either persistent or active disease.

Diagnosis is based on serologic markers: Hb_sAg+ denotes current infection and infectivity due to either acute or chronic disease, and Hb_eAg+ is a marker of high infectivity. *Anti-HB$_c$* is the first demonstration of an antibody response; it may be present in chronic carriers, and rises during flares of active disease, both acute and chronic. The presence of anti-HB$_s$ denotes recovery or previous immunization.

Treatment is symptomatic.

For *prevention*, passive immunization may be given effectively with hepatitis B immune globulin (0.06 mL/kg) and should be given as soon as possible after contact; active immunity may be conferred with recombinant vaccine given in three doses at 0, 1, and 6 mo, with anti-HB$_s$ drawn following completion of the cycle.

Hepatitis C

Hepatitis C is an RNA virus whose transmission is through tainted blood products. It has the worst prognosis of the viral hepatitides because it is more commonly associated with fulminant or chronic disease. Hepatitis C infection may lead to hepatocellular carcinoma and cirrhosis.

Hepatitis D

Hepatitis D is the RNA-containing delta virus. Disease is only associated with concurrent hepatitis B transmission. Infection with hepatitis D may lead to chronic hepatitis.

Other Causes

Hepatitis may also be caused by hepatitis E virus (a waterborne RNA-containing virus), Epstein–Barr virus, CMV, HSV, HIV, rubella, and coxsackieviruses.

ENTEROVIRUS INFECTIONS

Etiology and Epidemiology

Enteroviruses are single-stranded RNA picornaviruses. They are subdivided as polioviruses (3 antigenic types), coxsackie A (24 antigenic types), coxsackie B (1–6 antigenic types), and echoviruses (34 antigenic types). There is minor serologic cross-reactivity between several coxsackie and echovirus types, but no common group antigens of any diagnostic importance. Transmission is typically by the fecal–oral route, but they also may be spread by fomites or respiratory secretions. Children are the main susceptible cohort. Fetuses and neonates are affected more severely than older children. These viruses are distributed worldwide, with highest prevalence in summer and fall in temperate climates.

Clinical Manifestations

In general, severe illness with coxsackie A or echoviruses is rare. Polio can be severe, but rarely is seen as a result of immunization programs in this country. Coxsackie B infections have been implicated most commonly with severe and long-term disease. In general, severity is inversely related to age.

The most common manifestation of enteroviral infection is a nonspecific febrile illness that usually develops abruptly. Fever often is quite high (to 40°C), with the degree of fever commonly inversely proportional to age. Fever typically has a mean duration of 3 days but may be biphasic, occurring for 1 day, being absent for a day or two, and then recurring for another 2–4 days. Physical examination is often unremarkable except for a mild pharyngitis or conjunctivitis. Disease typically lasts 3–4 days.

Enteroviral infections also may lead to nonspecific gastroenteritis, with diarrhea and fever being the main symptoms. Respiratory symptoms may occur uncommonly: parotitis, croup, bronchitis, bronchiolitis, and pneumonia have been attributed to enteroviral infection.

Other clinical syndromes associated with enteroviral infection include the following.

ACUTE HEMORRHAGIC CONJUNCTIVITIS. Infection usually is attributed to enterovirus 70; it also has been described with coxsackie A24. Spread is by the eye–hand–fomite–hand–eye route. *Clinical manifestations* include sudden onset of painful conjunctivitis with photophobia, lacrimation, and blurred vision. Improvement begins after 3 days, with complete recovery after 7–12 days.

HERPANGINA. Herpangina is a common enteroviral infection that occurs in the summer and fall. It is predominantly caused by many subtypes of coxsackie A, and occasionally by coxsackie B and other enteroviral species. *Clinical manifestations* include sudden onset, acute febrile illness with papular, vesicular, and ulcerative lesions on the anterior tonsillar pillars, soft palate, tonsils, pharynx, and posterior buccal mucosa. The lesions typically are small and discreet in the posterior pharynx. They may be on the tip of the tongue, but if the lesions are primarily in the anterior oropharynx or >5 mm in size, they are not herpangina. Herpangina can occur as part of more widespread enteroviral disease with exanthem, meningitis, and other symptoms. The duration of illness is typically 3–6 days.

HAND–FOOT–MOUTH DISEASE. In this interesting disease there is the abrupt onset of high fever and rash in a characteristic acral distribution. The rash also may be found in the mouth and on the buttocks, although truncal sparing is the rule. The rash begins as scattered papules and then becomes vesicular. The lesions are typically 3–7 mm in size and may be painful or pruritic. The disease is typically caused by coxsackie A16 after a 3–5-day incubation period.

PLEURODYNIA. Also known as "Bornholm disease" or the "devil's grippe," pleurodynia is typically caused by coxsackie B3 and B5. Following an incubation period of 4–5 days, the patient experiences the sudden onset of fever and chest pain that often is excruciatingly severe, sudden, and stabbing. The pain is spasmodic and paroxysmal, with paroxysms lasting minutes to hours (usually 15–30 min) and coming minutes to hours apart. The disease typically lasts 2–3 days but may be biphasic. Chest roentgenograms typically are normal. Treatment is symptomatic, using nonsteroidal anti-inflammatory drugs for pain.

COMPLICATIONS WITH COXSACKIEVIRUS INFECTION. There are also a number of complications associated with coxsackievirus infection. Coxsackie B is the most common cause of viral carditis, causing 50% of all identifiable cases of viral carditis as a postviral complication. Adolescents and young adults are most commonly affected, with children spared for unclear reasons. Coxsackie B5 is most commonly implicated.

Coxsackie B also may be implicated in the development of chronic fatigue syndrome, adult-onset Still disease, and diabetes mellitis.

ROTAVIRUS

This member of the Reoviridae family is a double-stranded RNA virus and is the agent most commonly responsible for infant diarrhea worldwide. It is associated with outbreaks in the winter months and most commonly affects children less than 2 yr old. Because the virus undergoes frequent point mutations, patients may experience recurrent infections, and attempts to develop a long-term, effective vaccine have been unsuccessful.

Clinical manifestations include fever, watery diarrhea, and nonbilious emesis, all of which contribute to dramatic, rapid dehydration. The incubation period is 36–48 hr, and viral shedding typically continues for 2–5 days after the diarrhea stops.

Diagnosis is most commonly done by ELISA test.

Treatment is supportive, with special attention to hydration. Complications are rare.

RABIES

Etiology and Epidemiology

Rabies is a viral infection of the CNS caused by an RNA-containing rhabdovirus. It is widespread in distribution and is transmitted by infection of a wound with the saliva of an infected animal. The basic lesion in the brain is neuronal destruction in the brain stem and medulla after an incubation period that is extremely variable in duration, but typically 30–60 days.

Clinical Manifestations

Symptoms of rabies are those of an encephalitis that may be either furious or paralytic. Eighty percent of cases are furious, marked by periods of disorientation and combativeness alternating with periods of lucidity. Differential diagnosis includes encephalitis of any cause. Hydrophobia, the fear of water, is pathognomonic and results from recurrent aspiration whenever swallowing is attempted. Twenty percent of cases are paralytic and are marked by ascending paralysis that may be misdiagnosed as Guillain–Barré syndrome, poliomyelitis, myasthenia gravis, or botulism. Both forms are invariably fatal once symptoms begin.

Diagnosis

This is based on fluorescent antibody staining of corneal epithelial cells or sections of skin at the hairline.

Treatment and Prevention

Because prognosis is grave once symptoms have begun, management and control are based on prophylactic therapy. People at risk, such as veterinarians, should be actively immunized with three doses of human diploid cell vaccine. People who have been bitten by wild animals, especially those known to carry rabies (e.g., skunks, foxes, racoons, bats, and coyotes), should be treated with local cleansing, passive immunization with rabies immune globulin, and active immunization with human diploid cell vaccine. With unprovoked bites by domesticated animals, therapy may be withheld until the animal has been observed. If the animal acts abnormally, it should be sacrificed and tested for rabies, with therapy initiated if test results are positive.

HUMAN IMMUNODEFICIENCY VIRUS

Etiology and Epidemiology

There is no greater issue in medicine today than AIDS. Childhood AIDS is in the top 10 leading causes of childhood death and is on the rise: newborns and adolescents are two of the fastest growing populations affected. An RNA retrovirus capable of rapid antigenic variation, HIV is rapidly inactivated by detergents, heating, or drying. Transmission is only through intimate contact with body fluids. The virus has been isolated in tears, saliva, breast milk, semen, and blood, but transmission has been documented only in the last three.

Pathogenesis

HIV is attracted to cells expressing the CD4 antigen. These include T4 (helper) lymphocytes, monocytes, and macrophages. A membrane glycoprotein, gp120, interacts and binds to the CD4 antigen, enabling the RNA to enter the cytoplasm of the cell. The viral RNA is then transcribed into

DNA by reverse transcriptase and it is incorporated into the host cell genome. The host cells are then destroyed by a variety of mechanisms. Monocytes and macrophages are relatively resistant to cell killing; therefore, they serve as a reservoir for insidious viral replication. The infected monocyte is also a vehicle responsible for the transport of HIV into the CNS, where gp120 is a competitive inhibitor of neuroleukin, a neurotropic factor, leading to neurologic dysfunction.

Clinical Manifestations

Clinical manifestations of pediatric AIDS are summarized in Table 10–3. Laboratory findings typically include hypergam-

TABLE 10–3. CLINICAL MANIFESTATIONS OF PEDIATRIC AIDS*

Generalized
  Fever
  Failure to thrive
  Lymphadenopathy
  Recurrent infection
  Developmental delay
  Low birth weight (small for gestational age)

Specific
  Embryopathy
  Microcephaly
  Facial dysmorphism
  Hepatosplenomegaly
  Lymphocytic interstitial pneumonia
  Diarrhea
  Gastrointestinal bleeding
  Cardiomyopathy
  Arteriopathy
  Nephropathy
  Encephalopathy
  Parotitis
  Kaposi sarcoma
  Skin rashes

Infections
  Pneumocystis carinii
  Mycobacterium avium-intracellulare
  Cytomegalovirus
  Herpes simplex (types 1 and 2)
  Epstein–Barr virus
  Varicella–zoster virus
  Cryptococcus
  Cryptosporidium
  Aspergillus fumigatus
  Haemophilus influenzae type b
  Streptococcus pneumoniae
  Salmonella
  Shigella
  Moniliasis (oral and esophageal)
  Toxoplasmosis
  Giardiasis
  Amebiasis

* From Behrman RE (ed): Nelson Textbook of Pediatrics, 14th ed. Philadelphia, WB Saunders Company, 1992, p. 839.

maglobulinemia (with nonfunctional antibody formation), reversal of the T helper–suppressor cell ratio, reduced or absent cutaneous hypersensitivity tests, elevated erythrocyte sedimentation rate, and depression of any or all of the blood cell lines.

Diagnosis

This traditionally has been based on antibody identification using ELISA and western blot techniques. Because antibody may be transferred from mother to fetus and this antibody may be detectible for up to 15 mo diagnosis in the perinatal period always has been difficult. Infection is transferred from mother to fetus in 20–35% of exposures; discordant infection of monozygotic twins has been reported. In an effort to make rapid, accurate diagnosis of HIV infection in the newborn period, myriad techniques have been tried. Most promising are HIV antigen detection and polymerase chain reactions.

Treatment

Treatment of pediatric AIDS is currently aimed at limiting viral replication using drugs such as azidothymidine (AZT), dideoxycytidine (DDC), and dideoxyinosine (DDI) and prevention of infectious complications using monthly administration of intravenous gamma globulin (400 mg/kg) and antibiotics. Information on treatment of individual infectious complications can be found elsewhere in this chapter.

RICKETTSIAL DISEASE
(*NELSON TEXTBOOK*, SECS. 12.94–12.100)

Rickettsiae are small, pleomorphic coccobacilli that are Gram-stain negative and contain both DNA and RNA. They are transmitted to mammals by arthropod vectors and are obligate intracellular organisms. They cause a vasculitis in the mammalian host, and may lead to dramatic disease with associated shock and disseminated intravascular coagulation. Diagnosis may be made by a number of laboratory techniques, including the outdated Weil–Felix test and skin biopsy, but the most reliable and sensitive test in use today is indirect fluorescent antibody assay. Doxycycline, tetracycline, and chloramphenicol commonly are used in the treatment of rickettsial diseases. Duration of therapy is usually 7–10 days.

Rocky Mountain Spotted Fever

ETIOLOGY AND EPIDEMIOLOGY. Rocky Mountain spotted fever is the most common rickettsial disease in the United States; it accounts for nearly 90% of all rickettsial disease reported. The name is a misnomer because this disease is reported throughout the continental United States and only 5% of the cases are in the Rocky Mountain area. The agent is *R. rickettsii* and ticks are the arthropod vector.

CLINICAL MANIFESTATIONS. After a tick bite (50–60% of cases give a history of tick bite), the incubation period is 2–14 days, with a median of 7 days. The disease begins with nonspecific flu-like illness. One to 5 days after the onset of illness, the patient typically will get a rash that begins in the periphery and spreads centrally. The rash initially is maculopapular and then becomes petecchial or purpuric. It frequently involves the palms and soles. Hepatosplenomegaly is common, as are hyponatremia and thrombocytopenia. Complications may include necrosis and gangrene resulting from severe vasculitis. In uncomplicated cases, recovery takes place in the second week of illness.

Other Rickettsial Diseases

Other rickettsial diseases include those borne by ticks, Boutonneuse fever, ehrlichiosis, and Q fever. Rickettsialpox and scrub typhus (tsutsugamushi fever) are borne by mites. The three typhus diseases, epidemic, endemic, and flying squirrel associated, all are borne by fleas and lice.

MYCOTIC INFECTIONS
(*NELSON TEXTBOOK*, SECS. 12.103–12.109)

Fungi are a common cause of disease in children. In immunocompetent hosts, diseases caused by fungi largely are cutaneous or mucocutaneous, such as ringworm or thrush (see Chaps. 21 and 11), or localized pulmonary infections, such as cryptococcosis or histoplasmosis. Systemic infections are rare and usually are found in the immunocompromised host. These latter infections may be life threatening and must be treated with potent antifungal drugs such as amphotericin B.

HISTOPLASMOSIS

Etiology and Epidemiology

Histoplasma capsulatum, a dimorphic fungus, commonly is found in soils containing bird and bat excrement. It is the most common systemic mycosis in the United States and is endemic in the Mississippi, Missouri, and Ohio river valleys. Sporotrichosis and blastomycosis are other, less common fungal infections endemic to this area. Infection is caused by inhalation of airborne spores.

Clinical Manifestations

Skin test conversion and asymptomatic infection is the most common scenario. Clinical syndromes include an acute flu-like illness with pneumonitis and hilar adenopathy arising a few weeks after exposure. This disease persists for 3–4 wk and is self-limited, requiring no therapy. Re-exposure may lead to an identical syndrome, typically after a much shorter, 3-day incubation period.

Disseminated disease is uncommon, occurring in infants and immunosuppressed patients. Pneumonia often is complicated by infection of reticuloendothelial and hematopoietic organs. If left untreated, the disease is fatal.

Diagnosis

This usually is based on serum antibody response. Tissue cultures are diagnostic but are difficult to obtain. Skin testing is of limited value: positive tests may be indicative of acute or previous disease, and negative tests commonly are seen in patients with disseminated disease.

Treatment

Acute primary and secondary pulmonary infections are self-limited; no therapy is required. Amphotericin B is the treatment of choice with disseminated disease.

CRYPTOCOCCOSIS

Etiology and Epidemiology

Cryptococcus neoformans, an encapsulated budding yeast with a worldwide distribution, is the cause of this disease. Infection arises after inhalation of spores.

Clinical Manifestations

Cryptococcal meningitis is the most common form of life-threatening cryptococcal infection in children. It most commonly affects immunosuppressed patients and immigrants, presenting as a subacute or chronic meningitis. Pulmonary cryptococcosis is uncommon in children, presenting as a flu-like illness with pneumonitis following primary exposure.

Diagnosis

This is based on culture. Latex agglutination techniques also have been used to demonstrate cryptococcal antigen.

Treatment

Acute pulmonary infections in immunocompetent hosts are self-limited and rarely require treatment. Meningitis or systemic infections require therapy with amphotericin B and flucytosine.

COCCIDIOIDOMYCOSIS (Valley Fever, Desert Rheumatism)

Etiology and Epidemiology

Coccidioides immitis is a dimorphic fungus found in the soil of dry southwestern states. Spores are spread by inhalation.

Clinical Manifestations

After an incubation period of 10–16 days, the patient may develop a flu-like illness with associated rash, pneumonitis, and pleural effusions. The rash is variable in appearance and may be macular, urticarial, or erythema nodosum. Primary infection confers lifelong immunity, and 60% of primary infections are asymptomatic. Uncommon complications include a progressive or cavitary pneumonitis or disseminated infection, which is found most commonly in immunosuppressed patients.

Diagnosis

Culture of affected fluids and tissues is the definitive basis of diagnosis. Caution when handling specimens is advised because the spores are highly contagious. Although skin testing is available, it is of limited clinical utility: positive tests are indicative of current or previous infection, and patients with severe disease commonly have false-negative tests. Complement fixation tests have some utility because antibody response generally correlates with severity of disease.

Treatment

Primary infections are, in general, self-limited and require no therapy. Persistent or systemic disease should be treated with surgical excision where possible and amphotericin B.

PARASITIC INFECTIONS
(NELSON TEXTBOOK, SECS. 12.110–12.139)

Infections attributable to protozoa and helminths are the major infectious disease problem in many parts of the world. Protozoa are unicellular organisms that multiply within the host. Helminths are multicellular worms that usually do not divide within the human host. Both cause a variety of intestinal and systemic diseases.

PROTOZOAN INFECTIONS

Amebiasis

ETIOLOGY AND EPIDEMIOLOGY. *Entamoeba histolytica* is a protozoan transmitted as a cyst via contaminated food, water, or person-to-person contact. Distribution is worldwide, but the organism is more prevalent in areas of poor sanitation.

CLINICAL MANIFESTATIONS. Most infected individuals with amebiasis are asymptomatic. Disease occurs in less than 10% of those colonized and results from invasion of the intestinal mucosa, leading to characteristic flask-shaped ulcers. Clinical symptoms and signs include fever, crampy abdominal pain, and diarrhea that may contain blood or mucus. They may last from days to weeks and may recur.

Hepatic amebiasis is the most common form of disseminated disease and occurs in 1% of infected individuals. Manifestations include hepatic pain, distention, and fever.

DIAGNOSIS. Diagnosis of intestinal illness depends on demonstration of organisms in the stool or in biopsied tissue. Ultrasound or CT may be used to demonstrate hepatic abscess because stool examination frequently is negative for amebae.

TREATMENT. Metronidazole is the drug of choice for symptomatic disease, whereas diloxanide may be the drug of choice for intraluminal organisms.

Giardiasis

ETIOLOGY AND EPIDEMIOLOGY. *Giardia lamblia,* a flagellated protozoan, is transmitted as a cyst by person-to-person contact, by the fecal–oral route, or by drinking contaminated water. Infection is common in day-care centers.

CLINICAL MANIFESTATIONS. Colonized individuals may (1) be asymptomatic, (2) experience acute, explosive diarrhea with crampy distention and anorexia, or (3) experience chronic diarrhea with weight loss and malabsorption.

DIAGNOSIS. This is made by direct stool examination. Multiple stools must be obtained to rule out disease. Alternatively, duodenal specimens may be obtained using the "string test." ELISA can be used to detect *Giardia* antigen in the stool.

TREATMENT. Furazolidone, metronidazole, or quinacrine may be used in the treatment of giardiasis.

Cryptosporidiosis

ETIOLOGY AND EPIDEMIOLOGY. Cryptosporidium is a protozoan that is transmitted by person-to-person contact.

CLINICAL MANIFESTATIONS. Symptoms include watery diarrhea, cramps, and nausea that typically last 10–14 days but may be chronic.

DIAGNOSIS. Diagnosis is difficult, with special stool concentrating and staining methods required.

TREATMENT. No specific therapy is available.

Malaria

ETIOLOGY AND EPIDEMIOLOGY. One or more of the four *Plasmodium* species (*falciparum, vivax, ovale,* and *malariae*) cause disease after transmission by an infected female *Anopheles* mosquito. Disease also may be acquired transplacentally or through tainted blood products.

CLINICAL MANIFESTATIONS. Plasmodia invade the red blood cells, multiply, and rupture the infected cells, causing fever and hemolytic anemia. Associated symptoms may include headache, abdominal pain, and splenomegaly. *P. falciparum* may cause the most severe hemolysis and is the cause of "blackwater fever," so named because of the high concentration of hemoglobin and bile pigments found in the urine. Fever may be cyclic and associated with hemolysis, coming every 2–3 days when infection is caused by *P. vivax* or *P. malariae.*

TREATMENT. Chloroquine is the treatment of choice for malaria acquired in areas of low chloroquine resistance. In areas in which chloroquine resistance is high, quinine plus either tetracycline or pyrimethamine–sulfadoxine are indicated. Relapse with *P. ovale* or *P. vivax* infection may be prevented by using primaquine, which eradicates the hepatic phase of the parasite cycle. Because other species do not have a hepatic phase, primaquine is not indicated for them.

Prophylaxis of travelers includes the use of weekly doses of chloroquine and prevention of mosquito bites. Pyrimethamine–sulfadoxine should be available in case a febrile illness develops.

American Trypanosomiasis (Chagas Disease)

ETIOLOGY AND EPIDEMIOLOGY.   *Trypanosoma cruzi,* a protozoan hemoflagellate, is transmitted to humans by the blood-sucking reduviid bugs endemic to South and Central America. Infection also can be transmitted congenitally or through tainted blood products.

CLINICAL MANIFESTATIONS.   Disease in children typically is mild or asymptomatic. When acute symptoms occur, patients may note a nodular skin lesion (chagoma) at the site of inoculation. After hematogenous dissemination, symptoms include fever, rash, myalgias, and hepatosplenomegaly. Myocardial involvement is common and may lead to arrhythmias. Meningoencephalitis is less common.

Congenital disease is characterized by low birth weight, hepatomegaly, and meningoencephalitis. Infection may lead to chronic inflammation and fibrosis, resulting in cardiomyopathy.

DIAGNOSIS.   During acute disease trypanosomes can be demonstrated in the blood. Diagnosis of chronic disease is made serologically.

TREATMENT.   Nifurtimox is effective in the treatment of American trypanosomiasis.

Toxoplasmosis

ETIOLOGY AND EPIDEMIOLOGY.   *Toxoplasma gondii* is an intracellular protozoan acquired by the fecal–oral route from cat feces containing the infectious oocyte. Transmission also may occur by ingestion of undercooked meat, via blood transfusion or organ transplant, and transplacentally during acute infection of a pregnant woman.

CLINICAL MANIFESTATIONS.   Acquired infection usually is asymptomatic. Symptomatic infection occurs approximately 7 days after exposure and is characterized by a heterophil-negative, mononeucleosis-like syndrome with lymphadenopathy and hepatosplenomegaly. In immunosuppressed patients, disseminated infection involving the heart, lungs, and brain may be seen.

The incidence of congenital toxoplasmosis is 1–2:1,000 live births in the United States. Affected infants may have fever, rash, petechiae, hepatosplenomegaly, hydrocephalus or microcephaly, microphthalmia, chorioretinitis, thrombocytopenia, hyperbilirubinemia, and cerebral calcifications (see Chap. 7). Prognosis is guarded because infected patients may develop mental retardation and other neurologic disabilities years after birth.

DIAGNOSIS.   Serial serologic evaluation is the most common approach to diagnosis.

TREATMENT.   Pyrimethamine and sulfadiazine in conjunction with folinic acid may be used in the treatment of toxoplasmosis. This regimen has been shown to lessen risk of long-term disease and sequelae.

HELMINTH INFECTIONS

The helminths are classified into three groups, the round worms or nematodes and the flatworms: trematodes (flukes) and cestodes (tapeworms).

Ascariasis

ETIOLOGY AND EPIDEMIOLOGY. Affecting 1 billion people worldwide, this disease is caused by the nematode *Ascaris lumbricoides.* Human fecal–oral route is the usual mode of transmission.

CLINICAL MANIFESTATIONS. Asymptomatic infections are common. Clinical manifestations may depend on the organ affected by the worm. Small intestinal infection causes abdominal pain and distention; obstruction is a rare complication. Pulmonary infection leads to pneumonitis with eosinophilia and blood-tinged sputum production. Bile duct infection is rare, but may result in acute cholestasis with steatorrhea.

DIAGNOSIS. Stool examination is the basis for diagnosis.

TREATMENT. Pyrantel pamoate is the drug of choice and may be given as a single dose. Alternative agents are mebendazole or piperazine.

Hookworm Infections

ETIOLOGY AND EPIDEMIOLOGY. Although several species of hookworms may cause disease, *Necator americanus* is the most important in the western hemisphere and *Ancylostoma duodenale* is the predominant species in Europe. Larvae are found in appropriate soil conditions and infect hosts by skin penetration. From the skin, the larvae migrate to the lungs and ascend the trachea before being swallowed into the digestive tract for maturation.

CLINICAL MANIFESTATIONS. Infections usually are asymptomatic. Patients may experience intense itching at the site of skin penetration (ground itch). After migration to the gut, symptoms may include pain, distention, and diarrhea. Anemia invariably results from blood sucking by the offending worms.

DIAGNOSIS. Examination of the stool is diagnostic.

TREATMENT. Pyrantel pamoate or mebendazole should be used to treat infection. Iron therapy and, rarely, transfusion are necessary to treat anemia.

Enterobiasis (Pinworm)

ETIOLOGY AND EPIDEMIOLOGY. *Enterobius vermicularis* is a nematode with a worldwide distribution. Spread is by the fecal–oral route.

CLINICAL MANIFESTATIONS. Female worms live in the intestine and migrate to the perineum at night to lay their eggs. Worm irritation leads to the most common symp associated with pinworms: nocturnal pruritis ani. Vag salpingitis, and possibly appendicitis are associate pinworms.

DIAGNOSIS. Primary visualization of the worm, or the "Scotch tape test," results in diagnosis. The tape test is performed by placing a piece of clear adhesive on the perianal skin in the morning and then looking for eggs stuck to the tape under low-power microscopy.

TREATMENT. Pyrantel pamoate or mebendazole as a single dose usually is given. Because reinfection is common, a second dose 2 wk later or treatment of the entire family should be considered.

Visceral Larva Migrans

ETIOLOGY AND EPIDEMIOLOGY. Visceral larvae migrans is caused by ingestion of the eggs of *Toxocara* species (*canis, catii,* or *leonina*). Infection most commonly occurs in children with pica who have dogs or cats as pets. Mature worms reside in the dog or cat intestine; ingestion of the eggs in feces leads to human disease.

CLINICAL MANIFESTATIONS. After ingestion of eggs, the larva may migrate into any organ of the body and lead to disease. Symptoms depend on the organ affected. Nonspecific manifestations include fever, cough, rash, and adenopathy. Pulmonary signs include rales and wheezing. CNS infection may cause seizures. Visual symptoms and signs include decreased acuity, strabismus, and periorbital edema.

DIAGNOSIS. Biopsy is diagnostic, although not commonly done. ELISA may be helpful in diagnosis. Eosinophilia and hypergammaglobulinemia are common associated findings.

TREATMENT. Disease is self-limited. In severe disease, steroids and thiabendazole or diethylcarbamazine may be helpful.

Cutaneous Larva Migrans (Creeping Eruption)

ETIOLOGY AND EPIDEMIOLOGY. This syndrome is caused by skin contact with the larvae of many different species of nematodes found in soil, but is found most commonly with *Ancylostoma* species. The disease has a worldwide in distribution and is found predominantly in the southeastern states of the United States.

CLINICAL MANIFESTATIONS. Slow migration of the larvae at the dermal–epidermal junction leads to the main clinical feature: a serpiginous, raised, red track, typically found on the extremities.

DIAGNOSIS. This is made on clinical grounds.

TREATMENT. Treatment is not necessary because the syndrome resolves spontaneously in weeks to months. Alternatively, oral or topical thiabendazole or ethyl chloride spray may be used.

Schistosomiasis

ETIOLOGY AND EPIDEMIOLOGY. *Schistosoma* species (*haematobium, mansoni, japonicum, intercalatum,* and *mekongi*) are the cause of this disease. These agents are borne in contaminated water and penetrate intact skin. Once they ~ve gained entry, the worms migrate to known sites: *S.*

haematobium to the bladder and the others to the gut. Infection is uncommon in the United States.

CLINICAL MANIFESTATIONS. Symptoms and signs include nonspecific fever, rash, malaise, and cough as well as manifestations related to the organs affected. *S. haematobium* causes bladder granulomas and hematuria. Infection may lead to renal failure and bladder carcinoma. Infections caused by other species of *Schistosoma* cause intestinal ulceration, pain, and bloody diarrhea.

DIAGNOSIS. Eggs are typically found in the stool or urine.

TREATMENT. Praziquantel is the drug of choice.

Hydatid Disease

ETIOLOGY AND EPIDEMIOLOGY. Dogs become infected with these tapeworms, *Echinococcus granulosus*, by eating infected sheep or cattle. They then transmit disease to humans through the fecal–oral route. *Echinococcus* embryos pass through the intestines into the visceral organs and cause cystic disease. Distribution is worldwide, but disease in the Unites States is uncommon.

CLINICAL MANIFESTATIONS. Symptoms are related to the organs affected. Pulmonary cysts typically cause hemoptysis, cough, and respiratory distress. Liver cysts cause hepatomegaly and biliary stasis. Brain cysts cause focal neurologic findings and often are mistaken for tumors.

DIAGNOSIS. Serologic tests, ultrasonography, and more sensitive radiographic tests such as CT scan and MRI are essential in making the diagnosis.

TREATMENT. Surgical excision is required for large cysts. Mebendazole also may be effective.

11

THE DIGESTIVE SYSTEM

Much of the normal neurodevelopment of the gastrointestinal tract takes place in infancy, mimicking disease. Jaundice is common in the neonatal period because of the relative immaturity of the liver. During the 1st yr of life there may be great variation in appetite, stool color and output, and regurgitation. All may be due to normal day-to-day variation or symptomatic of underlying disease. More severe or long-lasting symptoms, such as dysphagia, anorexia, vomiting, diarrhea, constipation, gastrointestinal bleeding, abdominal distention, and pain, should be evaluated.

Dysphagia refers to disordered swallowing. Swallowing usually is well coordinated at birth; problems often are indicative of an oral or esophageal process. Neuromuscular disease may lead to transfer dysphagia. Esophageal obstruction resulting from intrinsic or extrinsic causes leads to dysphagia and regurgitation.

Anorexia is the loss of appetite. It is a common symptom of many disease processes, including those of the gastrointestinal tract.

Vomiting is a common symptom of many disease processes. It is caused by the violent contraction of gastrointestinal smooth muscle (unlike reflux, which is a more passive process). It may be a symptom of central nervous system disease, caused by stimulation of the emetic center in the medulla. Bile-stained vomitus is seen in cases in which there is obstruction or dysmotility distal to the second portion of the duodenum. The differential diagnosis of vomiting is listed in Table 11–1.

Diarrhea is the excessive loss of water and electrolytes in the stool. Diarrhea may be due to increased secretion of solute, increased motility through the intestines, decreased mucosal surface or function, and osmotic causes.

The causative mechanism of diarrhea varies with the disease. Secretory diarrhea is characteristic of cholera, toxigenic *Escherichia coli*, carcinoid, and neuroblastoma. Diarrhea resulting from increased motility is characteristic of irritable bowel syndrome, thyrotoxicosis, and the dumping syndrome. Mucosal invasion and disruption are characteristic of *Salmonella, Shigella, Yersinia,* and *Campylobacter*. Decreased mucosal surface leads to diarrhea in cases of bacterial overgrowth or the short bowel syndrome. Osmotic diarrhea is seen with malabsorption. A differential diagnosis of common causes of diarrhea is shown in Table 11–2.

Important causes of *constipation* and *abdominal* pain are listed in Tables 11–3 and 11–4, respectively.

Gastrointestinal bleeding is abnormal at any age. It may pres-

TABLE 11–1. DIFFERENTIAL DIAGNOSIS OF VOMITING DURING CHILDHOOD*

Infant	Child	Adolescent
Common		
Gastroenteritis	Gastroenteritis	Gastroenteritis
Gastroesophageal reflux	Systemic infection	Systemic infection
Overfeeding	Toxic ingestion	Toxic ingestion
Anatomic obstruction	Pertussis syndrome	Inflammatory bowel disease
Systemic infection	Medication	Appendicitis
		Migraine
		Pregnancy
		Medication
		Ipecac abuse/ bulimia
Rare		
Adrenogenital syndrome	Reye syndrome	Reye syndrome
Inborn error of metabolism	Hepatitis	Hepatitis
	Peptic ulcer	Peptic ulcer
	Pancreatitis	Pancreatitis
Brain tumor (increased intracranial pressure)	Brain tumor (Increased intracranial pressure)	Brain tumor (Increased intracranial pressure)
Subdural hemorrhage	Middle ear disease	Middle ear disease
Food poisoning	Chemotherapy	Chemotherapy
Rumination	Achalasia	Cyclic vomiting
Renal tubular acidosis	Cyclic vomiting	Biliary colic
	Esophageal stricture	Renal colic

* From Behrman RE (ed): Nelson Textbook of Pediatrics, 14th ed. Philadelphia, WB Saunders Company, 1992, p. 937.

TABLE 11–2. COMMON CAUSES OF DIARRHEA*

Infant	Child	Adolescent
Acute		
Gastroenteritis	Gastroenteritis	Gastroenteritis
Systemic infection	Food poisoning	Food poisoning
Antibiotic associated	Systemic infection	Antibiotic associated
	Antibiotic associated	
Chronic		
Postinfectious	Postinfectious	Inflammatory bowel disease
Secondary disaccharidase deficiency	Secondary disaccharidase deficiency	Lactose intolerance
Milk protein intolerance	Irritable colon syndrome	Giardiasis
Irritable colon syndrome	Celiac disease	Laxative abuse (anorexia nervosa)
Cystic fibrosis	Lactose intolerance	
Celiac disease	Giardiasis	
Short bowel syndrome		

* From Behrman RE (ed): Nelson Textbook of Pediatrics, 14th ed. Philadelphia, WB Saunders Company, 1992, p. 938.

TABLE 11–3. IMPORTANT CAUSES OF CONSTIPATION*

Nonorganic (functional)
Organic
  Intestinal
    Hirschsprung disease
    Anal–rectal stenosis
    Stricture
    Volvulus
    Pseudo-obstruction
    Chagas disease
  Drugs
    Narcotic
    Antidepressant
    Psychoactive (thorazine)
    Vincristine
  Metabolic
    Dehydration
    Cystic fibrosis (meconium ileus equivalent)
    Hypothyroidism
    Hypokalemia
    Renal tubular acidosis
    Hypercalcemia
  Neuromuscular
    Absent abdominal muscle
    Myotonic dystrophy
    Spinal cord lesions (tumors, spina bifida, diastematomyelia)
    Amyotonia congenita
  Psychiatric
    Anorexia nervosa

* From Behrman RE (ed): Nelson Textbook of Pediatrics, 14th ed. Philadelphia, WB Saunders Company, 1992, p. 938. (Adapted from Behrman RE, Kliegman RM: Nelson Essenbtials of Pediatrics. Philadelphia, WB Saunders, 1990.)

ent as hematemesis, melena, or hematochezia. Hematemesis is typical of esophageal bleeding, such as that due to severe esophagitis or varices. Melena is typical of upper gastrointestinal bleeding, such as that due to gastritis, ulcers, or swallowed blood. Hematochezia is more characteristic of lower gastrointestinal bleeding, such as that due to polyps or Meckel diverticulum, although it also may be seen with upper gastrointestinal bleeds in cases of increased motility.

DISEASES OF THE MOUTH
(*NELSON TEXTBOOK*, SECS. 13.1–13.11)

Diseases of the mouth are common in pediatrics and may be congenital or acquired. Any of the oral structures—the teeth, the soft tissues, the salivary glands, or the bones—may be affected, either alone or in combination.

THE TEETH

Development of the teeth begins at the 12th wk of gestation and continues into the teen years. Dental abnormalities are commonly first diagnosed by the pediatrician. Patients should be referred to a dentist by age 18–24 mo, with visits scheduled every 6–12 mo thereafter.

Congenital abnormalities of the teeth include those of abnormal number (anodontia, supernumary teeth), abnormal size (macrodontia, microdontia), and abnormal division (twinning). Patients also may experience dysplastic abnormalities of the dental anatomy, including those of the enamel or the dentin, as seen in cases of amelogenesis imperfecta, dentinogenesis imperfecta, and disturbances of calcification.

Natal teeth may occur in 1:2,000 live births and may run in families. The teeth most commonly found at birth are the two lower incisors. Because these teeth may interfere with feeding or may be aspirated, they often are removed.

Malocclusion refers to the malalignment of the upper and lower teeth such that the forces of mastication are not optimally distributed throughout the mouth. Malocclusion is a major cause of premature tooth loss. Examples of malocclusion include overbites and underbites, cross bites, and dental crowding.

Thumb sucking is a normal developmental phenomenon seen in more than half of children at some point in their childhood. If persistent, it may be associated with flaring of the central incisors. Although prognosis worsens in children greater than 6 yr of age, attempts at cessation are most successful in cases in which the child desires to stop.

Tooth decay is a common, preventable disease of childhood. The development of dental caries is due to a complex relationship between tooth surface, dietary carbohydrates (which are fermented into organic acids that erode the tooth surface), and oral bacteria (such as *Streptococcus mutans*). Frequent carbohydrate consumption seems to worsen the problem. Baby bottle tooth decay is due to prolonged exposure to carbohydrates occurring when the child is put to bed with a bottle of formula.

The prevalence of dental caries has decreased over the past few decades largely as a result of massive fluoridation programs. If the water supply is not fluoridated, supplemental fluoride should be given from birth into the teen years. The fluoride dose is 0.25 mg/24 hr for children less than 2 yr, 0.5 mg/24 hr for children 2–3 yr, and 1.0 mg/24 hr for children >3 yr. Early, regular dental care is also effective in the prevention of caries.

Oral injuries are very common in childhood, and the front incisors are affected most commonly in traumatic injuries involving the teeth. Fractures of the teeth may be complicated or uncomplicated depending on whether they involve the pulp. In general, pulp fractures are painful and may result in infection and necrosis. Displacement of the teeth also may occur and varies in severity from minor concussion to complete evulsion. Displaced teeth may be reimplanted and fixed with an acrylic splint, with varying long-term success. Rapid reimplantation and fixation correlates with better results.

TABLE 11-4. DISTINGUISHING FEATURES OF GASTROINTESTINAL TRACT PAIN IN CHILDHOOD*

Disease	Onset	Location	Referral	Quality	Comments
Functional: Irritable bowel syndrome	Recurrent	Periumbilical	None	Dull crampy, intermittent, 2-hr duration	Family stress, school phobia, onset about 5 yr old
Esophageal reflux	Recurrent, 1 hr after meal	Substernal	Chest	Burning	Sour taste in mouth; Sandifer syndrome
Duodenal ulcer	Recurrent, between meals, at night	Epigastric	Back	Severe burning, gnawing	Relieved by food, milk, antacids
Pancreatitis	Acute	Epigastric, left upper quadrant	Back	Constant, sharp, boring	Nausea, emesis, tenderness
Intestinal obstruction	Acute or gradual	Periumbilical—lower abdomen	Back	Alternating cramping (colic) and painless periods	Distention, obstipation, emesis, increased bowel sounds
Appendicitis	Acute	Periumbilical localized to RL quadrant	Back or pelvis if retrocecal	Sharp, steady	Nausea, emesis, local tenderness, fever

Meckel diverticulum	Recurrent	Periumbilical—lower abdomen	None	Sharp	Hematochezia
Inflammatory bowel disease	Recurrent	Lower abdomen	Back	Dull cramping, tenesmus	Fever, weight loss, hematochezia
Intussusception	Acute	Periumbilical—lower abdomen	None	Cramping, with painless periods	Hematochezia, knees in pulled up position
Lactose intolerance	Recurrent with milk products	Lower abdomen	None	Cramping	Distention, bloating, diarrhea
Urolithiasis	Acute, sudden	Back	Groin	Sharp, intermittent, cramping	Hematuria
Urinary tract infection	Acute, sudden	Back	Bladder	Dull to sharp	Fever, costochondral tenderness, dysuria, urinary frequency

* From Behrman RE (ed): Nelson Textbook of Pediatrics. 14th ed. Philadelphia, WB Saunders Company, 1992, p. 939. (Adapted from Behrman RE, Kliegman RM: Nelson Essentials of Pediatrics. Philadelphia, WB Saunders, 1990.)

THE SOFT TISSUES

Thrush, or oropharyngeal candidiasis, is probably the most common disease of the soft tissues of the mouth. Infection caused by the ubiquitous fungus *Candida albicans* appears as soft white plaques imbedded in the oral mucosa. Attempts at complete removal are unsuccessful and often hemorrhagic. Diagnosis is made by clinical appearance and confirmed by microscopic examination of the hyphae. Nystatin solution is effective therapy in most cases.

Aphthous ulcers, or canker sores, are painful ulcers of the mucosa that generally are <0.5 cm in diameter. They currently are thought to be due to an autoimmune process and are prone to recurrence. Lesions may heal more quickly with topical application of tetracycline. Differential diagnosis includes the gingival lesions of herpetic gingivostomatitis and herpangina.

Mucoceles are blue, raised vesicles that commonly appear on the lower lip and buccal mucosa. They are caused by minor traumatic rupture of a salivary duct, leading to a localized accumulation of mucus. Most resolve spontaneously, although recurrent lesions may require surgical excision.

CONGENITAL ANOMALIES THAT AFFECT THE MOUTH

A number of syndromes are associated with congenital oral anomalies, including Treacher Collins syndrome, Pierre Robin syndrome, Apert syndrome, and Crouzon disease. The most common major congenital anomalies of the mouth are clefts of the lip and palate.

Cleft lips result from hypoplasia of the embryonic mesenchyme found in the medial nasal and maxillary processes. They occur in 1:1,000 live births and may be associated with cleft palates and other anomalies. They may be unilateral and bilateral. Patients with isolated cleft lips may breast feed or drink from a bottle with minimal difficulty. Primary repair of cleft lip is typically undertaken at 2 mo, with plastic revision at 4–5 yr. Postoperative care must ensure a clean suture line with minimal stress on the tissues. Feedings should be given with a medicine dropper until there is good strength of the repair (usually 3 wk). Elbow cuffs should be used in an effort to keep the infant's hands away from the mouth.

Cleft palate occurs in 1:2,500 live births and results from poor fusion of the palate shelves. The cleft is usually in or near the midline and may connect the oropharynx with the nasopharynx either unilaterally or bilaterally. Feeding is difficult in patients with cleft palate and may be facilitated by the use of an obturator or bottle feeding through a soft nipple with a large hole. Closure is typically undertaken in the 1st yr of life, with revisions and orthodontic care as needed. Postoperative care is as with cleft lip. Recurrent otitis media, hearing, and phonation problems are common in patients with cleft palate.

DISEASES OF THE ESOPHAGUS
(*NELSON TEXTBOOK*, SECS. 13.15–13.25)

The esophagus is the organ responsible for the transport of food and liquids from the mouth to the stomach. Diseases of the esophagus may be congenital or acquired and essentially are of three types: obstructive diseases, motility diseases, and inflammatory diseases. Symptoms of esophageal disease include difficult or painful swallowing, choking, regurgitation or vomiting, and hematemesis.

TRACHEOESOPHAGEAL FISTULA AND ESOPHAGEAL ATRESIA

Esophageal atresia occurs in 1:3,000–4,000 births. In 85% of cases, there is also a fistula between the trachea and the distal esophagus; 30% of cases may have other associated anomalies, with cardiac anomalies the most common. Symptoms of esophageal atresia include excessive oral secretions, choking with feeds, and the inability to advance a feeding catheter into the stomach. As is true with any of the congenitally acquired high obstructions of the gastrointestinal tract, there is often a history of maternal polyhydramnios.

Diagnosis often is made on clinical grounds and may be confirmed by esophagram using a small amount of water-soluble contrast.

Treatment is surgical anastomosis of the two ends of the esophagus; this often must be done as a staged procedure if the two ends do not approximate each other.

ACHALASIA

Achalasia is an uncommon disease of adolescents and adults in which the lower esophageal sphincter fails to relax with swallowing. Symptoms include difficulty swallowing and regurgitation. Surgical correction involves ligation of the muscles at the cardioesophageal junction (Heller procedure).

CHALASIA

Gastroesophageal reflux, or chalasia, describes reflux across a dilated lower esophageal sphincter (LES) that is made worse by cough, crying, or other maneuvers that increase intra-abdominal pressure, and delayed gastric emptying. Eighty-five percent of infants with chalasia present with excessive reflux during the 1st wk of life. Symptoms improve in 60% of cases by age 2 yr as toddlers become more upright. Esophagitis may complicate the course, with the major symptom being hematemesis.

Diagnosis is suspected from the symptoms and may be confirmed by barium swallow or by placement of a pH probe in the distal end of the esophagus.

Medical *management* includes thickening feeds and postprandial placement in a prone position at a 30-degree angle. Cimetidine may be used for esophagitis, and metoclopramide may increase gastric motility while increasing LES tone.

In cases refractory to medical management, a surgical Nissen fundoplication may control reflux in 90% of cases.

ESOPHAGITIS

Esophagitis may occur secondary to repeated exposure to peptic acid or ingestion of corrosive substances, or as a result of infection, especially in immunocompromised patients. Infectious causes include viruses (herpes simplex virus [HSV], cytomegalovirus [CMV]), bacteria (diphtheria, tuberculosis, or secondary to downward extension of a retropharyngeal abscess), or fungi (*Candida*).

FOREIGN BODIES

Children commonly swallow any of a number of small objects that may become lodged in the esophagus. Symptoms include drooling, dysphagia, and occasionally dyspnea resulting from compression of the larynx.

Diagnosis usually is made radiographically and may require the instillation of a small amount of contrast material if the object is radiopaque.

Treatment involves esophagoscopic removal of objects trapped proximal to the LES. Objects distal to the LES require no intervention because they typically will pass in the stool without significant complication.

ESOPHAGEAL VARICES

Esophageal varices result from portal hypertension. The latter condition may result from obstruction, from thrombosis, as a sequela of umbilical venous catheterization, from infection, or from cirrhosis. Portosystemic shunts lead to varicosities in otherwise unimportant veins, such as those of the esophagus. Symptoms include massive hematemesis, ascites, and caput medusae. Bleeding can be life threatening and should be treated promptly. Plasma or vitamin K should be given in an effort to correct underlying coagulation defects, if present. Inflation of the balloon at the end of a Sengstaken–Blakemore tube placed in the esophagus may effectively tamponade the varices. Vasopressin may aid in hemostasis by vasoconstricting the blood vessels. Surgical interventions include sclerotherapy and splenorenal shunts.

OBSTRUCTIVE DISEASES OF THE STOMACH AND INTESTINES
(*NELSON TEXTBOOK*, SECS. 13.26–13.38)

The stomach and the intestines may become obstructed at any level as part of either congenital or acquired disease. Obstruction may be complete or partial, with complete lesions leading to more classic and dramatic presentations. High obstructive lesions tend to be associated with vomiting, which may be bilious if the site of obstruction is distal to the ampulla of Vater. Lower obstructions tend to lead to abdominal distention, often in association with constipation.

PYLORIC STENOSIS

Pyloric stenosis is the most common congenital obstruction of the stomach and intestines, occurring in 1:150 males and 1:750 females. It affects firstborn males more commonly and has a high concordance rate among monozygotic twins.

Clinical Manifestations

The clinical symptom of projectile vomiting, which usually presents in the 2nd or 3rd wk of life, is caused by hypertrophy and hyperplasia of the antrum of the stomach. The infants often appear wasted, with a fretful, "old man" appearance. Gastric peristaltic waves may be visible on physical exam, and a small, midepigastric "olive" may be palpable. Electrolyte abnormalities are common, with the patient often showing hyponatremia, hypokalemia, and a profound hypochloremic metabolic alkalosis.

Diagnosis

This is frequently made on clinical grounds if an olive is palpable. In more challenging cases, diagnosis may be suspected by the radiographic appearance of a large gastric bubble with a paucity of bowel gas seen distal to the obstruction. Abdominal ultrasound confirms the diagnosis. Differential diagnosis includes inexperienced parents, chalasia, hiatal hernia, duodenal stenosis, adrenal insufficiency, or inborn errors of metabolism.

Treatment

Surgical pyloromyotomy is indicated.

CONGENITAL DUODENAL OBSTRUCTION

Congenital causes of duodenal obstruction are duodenal atresia, malrotation of the intestines, annular pancreas, and duodenal webs. Duodenal atresia is the most common of these lesions and frequently is found among patients with Down syndrome.

Clinical Manifestations

Symptoms of duodenal obstruction include vomiting, which may be bilious or nonbilious depending on the site of the obstruction. The vomiting may be less projectile than that of pyloric stenosis and there is no palpable olive. On abdominal roentgenograms a "double bubble" sign is seen as a result of distention of the stomach and duodenum with a constricting pylorus between them.

Treatment

Therapy is surgical duodenoplasty, duodenoduodenostomy, or duodenojejunostomy in an effort to bypass the obstruction.

JEJUNAL, ILEAL OR COLON OBSTRUCTION

Obstructions of the jejunum or ileum may result from atresia or stenosis, meconium ileus, Hirschsprung disease, intussusception, Meckel diverticulum, intestinal duplication, or strangulated hernia.

Meconium Ileus

Meconium ileus is a syndrome most commonly associated with cystic fibrosis in which thick meconium is trapped in the terminal ileum. Symptoms include abdominal distention, vomiting, and constipation. On abdominal roentgenograms, a "ground glass" appearance may be seen in the right lower quadrant. Calcifications may be seen in cases with peritonitis. Treatment may include Gastrografin enema or surgical removal of meconium in refractory cases.

Hirschsprung Disease

Hirschsprung disease is the most common cause of neonatal obstruction of the colon. Males are affected more commonly than females. The disease is uncommon in premature infants. Hirschsprung disease results from the absence of ganglion cells in part or all of the wall of the colon, resulting in a state of chronic contraction. In 80% of cases, the aganglionic segment is limited to the rectosigmoid colon.

CLINICAL MANIFESTATIONS. Symptoms include constipation, distention, and bilious or feculent vomitus that typically presents in the newborn period. Cases with short-segment Hirschsprung disease may not become manifest until adolescence. Diagnosis may be suspected on barium enema by the appearance of a megacolon proximal to the aganglionic segment. Diagnosis is confirmed by the demonstration of an aganglionic segment of bowel on punch biopsy.

TREATMENT. Surgical resection of the aganglionic segment is indicated. This usually is done in two stages, with a colostomy and eventual reanastomosis.

Meckel Diverticulum

Diverticula and duplications may lead to obstruction of the intestines, with the most common of these being a Meckel diverticulum. Meckel diverticulum is the persistent remnant of the vitellointestinal duct. It occurs in 2–3% of individuals. Although this remnant may lead to diverticulitis, intussusception, or hernia, the most common complication is that of painless rectal bleeding resulting from gastric acid–secreting cells at the tip of the diverticulum that lead to ulceration and hemorrhage. Symptoms may occur at any age, but are most common in the first 2 yr of life. Diagnosis is made by a Meckel scan in which a radioisotope, 99m-technetium, localizes to gastric mucosa from which it is excreted. Treatment is surgical resection.

Acquired Obstructions

Acquired causes of intestinal obstruction include paralytic ileus resulting from infection, electrolyte imbalance, or uremia. Intussusception, cystic fibrosis, masses of round-worms, foreign bodies, bezoars, or tumors also may lead to acquired intestinal obstruction.

INTUSSUSCEPTION

Intussusception occurs when a segment of bowel is tele-scoped into another segment of bowel just distal to it. It is the most common cause of intestinal obstruction between 3 mo and 6 yr; it is more common in males.

Intussusceptions tend to occur in areas in which a peristaltic intestine abuts an aperistaltic segment. Aperistaltic segments are frequently found to be areas of enlarged Peyer patches, Meckel diverticulum, tumors, or hematomas complicating Henoch–Schönlein purpura. Intussusceptions most often are ileocolic or ileoileocolic.

Clinical Manifestations

Symptoms include sudden onset of paroxysmal colicky abdominal pain and vomiting that may progress to a shock-like state or bloody, "currant jelly" stools. Physical examination may reveal a sausage-shaped mass in the right upper abdomen.

Diagnosis and Treatment

These may be achieved with a barium enema, in which a "coiled spring"–appearing area of intussusception may be seen and reduction is achieved by hydrostatic pressure. If enema is unsuccessful in reducing the intussusception, surgical reduction must be performed. Left untreated, intussusception invariably leads to perforation, peritonitis, and death.

INFLAMMATORY GASTROINTESTINAL DISEASE
(*NELSON TEXTBOOK*, SECS. 13.39–13.48)

The noninfectious inflammatory gastrointestinal diseases include ulcers, ulcerative colitis, Crohn disease, Behçet disease, and food allergy.

ULCERS

There are two major types of ulcer disease in children, primary (peptic) ulcers and secondary (stress) ulcers. They are treated in a similar fashion.

Peptic Ulcers

Peptic ulcers occur primarily in the duodenum, although primary gastric ulcers are common in the first 2 yr of life. Their pathogenesis is not completely understood, but there is a family history of ulcers in 25–50% of patients, implying a genetic predisposition. Environmental exposures, drugs, the presence of gastric acidity, and an ill-understood relationship with *Helicobacter pylori,* which frequently is cultured from biopsy specimens, all seem to play a role.

CLINICAL MANIFESTATIONS AND DIAGNOSIS. Symptoms of peptic ulcer disease include vomiting, gastrointestinal blood loss, and dull, aching, or nocturnal abdominal pain. Diagnosis may be suspected in cases with a positive family history and may be made roentgenographically or by direct visualization with gastroduodenoscopy.

TREATMENT. Products that enhance ulcer formation, such as tobacco, caffeine, alcohol, and nonsteroidal anti-inflammatory drugs, should be avoided. Antacids containing magnesium, aluminum, or calcium buffers may be used to neutralize excess acid. Acid secretion may be inhibited with histamine-2 (H_2) blockers such as cimetidine and ranitidine or omeprazole, a hydrogen–potassium pump inhibitor. Sucralfate may be used to coat the ulcers locally.

Stress Ulcers

Stress ulcers usually are acute and occur in association with physical trauma, burns, shock and sepsis, or other critical illness. Treatment is as detailed above for peptic ulcers.

ULCERATIVE COLITIS

Ulcerative colitis (UC) is a disease characterized by recurrent bouts of profuse, explosive bloody diarrhea. Approximately 20% of cases begin in childhood or adolescence, with the peak age of onset being 15–25 yr. The cause is unknown, but it is presumed that the disease begins following exposure to some antigenic trigger in genetically predisposed individuals. The antibody response leads to inflammation of the terminal colon. It is marked by distorted crypt architecture, crypt abscesses, and infiltration of the lamina propria that may extend proximally to involve the whole colon.

Clinical Manifestations

Symptoms include bloody diarrhea with mucus, fecal urgency, tenesmus, and crampy abdominal pain, particularly just before defecation. Systemic signs and symptoms include weight loss, anorexia, arthritis, erythema nodosum, pyoderma gangrenosum, iritis, hepatitis, clubbing of the fingers, and hemolytic anemia, although these complaints are seen less commonly than with Crohn disease. The most serious complications of UC are profuse hemorrhage, toxic megacolon, and colon cancer, which may occur in 20% of patients after 10 years of disease.

Diagnosis

This is typically made by colonoscopy. Friable, inflamed mucosa is seen, with inflammatory cells and crypt abscesses seen on biopsy.

Treatment

In general, diet should be left unrestricted and nutritious. Sulfasalazine is used to reduce inflammatory activity in the colon and limit exacerbations. Corticosteroids are effective in the treatment of acute disease flares. The disease may be cured by resection of the entire colon. This is commonly considered during the second decade of disease as the risk of cancer grows.

CROHN DISEASE

Crohn disease is a segmental, transmural inflammatory disease that typically affects the distal ileum and colon. Some 25–40% of cases begin before the age of 20 yr. The cause of the disease is unknown, but is presumed to be similar to that of UC. The inflammatory process is characterized by regional noncaseating granulomas. Fistula formation between loops of bowel and adjoining structures is common.

Clinical Manifestations

Symptoms include crampy abdominal pain and diarrhea that is typically less explosive than that seen in UC. Systemic symptoms are common, and include fever, anorexia, weight loss, arthritis, and finger clubbing. Erythema nodosum, iritis, hepatitis, and phlebitis are rare.

Diagnosis

This is suggested by clinical features and a high erythrocyte sedimentation rate. Diagnosis usually is confirmed by the appearance of segmental disease with bowel wall thickening, irregular cobblestone appearance, and fistula formation on barium contrast roentgenograms.

Treatment

Diet should be left unrestricted and nutritious except during periods of acute exacerbations. During flares, bowel rest using hyperalimentation or an elemental diet usually diminishes disease activity. Corticosteroids also have been found to be helpful during disease flares. More chronic therapy using azathioprine, 6-mercaptopurine, metronidazole, methotrexate, or cyclosporine has been advocated in severe cases.

FOOD ALLERGIES

Food protein intolerance may lead to chronic gastrointestinal symptoms by any of the antigenically mediated hypersensitivity pathways. Manifestations may include oral ulceration, abdominal pain, vomiting, and diarrhea that may be bloody. Diagnosis is made clinically by elimination of the offending allergen and demonstration of symptomatic improvement. Most cases of food protein intolerance are transitory: 50% of cases will resolve within 1 yr, with the remainder typically resolving in 2 yr.

IRRITABLE BOWEL SYNDROME

Although this is not an inflammatory disease of the bowel, it is a common cause of recurrent or chronic gastrointestinal symptoms, particularly among teenagers. In children <2 yr of age, the cause usually is organic. In older children, an organic cause is identified in <10% of patients.

Clinical Manifestations

Signs and symptoms are nonspecific and inconsistent. Patients tend to look well. Attacks of pain are variable in their relationship to food or activity. Tenderness on examination often is variable in location and degree. It is not consistently reproducible among observers. A history of psychological disturbances may be present.

Diagnosis

This relies more on clinical judgment than on the laboratory. Urine and stool assays for infection often are the most useful tests, and gynecologic assessment, including pregnancy testing, should be considered where appropriate. Other tests, including ultrasonography, barium contrast studies, and endoscopy, are not generally helpful and should be reserved for atypical or severe cases.

Treatment

This consists primarily of reassurance and promotion of a normal sense of health.

MALABSORPTIVE DISORDERS
(*NELSON TEXTBOOK*, SECS. 13.49–13.64)

Malabsorptive disorders of the digestive tract may occur for any of a variety of reasons. Despite these myriad causes, clinical manifestations of malabsorption are strikingly similar: abdominal distention, wasting of the proximal muscle groups, failure to thrive, and pale, foul, or bulky stools commonly are noted. Evaluation begins with a history and physical examination, of which the rectal examination is among the most important components. Laboratory evaluation involves identifying those substances that are being malabsorbed and then identifying the anatomic site responsible.

Fat malabsorption is best diagnosed by quantitation of fecal fat relative to dietary fat intake. In a sample of stool collected for 3–4 days, stool fat excretion should not exceed 15% of dietary fat in an infant and 10% of dietary fat in older children. Because this method is cumbersome, other tests, such as fasting serum carotene levels, may be performed, although these lack the sensitivity and specificity of fecal fat assays.

Carbohydrate malabsorption is more easily assayed. The normal stool typically is carbohydrate free. The presence of reducing sugars (most dietary sugars, except sucrose) in the stool may be assayed easily at the bedside. Sucrose can be assayed only after hydrolysis with HCl. Intraluminal carbohydrates are fermented into organic acids by the intestinal flora, leading to more acidic stools (pH < 6.0) and the liberation of hydrogen gas in the breath. Both of these may be assayed readily.

Protein malabsorption may be diagnosed by the fecal clearance of α_1-antitrypsin.

Localization of the affected area of intestine may be inferred from the profile of substances being malabsorbed, or by more specific methods.

D-Xylose is absorbed exclusively by the upper small bowel. Low *urinary levels of xylose* after a dietary challenge implies a proximal intestinal lesion.

The *Schilling test* assays for the absorption of vitamin B_{12} with and without supplemental intrinsic factor. Poor absorption after dietary administration of B_{12} when given with supplemental intrinsic factor implies disease in the terminal ileum.

Disease also may be localized by *radiographic methods* using barium contrast roentgenograms, ultrasonography, and peroral biopsy techniques.

BACTERIAL OVERGROWTH SYNDROME

This syndrome typically occurs in conjunction with partial obstructions of the proximal bowel, which lead to dysmotility, mucosal interruption, and overcolonization with enteric flora. These bacteria deconjugate bile salts, leading to fat malabsorption. They also may damage the microvillus brush border, interfering with disaccharidase activity and leading to carbohydrate intolerance. Treatment involves correction of the partial obstruction and the use of oral antibiotics in an effort to limit bacterial growth.

SHORT BOWEL SYNDROME

Short bowel syndrome arises in congenital or acquired conditions in which a large segment of the small intestine is missing. It is most commonly seen as a complication of surgical resection. Absorption is compromised by loss of mucosa, bacterial overgrowth, and gastric hyperacidity. In cases in which the ileum is lost, malabsorption of bile salts leads to particularly profound water loss and steatorrhea.

Treatment involves limitation of dietary fats and supplementation with medium-chain triglycerides. Cholestyramine may be used to bind bile salts in cases of severe steatorrhea. Simple sugars may be better tolerated than complex carbohydrates. Vitamin supplements usually are necessary. Antidiarrheal medicines are of no value in the treatment of this disease.

CELIAC DISEASE (Gluten-Sensitive Enteropathy)

Celiac disease is a lifelong intolerance to gliadin, a protein contained in wheat, rye, and barley. Eighty to 90% of patients are HLA-B8 positive, and enteric infection with adenovirus 12 may trigger the disease in a susceptible host. Intestinal damage is mediated by both cellular and humoral immune mechanisms, with antigliadin, antireticulin, and antimysium antibodies being indicators of sensitization to gluten.

Clinical Manifestations

Signs and symptoms of celiac disease vary in severity and include failure to thrive, anorexia, diarrhea, vomiting, wasted proximal muscle groups, and abdominal distention. Selective immunoglobulin A (IgA) deficiency and diabetes mellitus are associated with celiac disease.

Diagnosis

This is made by intestinal biopsy, in which short, flat villi with deep crypts and lymphocytic infiltration are seen. All other tests may support the diagnosis, but lack specificity and sensitivity. Mucosal damage may be diagnosed with D-xylose challenge test. Serum antibodies to gliadin may be detected. Anemia commonly is associated, and vitamin B_{12} deficiency and hypoalbuminemia also may occur.

Treatment

Therapy requires lifelong elimination of all wheat, rye, and barley from the diet. Maize, rice, and a small amount of oats are tolerated well. Early treatment should include simple carbohydrates and fat supplementation, because mucosal damage early in therapy will interfere with absorption.

CHRONIC PERSISTENT DIARRHEA

This syndrome typically occurs in children after an acute infectious diarrhea, and commonly complicates acute gastroenteritis in the developing world. Predisposing factors include poverty, immunosuppression, malnutrition, lack of breast feeding, and antecedent bacterial enteritis. Carbohydrates and, to a lesser extent, fats and proteins are malabsorbed.

Diagnosis is made by demonstration of reducing substances and low pH in the stool consistent with carbohydrate malabsorption. Fat and protein malabsorption also may be detected. Differential diagnosis includes parasitic infections and any of the other malabsorption syndromes discussed in this section.

Treatment includes rehydration, by the oral route if possible. Breast milk, if available, is the best source of nutrition for these children; otherwise elemental formulas should be used.

TODDLER DIARRHEA

Toddler diarrhea is a chronic diarrhea occurring in children 6–30 mo of age. It usually is seen in otherwise healthy children, without associated weight loss, malabsorption, or dehydration. All laboratory tests are normal. It is probably a variant or early manifestation of irritable bowel syndrome and should be treated with reassurance.

OTHER MALABSORPTION SYNDROMES

Other malabsorption syndromes include *intractable diarrhea of infancy*, which is probably similar in pathogenesis to chronic persistent diarrhea. *Tropical sprue* is a syndrome of general malabsorption confined to certain tropical regions that usually responds to antibiotics and nutritional supplementation, thereby implicating the intestinal flora in its pathogenesis. *Whipple syndrome, intestinal lymphangiectasia,* and *Wolman disease* are other rare causes of malabsorption in childhood.

Specific Enzyme Deficiencies That Lead to Malabsorption

Of the specific enzymatic deficiencies that lead to malabsorption, the most commonly seen in *lactase deficiency*. This may be seen as a normal variant in some ethnic groups or may transiently complicate infection or celiac disease. Symptoms include bloating, borborygmi, abdominal pain, and diarrhea. Diagnosis is made by detection of reducing substances in the stool. Treatment may include reduction in the intake of milk products and lactase supplementation.

Other enzymatic deficiencies that may lead to malabsorption are rare and, for the most part, congenitally acquired. Symptoms vary with the protein, vitamin, or ion that is not absorbed. Treatment is through nutritional supplementation. Examples of such diseases include acrodermatitis enteropathica, which is due to zinc malabsorption; Menkes kinky hair syndrome, which is due to copper malabsorption; and pernicious anemia.

ACUTE APPENDICITIS
(*NELSON TEXTBOOK*, SEC. 13.66)

Acute appendicitis is the most common cause of abdominal surgery in childhood. The disease typically is caused by some obstruction of the lumen of the appendix that leads to inspissation of mucus, ischemia of the mucosal tissues, bacterial invasion and infection of the deteriorating appendiceal tissue, and ultimate perforation. Examples of such obstructions include fecoliths, calculi, submucosal lymphoid tissue, and tumors.

CLINICAL MANIFESTATIONS

Symptoms include abdominal pain that begins as cramps in the periumbilical region as a result of stimulation of the visceral pain fibers. As the inflammation grows to involve the parietal nerve fibers, the pain localizes to the area overlying the appendix. In most cases this is the "McBurney point," which is located in the lateral third of an imaginary line drawn between the umbilicus and the anterior superior iliac spine. If the appendix is retrocecal, pain may be elicited best on rectal examination or by extension or abduction of the hip (psoas and obturator signs, respectively). Associated symptoms include fever, tachycardia, vomiting, and anorexia.

DIAGNOSIS

This is suspected by clinical examination. Abdominal ultrasound is helpful in cases without perforation, reliably demonstrating an enlarged, edematous appendix. Abdominal roentgenograms are typically nonspecific and should not be routinely done. Associated lab findings include a high white blood cell count and pyuria in cases in which the inflamed appendix overlies the right ureter.

COMPLICATIONS

These include rupture and peritonitis, which are seen more commonly in young children and in those whose diagnosis has been delayed. Postoperative complications include wound infection and intestinal obstruction resulting from adhesion formation.

TREATMENT

Surgical removal of the inflamed appendix is required. Preoperative antibiotics are routinely used, with postoperative continuation if a perforation is found.

TUMORS OF THE INTESTINAL TRACT
(*NELSON TEXTBOOK*, SEC. 13.68)

Because primary malignancy of the gastrointestinal tract is rare in childhood, tumors of the intestinal tract may be best thought of as benign or premalignant.

JUVENILE COLONIC POLYPS

These benign lesions are the most common tumor of the bowel in childhood, affecting 3–4% of people before age 21 yr. The lesions are hamartomas that are most often solitary and located in the sigmoid region. Multiple juvenile colonic polyps may be found in families, inherited as an autosomal dominant trait. This latter variant also is benign but must be distinguished from the similarly inherited premalignant conditions listed below.

Symptoms include painless rectal bleeding during or immediately after a bowel movement. Diagnosis is made by rectal examination or by colonoscopy, during which the lesion usually is removed. Recurrences are unusual.

FAMILIAL ADENOMATOUS POLYPOSIS COLI

This premalignant condition is inherited as an autosomal dominant condition with reduced penetrance and is characterized by a large number of adenomatous polyps in the distal colon. The gene coding for this lesion is found on the long arm of chromosome 5. Symptoms include hematochezia, cramps, and, rarely, diarrhea. Diagnosis is made by colonoscopy. Management includes colonoscopy every 2 yr in children >12 yr, monitoring for malignant change. Malignancy is treated with pancolectomy.

OTHER TUMORS OF THE GASTROINTESTINAL TRACT

Rare tumors of the gastrointestinal tract include the benign hamartomas seen with the Peutz-Jeghers syndrome, the premalignant polyps seen with Gardner syndrome, and the low-grade malignant carcinoid tumors, which most commonly occur in the appendix and may lead to appendicitis.

DISEASES OF THE PANCREAS
(*NELSON TEXTBOOK*, SECS. 13.70–13.80)

The exocrine pancreas is responsible for the elaboration of numerous enzymes important for digestion. The main pancreatic disorder of childhood is cystic fibrosis (see Chap. 12). Other diseases of the pancreas are less common, and are due to anatomic, metabolic, congenital, autoimmune, or inflammatory pathology. These diseases may be detected anatomically through the use of abdominal ultrasonography or computerized tomography (CT) scans. Pancreatic function usually is assayed by fecal fat analysis or by direct measurement of the pancreatic enzyme activity in the stool or duodenal contents.

ANATOMIC DISEASE

Anatomic diseases of the pancreas include *pancreas divisum*, which occurs in 5–15% of the population. This normal variant results from failure of the dorsal and ventral pancreatic anlagen to fuse and may be associated with recurrent pancreatitis. *Annular pancreas* results from incomplete rotation of the ventral pancreatic anlage and usually presents as a partial small bowel obstruction in infancy. Choledochal cysts are dilations of the biliary tract that typically cause biliary symptoms but may mimic acute pancreatitis.

PANCREATIC INSUFFICIENCY

Cystic fibrosis is the main cause of pancreatic insufficiency in childhood. Other causes are rare and include Shwachman-Diamond syndrome, enzymatic defects, and chronic pancreatitis.

Shwachman-Diamond syndrome is an autosomal recessive condition in which there is pancreatic insufficiency, neutropenia, metaphyseal dysostosis, failure to thrive, and short stature. Patients present in infancy with symptoms of malabsorption, normal sweat chloride levels, and characteristic bony changes. Recurrent pyogenic infections, anemia, and thrombocytopenia may complicate this disease.

Treatment of pancreatic insufficiency consists of enzymatic replacement with commercially available preparations. Dosage varies with meal size and fat content and should be titrated to normalize stools. Supplementation with fat-soluble vitamins may be necessary.

ACUTE PANCREATITIS

Acute pancreatitis may result from mumps or other viral infection, drugs, or blunt trauma. After the initial insult, pancreatic enzymes leak from the acinar structures into the pancreatic tissue, resulting in autodigestion of the organ.

Clinical Manifestations

Symptoms are epigastric pain, vomiting, and fever. Diagnosis usually is based on clinical symptoms and serum amylase levels. Serum lipase or immunoreactive trypsin also are elevated. Anatomic changes may be appreciated on abdominal ultrasound or CT scan.

Treatment

This involves pain relief with meperidine and restoration of metabolic homeostasis with judicious use of intravenous fluids. Patients should not be fed until the serum amylase returns to normal, which is typically 2–4 days. Vomiting patients should have nasogastric suction.

Complications

These are uncommon and include pancreatic hemorrhage and pancreatic pseudocyst formation. The former is rare in children, but carries a mortality of 50%. The latter also is uncommon and should be treated with either surgical or percutaneous drainage.

CHRONIC PANCREATITIS

Chronic relapsing pancreatitis may be inherited as an autosomal dominant condition or may be due to congenital anomalies of the biliary tract or pancreas. It also may be associated with hyperlipidemia, hyperparathyroidism, ascariasis, or cystic fibrosis. Manifestations are recurrent attacks of abdominal pain, vomiting, and fever lasting 4–7 days, and typically worsening in their severity over time. Therapy is supportive, with correction of the underlying defect where possible.

DISEASES OF THE LIVER AND BILIARY SYSTEM
(NELSON TEXTBOOK, SECS. 13.81–13.102)

The liver performs a number of important bodily functions. The organ is important in carbohydrate metabolism, storing excess carbohydrate as glycogen when excess substrate is available and liberating carbohydrate during times of fast. A number of proteins are synthesized by the liver, including albumin, α-fetoprotein, fibrinogen, transferrin, ceruloplasmin, and the factors of the coagulation and complement cascades. Lipids are metabolized by the liver as an emergency energy source. Fat absorption relies on bile salts synthesized by the liver. The liver is also the most important organ in the metabolism and detoxification of drugs and toxins.

CLINICAL MANIFESTATIONS OF DISEASE

Signs of liver disease include hepatomegaly and right upper quadrant tenderness, which are best assessed by clinical examination. Jaundice may be the only manifestation of liver disease and is due to the accumulation of bilirubin. Pruritus occurs in patients with cholestasis and probably is due to retention of bile salts. Xanthomata are intradermal subcutaneous collections of cholesterol and are seen with chronic cholestasis. Spider angiomata reflect altered estrogen metabolism. Ascites may be due to increases in portal venous pressure or hypoalbuminemia. Palmar erythema may be due to vasodilation and increased blood flow. Nonspecific symptoms of liver disease include anorexia, abdominal pain, and bleeding resulting from altered synthesis of coagulation factors.

The central nervous system may be involved in severe cases. Hepatic encephalopathy may produce neuromuscular dysfunction, altered mentation, or alterations in consciousness, including coma. Changes may be due to profound inhibition caused by increases in γ-aminobutyric acid or decreases in other neuroactive compounds, such as glycine.

Renal dysfunction also may accompany severe liver disease. The **hepatorenal syndrome** is defined as otherwise unexplainable renal failure in a patient with cirrhosis. Although the reasons for this complication are not completely understood, alterations in renal blood flow seem to be involved.

LABORATORY EVALUATION

Liver dysfunction may be evaluated by a number of serologic tests. Assays of the blood include serum bilirubin, aminotransferases, alkaline phosphatase, prothrombin time, and albumin. Bilirubin most commonly is assayed as total bilirubin, with assays of direct (conjugated or glucuronidated) and indirect (albumin-bound) fractions available. The direct fraction commonly is elevated in hepatic or cholestatic disease. Aminotransferases are sensitive indicators of hepatocellular disease, with alanine aminotransferase (ALT, SGPT) being more specific than aspartate aminotransferase (AST, SGPT). Alkaline phosphatase and 5'-nucleotidase levels are sensitive indicators of obstructive processes of the biliary tract. Elevation of prothrombin times may be an early indicator of impaired synthesis in the liver, whereas depressed albumin levels reflect longer standing disease. Hypoglycemia, electrolyte abnormalities, and hyperammonemia are nonspecifically found in hepatic disease.

IMAGING PROCEDURES

The liver may be visualized radiographically. Ultrasonography provides information about the size, composition, and blood flow of the liver. A hyperechogenic liver may be seen with metabolic diseases, with fatty infiltration, or following corticosteroid therapy. Mass lesions as small as 1–2 cm may be detected. Information about the gallbladder and bile ducts may be shown. CT scans or magnetic resonance imaging may provide more precise anatomic detail.

Radionuclide scans using various radioisotopes are available. Perhaps most helpful is scanning with 99m-technetium–labeled iminodiacetic acid, which is taken up by hepatocytes and excreted into the bile. In cases of intrahepatic cholestasis, there is poor uptake of the radioisotope with fairly normal excretion, whereas in cases of extrahepatic obstruction, there is normal uptake and delayed excretion.

Cholangiography, endoscopic retrograde cholangiopancreatograpy (ERCP), and selective angiography are other ways of visualizing the hepatobiliary tree.

NEONATAL CHOLESTASIS

Neonatal cholestasis may be due to infections, genetic causes, metabolic diseases, or functional impairment of bile flow. Symptoms include dark urine, clay-colored (acholic) stools, hepatomegaly, and jaundice. The first step in evaluation is the differentiation of conjugated from unconjugated bilirubin, the former being less common and more indicative of hepatobiliary disease. Next, the physician must recognize and begin treatment for any treatable causes of secondary direct hyperbilirubinemia, including sepsis, hypothyroidism, or specific metabolic disease such as galactosemia or tyrosinemia. Finally, primary causes of direct hyperbilirubinemia should be sought. These include infectious causes and intrahepatic and extrahepatic obstructions.

Intrahepatic Bile Duct Paucity

Alagille syndrome is the most common syndrome in which there is intrahepatic bile duct paucity. Clinical features of the syndrome include unusual facies, ocular anomalies, cardiovascular anomalies, vertebral arch defects, and nephropathy. Although survival may be prolonged, the disease is marked by progressive destruction of the bile ducts and increasing features of cholestasis.

Zellweger (*cerebrohepatorenal*) *syndrome* is marked by unusual facies, hepatomegaly, renal cortical cysts, ocular abnormalities, and stippled calcifications of the patella and greater trochanter. The disease is inherited as an autosomal recessive trait. Absence of peroxisomes is seen on microscopic assessment of the liver.

Extrahepatic Biliary Atresia

The most common variant of this disease (85%) shows obstruction of the bile ducts at or above the portal hepatis. Distal atresia is less common and more easily treated. The disease occurs in 1:10,000–15,000 live births.

CLINICAL MANIFESTATIONS AND DIAGNOSIS. Symptoms suggestive of cholestasis become present in the 1st wk of life. Evaluation should include ultrasound in an effort to rule out more readily treatable causes of chole-stasis, such as choledochal cyst. Radionuclide scan using iminodiacetic acid analogues may be helpful in differentiating between neonatal hepatitis and biliary atresia. Liver biopsy usually is diagnostic.

TREATMENT. Therapy includes laparoscopy with surgical correction in cases of distal atresia and the Kasai (hepatoportoenterostomy) procedure in cases in which direct drainage cannot be accomplished easily. Liver transplant often ultimately is necessary in these latter cases.

Long-term medical management of patients with cholestasis includes supplementation with fat-soluble vitamins. Normal dietary fats should be replaced or supplemented with medium-chain triglycerides. Protein intake should be limited in an effort to maintain nitrogen balance without hyperammonemia. Minerals such as calcium, phosphorus, and zinc and water-soluble vitamins should be provided. Phenobarbital may act as a choleretic and cholestyramine binds bile acids. Ascites should be treated with salt restriction and diuretics, using paracentesis and albumin infusion in extreme cases.

ACUTE HEPATIC DISEASES

Although acute hepatic disease may occur alone or as part of systemic disease, the most common cause of acute hepatic disease in children is infection. In addition to the five known hepatotrophic viruses outlined in Table 11–5, CMV and Epstein-Barr virus commonly may lead to hepatitis. Other infections of the liver include hepatic abscesses, most commonly the result of infection with *Staphylococcus aureus*, *E. coli*, *Salmonella* species, anaerobic organisms, or *Entamoeba histolytica*.

Liver disease also may complicate diseases of other organ systems. UC and Crohn disease may be complicated by hepatobiliary complications. Bacterial sepsis, most commonly due to *E. coli*, *Klebsiella pneumoniae*, and *Pseudomonas aeruginosa*, may lead to an endotoxin-mediated cholestasis. Congestive heart failure and cyanosis each may lead to liver disease. Total parenteral nutrition commonly leads to cholestasis, especially among low-birth-weight infants. Veno-occlusive disease and graft-versus-host disease commonly may complicate bone marrow transplants.

Reye Syndrome

This acute disease of the liver is associated with antecedent viral infection and use of salicylates. The incidence of Reye syndrome has dropped from a peak of 400 cases in 1974 to 20 cases in 1988, largely as a result of reduction in salicylate use.

Clinical Manifestations

These begin 5–7 days after the onset of a viral illness and include vomiting and rapidly progressive global neurologic symptoms. Laboratory findings include hyperammonemia and elevated liver and muscle enzymes, such as ALT, AST,

TABLE 11–5. CHARACTERISTICS OF THE AGENTS CAUSING ACUTE VIRAL HEPATITIS*

	Hepatitis A Virus (HAV; Enterovirus 72)	Hepatitis B† Virus (HBV)	Hepatitis C‡ Virus (HCV; formerly post-transfusion non-A, non-B virus)	Hepatitis D Virus (HDV)	Hepatitis E Virus (HEV; formerly enteral non-A, non-B virus)
Agent	27-nm RNA virus	42-nm DNA virus	60–70-nm RNA virus Similar to flaviviruses	36-nm RNA hybrid particle with HB$_s$Ag coat	32–34-nm RNA virus Similar to Norwalk type viruses
Transmission	Fecal–oral Food–water	Transfusion, sexual, inoculation, vertical	Parenteral, transfusion, vertical (sexual?)	Similar to HBV	Enteral: endemic and epidemic
Incubation period	30 days	60–180 days	30–60 days		25–60 days
Serum markers	Anti-HIV	Antigens†, Anti-HB$_s$ Anti-HB$_c$	Anti-HCV (IgG, IgM)	Similar to HBV Anti-HDV, RNA	Anti-HEV
Fulminant liver failure	Rare	Uncommon unless with δ agent§	Uncommon	Yes	Yes in pregnancy

230

Chronic liver disease	No	Yes	Yes	Yes	Uncommon
Carrier state	No	Yes||	Yes	Yes	No
Risk of hepatocellular cancer	No	Yes	Yes	No	No
Prophylaxis against	Immune serum globulin; hygiene	Hepatitis B immune globulin vaccine; Screen blood products for HBsAg	Screen blood for antibody appearing 4 mo postinfection (6 mo post-transfusion)	Screen blood for HBV markers	Screen blood for IgM, IgG antibody

* From Behrman RE (ed): Nelson Textbook of Pediatrics, 14th ed. Philadelphia, WB Saunders Company, 1992, p. 1017.
† Hepatitis B whole virus particle is the Dane particle, which consists of a surface antigen HBsAg, a core antigen HBcAg, an e antigen HBeAg, and DNA with a DNA polymerase.
‡ An unknown number of post-transfusion hepatitis cases are due to viruses other than HBV, HCV or cytomegalovirus, Epstein-Barr virus, human herpesvirus-6, or known agents and remain designated as caused by a non-A, non-B hepatitis agent.
§ The δ agent or hepatitis D virus requires hepatitis B virus coinfection or superinfection of a chronic HBV carrier for replication.
|| Chronic carrier state common in Afro-Asian, Haitian, Eskimo, South Pacific immigrants, drug abusers, Down syndrome, multiply transfused patients, homosexuals, patients on hemodialysis, and dental workers.

creatine phosphokinase, and lactate dehydrogenase. The mitochondrial enzyme glutamate dehydrogenase is greatly elevated.

Treatment

Reye syndrome management relies on supportive care, including maneuvers attempting to control elevations in intracranial pressure, such as fluid restriction, hyperventilation, osmotherapy, and pentobarbital. Blood pressure should be supported with intravenous fluids and cardiotonic drugs. Coagulopathies should be treated with plasma.

CHRONIC HEPATIC DISEASE

Chronic diseases of the liver may be due to (1) chronic hepatocyte injury; (2) storage of lipid, glycogen, or other products; (3) metabolic defects; or (4) chronic infection.

Metabolic Diseases of the Liver

Glucuronyl transferase deficiency leads to *Crigler-Najjar syndrome,* which has two types: the severe, autosomal recessive type; and the more common, less severe, autosomal dominant type. The former is marked by severe unconjugated hyperbilirubinemia and pale yellow stools during the first days of life. The disease is diagnosed by biopsy and measurement of hepatic glucuronyl transferase activity. It usually progresses to kernicterus by young adulthood. The latter is marked by a lesser degree of unconjugated hyperbilirubinemia, which usually declines in response to low-dose phenobarbital. It rarely causes kernicterus.

Enzyme defects causing conjugated hyperbilirubinemia include *Dubin-Johnson syndrome* and *Rotor syndrome.* Both are inherited as autosomal recessive traits and lead to a mild conjugated hyperbilirubinemia that usually is diagnosed in adolescence or young adulthood. Other liver function tests are typically normal.

Wilson disease (hepatolenticular degeneration) is an autosomal recessive disorder characterized by degenerative changes in the brain, cirrhosis, and Kayser–Fleischer rings in the cornea. The disease is caused by improper copper excretion resulting from low ceruloplasmin levels. Clinical manifestations include neurologic or behavioral changes, liver disease, and acute hemolysis. Demonstration of a low serum ceruloplasmin level, high concentrations of urinary copper, or liver biopsy confirm the diagnosis. Treatment includes avoidance of foods containing high levels of copper, such as liver, shellfish, nuts, and chocolate. Chelation therapy with either penicillamine or triethylene tetramine dihydrochloride should be used. Vitamin B_6 should be supplemented in patients taking penicillamine.

α_1-*Antitrypsin deficiency* may lead to neonatal cholestasis and ultimately childhood cirrhosis. Although 20 different codominant alleles code for the protease inhibitor, it is usually only the PiZZ genotype that causes liver disease. Diagnosis is made by determination of the α_1-antitrypsin phenotype and is confirmed by liver biopsy. Liver transplantation is curative.

Chronic Hepatitis

Chronic hepatitis may be due to infection (hepatitis B, C, and D), drugs (such as isoniazid, aldomet, and sulfonamides), or an idiopathic, probably autoimmune, mechanism. The majority of cases fit into the last group and commonly are associated with other autoimmune diseases. The symptoms and prognosis may be mild or severe, correlating with changes in liver morphology, and the condition is classified as chronic persistent hepatitis and chronic active hepatitis.

Chronic persistent hepatitis typically runs a benign course in childhood. On pathologic specimen, inflammation is limited to the portal triads, without significant fibrosis or cirrhosis. Manifestations include right upper quadrant tenderness and hepatomegaly as well as mild systemic complaints such as anorexia and fatigue. There may be mild elevations of the transaminases and bilirubin. The prognosis in childhood is good, although adults with chronic persistent hepatitis due to hepatitis B or C may progress to cirrhosis or hepatocellular carcinoma.

Chronic active hepatitis is characterized by unresolving inflammation, necrosis, and fibrosis of the liver that leads to progressive symptoms. On pathologic specimen, there is destruction of the normal liver architecture with extensive inflammation, fibrosis, and piecemeal or bridging necrosis. Symptoms may appear suddenly or insidiously, with the former presentation mimicking acute hepatitis. In addition to the signs and symptoms of hepatitis, patients also may show other manifestations of autoimmune disease, including arthritis, vasculitis, nephritis, thyroiditis, or Coombs-positive anemia.

On laboratory assessment, there often is moderate elevation of the transaminases and direct bilirubin, with normal or slightly elevated alkaline phosphatase and γ-glutamyl transpeptidase. Hypergammaglobulinemia, hypoalbuminemia, and prolongation of the prothrombin time are common.

Treatment seeks to limit the progression of disease with minimal side effects while maintaining optimal liver function. Prednisone and azathioprine have been used to counter the autoimmune process. Interferon-α may be helpful in cases resulting from hepatitis B or C.

DISEASES OF THE GALLBLADDER
(*NELSON TEXTBOOK*, SEC. 13.101)

Cholelithiasis and *cholecystitis* are the two most common diseases of the gallbladder in childhood. Both are relatively rare in otherwise healthy children. Cholelithiasis most commonly is seen in patients with hemolytic anemias and is due to increased bile pigments. Cholesterol cholelithiasis most commonly affects obese adolescent girls and those with impaired enterohepatic circulation of bile acids. Symptoms include right upper quadrant pain, especially with ingestion of fatty foods. Diagnosis is made with abdominal ultrasound. Cholecystectomy is curative.

PERITONITIS
(NELSON TEXTBOOK, SEC. 13.103)

Acute infections of the peritoneum may be associated with intra-abdominal or distant infection. Primary peritonitis is a bacterial infection entering the peritoneum by a hematogenous or lymphatic route. Pneumococci and group A streptococci are most commonly implicated. Most cases occur in children less than 6 yr. Symptoms progress rapidly and include fever, toxic appearance, vomiting, abdominal pain, and distention. Bowel sounds are hypoactive or absent. Diagnosis is made by paracentesis, which shows high protein and many white blood cells. Treatment is initially empiric, with ampicillin and gentamycin, pending culture and sensitivity results.

Secondary peritonitis and peritoneal abscesses are associated with rupture of an intraperitoneal viscus, most commonly the appendix. Antibiotics are chosen to cover the enteric flora; ampicillin, gentamycin, and clindamycin or metronidazole commonly are chosen.

12

THE RESPIRATORY SYSTEM

GENERAL CONSIDERATIONS
(*NELSON TEXTBOOK*, SECS. 14.1–14.18)

DEVELOPMENT

The development of the lung begins in the 4th wk of gestation and continues into mid-childhood. The embryonic period is marked by progressive arborization of the pulmonary structures, with alveolar development and multiplication occurring during the 3rd trimester. It is during the latter half of the 3rd trimester that surfactant is made by the type II pneumocytes, thereby preparing these new alveoli for optimal postnatal function. After birth, lung development is limited to the production of new alveoli, which continues until age 5–8 yr. After this age, pulmonary structures grow only by alveolar expansion.

PHYSIOLOGY

The primary role of the lungs is gas exchange, taking place at the alveolar level. The lungs are encased in the two-layered pleural sack. The visceral pleura lines the lungs and the parietal pleural lines the chest wall. Between the two layers of this sack is a potential vacuum such that the lungs are expanded with increases in the size of the thoracic cavity. Active expansion of the chest wall draws air into the alveoli such that gas exchange can occur. Exhalation occurs by passive relaxation of the chest wall. The normal respiratory cycle is shown in Figure 12–1.

The pulmonary structures perform numerous functions in addition to their role in respiratory gas exchange. The nose and oropharynx are responsible for warming, humidifying, and filtering inspired air. Particles greater than 5 μ usually are trapped on the nasal surface. Particles of the size 1–5 μ typically are trapped in the mucociliary blanket of the trachea and bronchi. Smaller particles are immunologically cleared by secretory immunoglobulin (IgA) and phagocytosis.

The lungs also have numerous metabolic functions. They are able to synthesize many of the lipids and glycoproteins important in their protection and repair. Additionally, they are responsible for the metabolism of numerous vasoactive hormones produced by other organs in the body, such as angiotensin II, bradykinin, and many of the prostaglandins.

PATHOPHYSIOLOGY

Respiratory function may be impaired by several different types of processes.

235

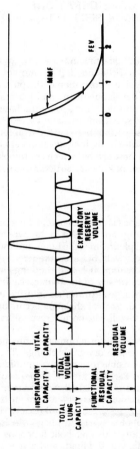

Figure 12–1. *Left,* Functional division of total lung capacity. *Right,* Flow–time relationship during a forced expiration from vital capacity. FEV represents the volume expired for a given period of time and is often measured at 1 sec. MMF represents the maximal midexpiratory flow rate and is calculated as the average flow for the middle 50% of the forced vital capacity (as shown by the cord in the drawing). (From Doershuk CF, Lough MD: *In* Lough MD, Doershuk CF, Stern RC [eds]: Pediatric Respiratory Therapy. Chicago, Year Book Medical Publishers, 1974.)

Restrictive Lung Diseases

Restrictive lung diseases are those in which the alveoli are unable to expand fully. Causes of restrictive lung disease include diseases of the pulmonary parenchyma, such as pneumonia, fibrosis, and consolidation. Diseases affecting the pleura, such as pneumothorax, hemothorax, or pleural effusions, may lead to restrictive lung disease by interfering with pulmonary expansion. Chest wall expansion may be affected by processes that affect the musculoskeletal components of respiration, such as neuromuscular diseases, scoliosis, or flail chest.

Patients with restrictive lung disease typically take *rapid shallow breaths*. Additionally, they may *grunt*, the sound made by air expired against a partially closed glottis in an effort to increase end-expiratory pressure and functional residual capacity. This keeps the lungs partially expanded, minimizing the work of breathing. The lungs typically are dull to percussion.

Obstructive Lung Diseases

Obstructive lung diseases are those in which the flow of gases through the airways is inhibited. Extrathoracic obstructions typically cause *stridor*, a harsh, high-pitched respiratory sound heard best in inspiration. Intrathoracic obstruction typically causes *wheezing*, a whistling respiratory sound that is typically heard best in expiration. Patients with obstructive lung disease typically take *long, deep breaths*. The lungs typically are hyperinflated and tympanitic to percussion.

DIAGNOSTIC PROCEDURES IN PULMONARY MEDICINE

A number of different techniques are used when evaluating the respiratory system. Anatomic information is primarily gleaned by *radiologic and endoscopic techniques*. Radiographic techniques include roentgenograms of the chest, upper airway, and sinuses; contrast studies of the airway and blood vessels; computerized tomography (CT) scans; and radionuclide ventilation scans. Endoscopic techniques include laryngoscopy and bronchoscopy.

Microanatomic and microbiologic data usually are obtained from direct sampling of the tissues. *Thoracentesis* is the removal of fluid from the pleura of fluid that then can be assessed as a transudate, exudate, or empyema. *Lung biopsies* usually are done either as an open procedure or via a transtracheal route.

Pulmonary function is assessed best by blood gas analysis or through pulmonary function testing (see Figure 12–1). In patients with restrictive lung disease, total lung capacity, residual volume, and vital capacity all tend to be low. In patients with obstructive lung disease, there is gas trapping, which leads to increases in residual volume and functional residual capacity. Measurements of forced expiratory volume are low with obstructive lung disease.

DISEASES OF THE NOSE
(*NELSON TEXTBOOK*, SECS. 14.19–14.23)

CHOANAL ATRESIA

Choanal atresia is the most common congenital anomaly of the nose. This lesion consists of a bony or membranous septum between the nose and the pharynx that may be unilateral or bilateral. It usually is diagnosed by the inability to pass a 5.0-French feeding tube from the nose into the oropharynx or stomach.

When choanal atresia is *unilateral*, the infant is relatively asymptomatic but may show a unilateral nasal discharge. Respiratory distress typically occurs when there is blockage of the unaffected nares, as is seen with concomitant upper respiratory tract infection or allergic rhinitis.

Bilateral choanal atresia typically results in newborn infants having difficulty breathing. They may exhibit cyanosis when efforts at mouth breathing are inhibited, such as during feeds. Infants typically will respond to cyanosis by crying, thereby relieving the cyanosis and causing them to be more calm.

Treatment consists of surgical removal of the septum. This typically is done as an elective procedure. Newborns with bilateral choanal atresia may be treated with an oral airway in an effort to maintain the mouth in an open position. Nutrition may be supported either by orogastric tube feeding or by use of a feeding nipple with large holes at the tip.

ACQUIRED DISORDERS OF THE NOSE

The most common acquired disorders of the nose are foreign bodies, epistaxis, and acute nasopharyngitis.

Foreign Bodies

These are common in childhood and usually are suspected by the appearance of a purulent or mucopurulent discharge from one of the nares. The foreign body usually can be visualized with a nasal speculum and should be removed with forceps or nasal suction in an effort to minimize local tissue necrosis.

Epistaxis

Although nosebleeds may be seen with congenital vascular abnormalities, platelet disorders, or hypertension, they most commonly are seen following trauma or with concurrent upper respiratory infection. The source of bleeding usually is the anterior portion of the nares, arising from the septum (Kiesselbach plexus) or the turbinates.

Primary treatment of nosebleeds involves local compression and placement of the child in an erect position such that the nose is superior to the heart. Local vasoconstrictors such as Neo-Synephrine and cocaine, topical thrombin, or anterior nasal packing may be useful in severe cases.

Acute Nasopharyngitis

Acute nasopharyngitis (the common cold) is the most common infection of childhood. The illness is caused by several hundred serologically distinct viruses, with rhinoviruses and coronaviruses most common among them. Group A streptococci are the most common bacterial cause of acute nasopharyngitis.

Clinical manifestations usually last for less than 1 wk and begin with fever, irritability, restlessness, and sneezing. The mucous membranes of the nose typically are inflamed. The nasal smear reveals numerous polymorphonuclear leukocytes. Complications are common, with otitis media being the most prevalent among them. Nasopharyngitis also may trigger asthma exacerbations.

Treatment should consist primarily of supportive care. Fever should be treated with non–salicylate-containing antipyretics. Nasal obstruction may be treated with saline nose drops or α-adrenergic agents. The use of antihistamines is controversial, although many over-the-counter preparations combine antihistamines and α-adrenergic decongestants.

DISEASES OF THE OROPHARYNX
(*NELSON TEXTBOOK*, SECS. 14.24–14.29)

ACUTE PHARYNGITIS

Acute pharyngitis typically is due to viral infection. Disease usually lasts less than 5 days and begins insidiously with early signs including fever, malaise, anorexia, and sore throat. Tonsils may be large and inflamed, and there may be an associated exudate. Anterior cervical lymph nodes are enlarged and may be tender. Bacterial pharyngitis may be caused by group A streptococci, pneumococci, *Haemophilus influenzae,* or gonococci.

Infection due to group A streptococcus commonly occurs in children over 2 yr of age and often is associated with a high fever, tonsilar enlargement, exudate, and tender anterior cervical lymphadenopathy. Diagnosis is made by throat culture or by rapid antigen detection tests. Because rapid strep tests lack sensitivity, antigen-negative swabs always should be followed by throat culture. Complications of strep throat include glomerulonephritis and rheumatic fever.

Treatment of all acute pharyngitis should be supportive. Non–salicylate-containing antipyretics should be used in an effort to control fever. Warm saline gargles or throat lozenges may be used in an effort to control pain. Acute pharyngitis caused by streptococci should be treated with penicillin or erythromycin.

RETROPHARYNGEAL AND PERITONSILLAR ABSCESS

Retropharyngeal Abscess

This results from an infection in the potential space between the posterior pharyngeal wall and the prevertebral fascia. It is most typically a complication of bacterial pharyngitis with group A streptococci, oral anaerobes, and *Staphylococcus aureus*.

Clinical manifestations include sore throat, fever, difficulty swallowing, and noisy respirations. On physical examination, a bulging posterior pharyngeal wall usually is apparent.

Diagnosis may be supported by lateral neck roentgenogram, on which an increase in the retropharyngeal soft tissue is apparent.

Treatment includes incision and drainage and the use of either parenteral penicillin G or a semisynthetic penicillin to cover *S. aureus*.

Peritonsillar Abscess

This typically is caused by group A streptococci or oral anaerobes, which lead to abscess formation in the potential space between the superior constrictor muscle and the tonsil.

Clinical manifestations include fever, severe throat pain, and difficulty in swallowing and phonation. On physical examination, there is unilateral swelling of the peritonsillar area with displacement of the uvula to the opposite side.

Treatment consists of incision and drainage and penicillin G.

SINUSITIS

Development of the Sinuses

The sinuses begin to develop in the bones of the face during the 3rd to 5th mo of gestation but do not become radiographically or clinically significant until later in childhood. The maxillary and ethmoid sinuses are the first to develop. They typically are radiographically apparent by age 1–2 yr. They account for most of the sinus infections of early childhood and infancy. The sphenoid sinuses become radiographically apparent at 5–6 yr and may become infected beginning in the toddler years. The last sinuses to develop are the frontal sinuses. They typically are fully radiographically apparent by age 10 yr and commonly are infected later in childhood.

Sinus Infections

Sinusitis is a common infection of childhood that may be acute or chronic. It usually is a complication of upper respiratory tract infection or other conditions in which sinus drainage may be impaired. Chronic sinusitis is commonly associated with nasal polyps, nasal septal deviation, or adenoidal hypertrophy. It also is associated with conditions such as cystic fibrosis and Kartagener syndrome, in which mucociliary clearance is impaired by other mechanisms. Bacteria causing sinusitis are the same as those found in acute otitis media: *Streptococcus pneumoniae*, *Moraxella catarrhalis*, and nontypable *H. influenzae*.

Clinical Manifestations

Symptoms of sinusitis include purulent nasal drainage, headache, and fever. Periorbital cellulitis may complicate ethmoidal sinusitis in young children.

Diagnosis

This is based on clinical findings, which may be accompanied by radiographic changes. Although sinus roentgenograms historically have been the gold standard of diagnosis, they may be difficult to interpret in children because of asymmetric development of the sinuses. In many centers, CT scan and ultrasound are being used increasingly in the diagnosis of sinusitis.

Treatment

This consists of 14–21 days of oral antimicrobial therapy. Decongestants and antihistamines are not helpful in the treatment of sinusitis. Surgical sinus drainage and irrigation typically are reserved for patients with chronic sinusitis or those who have failed therapy.

DISEASES OF THE AIRWAYS
(*NELSON TEXTBOOK*, SECS. 14.34–14.55)

CONGENITAL

Tracheomalacia and Laryngomalacia

These are the most common causes of congenital stridor. Other common causes include tracheoesophageal fistula and vascular rings.

Patients with tracheomalacia or laryngomalacia usually present with stridor in the neonatal period. Stridor is worse when the infant is in the supine position or agitated. Symptoms include a noisy, crowing sound during inspiration that is due to excessive flabbiness or weakness of the upper airway walls. Diagnosis usually is made clinically and may be supported by direct laryngoscopy. The condition usually resolves spontaneously by 18 mo. Rarely is tracheostomy required. Feedings may be difficult in patients with these anomalies: parents should be counseled to feed slowly and carefully, using a small-holed nipple or gavage feeding if necessary.

ACQUIRED

Acquired conditions affecting the lower airways typically fall into three categories: those due to infection, allergy, or foreign body. Infectious diseases include epiglottitis, laryngitis, laryngotracheobronchitis, abscess, and bacterial tracheitis. Allergic causes include anaphylaxis, angioedema, and possibly spasmodic croup. Foreign bodies or laryngeal tumors such as papillomas or nodules also may cause symptoms.

Clinical manifestations depend on the area of the airway affected. Conditions affecting the glottic region typically cause hoarseness, brassy cough, and inspiratory stridor. Conditions affecting the trachea or bronchi may lead to inspiratory or expiratory stridor, productive cough, or wheezing if the lumen is sufficiently narrowed. Conditions affecting the smaller airways produce wheezing.

Epiglottitis

Epiglottitis is an acute swelling of the epiglottis caused by *H. influenzae* type B infection. It is typically seen in children age 2–7 yr (peak: 3½ yr).

Clinical manifestations appear suddenly and include high fever, toxic appearance, and respiratory distress. The patient prefers to sit upright, leaning forward in an effort to maintain patency of the airway (tripod position). Associated symptoms include aphonia, drooling, and dysphagia. Physical examination may reveal a cherry red epiglottis, although direct laryngoscopy is not recommended because it may precipitate spasm and closure of the airway. Lateral neck roengenograms may show an enlarged epiglottic shadow (thumbprint sign).

Because this disease is rapidly progressive, *treatment* includes emergency placement of an endotracheal tube and intravenous antibiotics against *H. influenzae*. α-Adrenergic drugs, mist, and corticosteroids have no place in the treatment of this disease.

Laryngitis

Laryngitis typically is caused by viral infection. Clinical manifestations include sore throat, hoarseness, cough, and low-grade fever. Physical examination may reveal erythema of the pharynx and stridor. Laryngoscopy may show edema of the vocal cords. Treatment is supportive.

Croup

Although it may be caused by many different viruses, acute laryngotracheobronchitis, or the croup, is most commonly the result of infection with the parainfluenza virus. It commonly occurs in children age 3 mo to 5 yr following a few days of upper respiratory complaints. Temperature is mildly elevated. Other manifestations include sore throat, a "seal bark" brassy cough, and inspiratory stridor. Symptoms are characteristically worse at night.

Spasmodic croup has similar clinical manifestations, although the infectious upper respiratory prodrome is absent.

Anterior–posterior neck roentgenograms may reveal narrowing of the tracheal silhouette ("steeple sign").

Treatment consists of mist and oxygen. Corticosteroids may be of some benefit because they may moderate the edema. Vaponephrine, an α-adrenergic agent, may decrease the edema by vasoconstriction.

Bacterial Tracheitis

Bacterial tracheitis is an acute bacterial infection of the upper airway that usually is caused by *S. aureus*. It may follow croup and is suspected clinically when a patient with croup experiences progressive deterioration with increasing cough, sputum, fever, and toxicity. The disease usually is treated with antistaphylococcal antibiotics. Intubation usually is necessary because the swelling of the trachea is progressive.

Bronchitis

Bronchitis is a commonly diagnosed disease of childhood. It may be acute or chronic and probably is multifactorial in etiology. Infections, allergens, and air pollutants probably all play a role in the pathogenesis of acute bronchitis. Symptoms include productive cough, rhonchi, and soreness of the chest. Immunodeficiencies, immotile cilia, asthma, and cystic fibrosis all should be suspected in patients with chronic bronchitis. Treatment decisions should be based on the underlying etiology.

Bronchiolitis

Bronchiolitis is a common viral infection of the first 2 yr of life. It is attributed most often to the respiratory syncytial virus (RSV), although many other viruses may lead to a similar illness.

Clinical manifestations include an upper respiratory viral prodrome after which wheezing and respiratory distress appear. Complications may include apnea or respiratory failure; the latter is more common in patients with underlying cardiopulmonary disease.

Treatment of bronchiolitis is largely symptomatic, with provision of oxygen when needed. Bronchodilators may be of some value in this disease, although their utility is unpredictable. Corticosteroids are not effective in the treatment of bronchiolitis.

Although most bronchiolitis is self-limited and conservative therapy is all that is needed, *ribavirin* is an effective antiviral drug useful against RSV. It usually is delivered via a small-particle aerosol generator (SPAG) for 12–24 hr/day. Because ribavirin is a known teratogen and its use may aggravate pre-existing lung conditions in health care workers, its use has been limited to those patients with or at risk for severe disease, such as patients with underlying cardiorespiratory disease.

Foreign Body

Clinical manifestations related to a foreign body depend on the location in which it is lodged. Laryngeal or tracheal foreign bodies cause stridor. Sputum production often is increased and may be bloody. Bronchial foreign bodies lead to wheezing and air trapping. They usually are suspected in toddlers with unilateral wheezing. Diagnosis often is made by comparing end-inspiratory and end-expiratory chest roentgenograms, which show unilateral air trapping with shift of the mediastinal structures to the contralateral side.

PNEUMONIA
(NELSON TEXTBOOK, SECS. 14.56–14.74)

Pneumonia refers to any of a number conditions that cause inflammatory changes to the lung parenchyma. The *diagnosis* may be made clinically in a patient who experiences any or all of the following manifestations: tachypnea, dyspnea, cough, wheezing, grunting, flaring of the alae nasae, retractions of the accessory muscles of respiration, or cyanosis. Radiographic diagnosis is based on the demonstration of an abnormal density of tissue not found in the normal lung parenchyma.

The most common etiology of pneumonia in children is viral infection. Bacteria are the next most common cause of pneumonia in children. Bacterial invasion typically follows a viral prodrome in which local defense mechanisms are altered. Parasitic and fungal infections are much less common; they are found most commonly in children with risk factors such as immunosuppression or life in an endemic area. Aspiration pneumonia may be found in children who have impaired ability to handle oral secretions.

VIRAL PNEUMONIA

Although a number of viruses may cause pneumonia, the viruses most commonly associated are RSV, one of the parainfluenza viruses, adenovirus, or enterovirus.

Clinical manifestations of pneumonia typically are preceded by several days of rhinitis and cough. Symptoms then progress over the course of days to dyspnea, tachypnea, retractions, and other signs of lower respiratory tract disease. Wheezing is commonly heard with pneumonia caused by RSV and parainfluenza.

Chest roentgenograms typically are characterized by a diffuse infiltrate in the perihilar areas, although lobar infiltrates also may be seen. Hyperinflation is common. Specific viruses implicated may be diagnosed by culture or fluorescent antibody techniques.

Treatment of viral pneumonia is nonspecific. Intravenous fluids, oxygen, and respiratory assistance are provided as necessary. Antibiotics frequently are given initially if bacterial pneumonia is suspected. The antiviral drug ribavirin has been shown to be effective in some patients with infection caused by RSV.

Although most children with viral pneumonia recover uneventfully, some children may progress to fulminant disease. Adenovirus is most commonly implicated in more severe disease.

PNEUMOCOCCAL PNEUMONIA

The pneumococcus accounts for over 90% of childhood bacterial pneumonia.

Clinical manifestations often begin with a relatively mild upper respiratory tract infection that progresses suddenly to tachypnea, dyspnea, and cyanosis. Respiratory symptoms often are associated with high fever and mental status changes. Chest examination may reveal localized rales, dullness to percussion, and tactile and vocal fremitus in the affected lobes. Complications are relatively uncommon and include empyema, lung abscess, and pneumatoceles.

Chest roentgenograms classically show a lobar pneumonia

with gross consolidation, although this is seen less commonly in young children. On pathologic specimen, the pneumococcus produces an inflammatory mucosal lesion and alveolar exudate, usually without intense destruction of the surrounding tissues.

Diagnosis is suspected by the classic presentation and confirmed by isolation of the bacteria from the trachea, blood, or pleural fluid. Latex agglutination of the blood, urine, or plural fluid may be helpful in establishing a diagnosis. The white blood cell count typically is elevated to 15,000–40,000 cells/mm^3, and white blood counts less than 5,000/mm^3 often are associated with grave prognosis.

Treatment consists of appropriate use of supportive care and antimicrobial therapy. Liberal intake of fluid should be stressed because insensible water losses resulting from tachypnea may be great. Nonsalicylate antipyretics should be used to relieve fever. Oxygen therapy should be provided as necessary. Decisions to hospitalize are based on individual cases, with important factors being patient respiratory status, oxygen requirement, and reliability of parental care. Appropriate antibiotics include penicillin and first- or second-generation cephalosporins.

STREPTOCOCCAL PNEUMONIA

Streptococci typically cause disease limited to the upper respiratory tract, but also may be responsible for lower respiratory tract disease. Streptococci may invade the mucous membranes and produce bronchiolitis, peribronchiolitis, and interstitial disease. Lobar pneumonia is uncommon. Infection also may involve the lymphatics or lead to inflammation of the pleural surfaces.

Clinical manifestations most commonly appear suddenly, with the abrupt onset of high fever and respiratory distress. Complications include empyema, which occurs in 20% of children, and a rare association with acute glomerulonephritis.

Diagnosis is based on the recovery of streptococcus in the blood, pleural fluid, or lung aspirates. Associated laboratory findings include a high white blood cell count and a rise in the antistreptolysin O titer. Chest roentgenograms usually reveal a diffuse bronchopneumonia with large pleural effusions.

Treatment includes antibiotics and supportive care as for other causes of pneumonia. Penicillin G is effective in the treatment of streptococcal disease. Thoracentesis may be necessary for the removal of pleural fluid.

STAPHYLOCOCCAL PNEUMONIA

Staphylococcus aureus may cause pneumonia in childhood; it is most commonly seen in the 1st yr of life. Disease may be associated with a patient history or family history of staphylococcal skin lesions.

Clinical manifestations include an antecedent upper respiratory tract infection followed by the abrupt onset of high fever, cough, and evidence of respiratory distress. Mental status changes and shock are common. The disease is rapidly progressive. Chest roentgenograms may show a nonspecific bronchiopneumonia early in the illness that then rapidly progresses to lobar or complete hemithorax involvement. Pleural effusion, empyema, or pneumatoceles are common complications.

Treatment includes antibiotics and supportive care as for other causes of pneumonia, although hospitalization is mandatory because of the rapid progression of this disease. Antibiotic choices include first-generation cephalosporins and penicillinase-resistant penicillins. Chest tube drainage of empyema is frequently necessary. Therapy is usually prolonged, with hospitalizations not uncommonly lasting 2–3 mo.

Mortality is high, ranging from 10 to 30%.

PNEUMONIA CAUSED BY *HAEMOPHILUS INFLUENZAE*

Haemophilus influenzae type B is a frequent cause of bacterial infection in children and may cause bacterial pneumonia. Pneumonia due to *H. influenzae* typically has an insidious presentation. The pneumonia usually is lobar in distribution, with extensive destruction of the small airways and interstitium. Pulmonary complications are common and include pleural effusion and empyema. Extrapulmonary complications include meningitis (seen in up to 15% of younger patients), joint infections, bone infections, and pericarditis.

Diagnosis is based on the isolation of *H. influenzae* from the blood, tracheal aspirates, or pleural fluid. Latex agglutination of the blood, urine, or pleural fluid may aid in diagnosis. The white blood cell count usually is moderately elevated.

Treatment includes antibiotics and supportive care as for other causes of bacterial pneumonia. Hospitalization and intravenous antibiotics are mandatory because of the invasive nature of the bacteria. Second- and third-generation cephalosporins commonly are used in the treatment of disease due to *H. influenzae*. Thoracentesis or chest tube placement should be considered for effusions and empyema.

NOSOCOMIAL PNEUMONIA

Klebsiella pneumoniae and *Pseudomonas aeruginosa* are increasingly common causes of pneumonia in children, especially in those chronically hospitalized and those immunosuppressed. *Klebsiella* has been associated with neonatal disease and *Pseudomonas* is responsible for much of the pneumonia experienced by children with cystic fibrosis. Both may cause a severe progressive pneumonia with widespread tissue destruction. *Klebsiella* is especially invasive and commonly may cause pulmonary abscesses and cavitations. Treatment includes intravenous antibiotics with supportive care and thoracentesis as necessary.

PNEUMOCYSTIS CARINII PNEUMONIA

Pneumonia caused by *Pneumocystis carinii* most commonly is seen in immunosuppressed patients or those patients with chronic debilitated states. In pediatric patients, it usually is seen as a complication of the treatment of malignancy or in patients with acquired immunodeficiency syndrome (AIDS). Infection with this fungus produces a characteristic intra-alveolar exudate that contains histiocytes, lymphocytes, plasma cells, and cysts.

The *clinical manifestations* usually begin insidiously with low-grade fever and tachypnea that progress to severe respiratory distress. Chest roentgenograms typically show hyperexpansion of the lung fields with bilateral granular pulmonary infiltrates that originate at the hilum and extend to the periphery.

Definitive *diagnosis* is made by demonstration of the fungus in tracheal aspirates, bronchial washings, or lung biopsy specimens.

If left untreated, the disease is often fatal. Trimethoprim–sulfamethoxazole or pentamidine is recommended in the prophylactic prevention and treatment of this disease.

ASPIRATION PNEUMONIA

Aspiration pneumonia is a common problem in children. It usually is seen in infants and in patients with impaired ability to handle gastric contents, such as those with altered mental status or impaired gastrointestinal motility.

Clinical manifestations typically begin soon after an aspiration event with fever, tachypnea, and cough. Physical examination usually reveals diffuse rales, rhonchi, and wheezing. Cyanosis is common. Chest roentgenograms may reveal infiltrates that often are limited to the right lower lobe; infiltrates may be bilateral. Lung injury probably is due to both oral anaerobic bacteria and aspiration of hydrochloric acid.

Treatment includes immediate suctioning of the airway and oxygen supplementation. Penicillin and clindamycin are commonly used antibiotics because they are effective against most oral flora. In chronically hospitalized children, in whom oral gram-negative species are common, the addition of an aminoglycoside should be considered. The use of corticosteroids in patients with aspiration pneumonia is controversial but is thought by some to ameliorate the inflammatory response.

PULMONARY ASPERGILLOSIS

A number of species of the fungal genus *Aspergillus* may be responsible for lung disease in humans. Allergic bronchopulmonary aspergillosis (ABPA) has been found to occur in children with pre-existing pulmonary conditions such as asthma and cystic fibrosis.

The *diagnosis* of ABPA should be suspected in a chronically ill child who has an acute onset of cough, wheezing, and low-grade fever. Diagnosis is based on a positive skin test, elevated IgE level, peripheral blood eosinophilia, or the demonstration of *Aspergillus*-specific IgE or IgG in patient serum.

Treatment includes aerosolized amphotericin or systemic corticosteroids.

Aspergillomas (fungus balls) or invasive aspergillosis are less common presentations of disease caused by this fungus and occur in immunocompromised patients.

PULMONARY HEMOSIDEROSIS

Pulmonary hemosiderosis is a chronic pneumonia diagnosed by finding hemosiderin-laden macrophages in the lungs. Pulmonary hemosiderosis may be primary or secondary. There are four types of primary pulmonary hemosiderosis: (1) the idiopathic form, (2) the form associated with cow's milk hypersensitivity (Heiner syndrome), (3) the form associated with myocarditis, and (4) the form associated with progressive glomerulonephritis (Goodpasture syndrome). Secondary pulmonary hemosiderosis has been associated with obstructive left-heart lesions, collagen vascular diseases, and hemorrhagic diseases.

Clinical manifestations include chronic, progressive pneumonia and anemia. Cough, dyspnea, cyanosis, digital clubbing, and hemoptysis frequently are seen. The anemia typically is microcytic and hypochromic, with low serum iron concentrations.

Corticosteroids may be of some benefit to patients with primary idiopathic pulmonary hemosiderosis. Patients with Heiner syndrome should be placed on a milk-free diet.

OTHER DISEASES OF THE LUNGS
(*NELSON TEXTBOOK*, SECS. 14.75–14.87)

CONGENITAL DISEASES

The most common congenital anomaly of the lungs is *congenital lobar emphysema*. In this disease, there is irreversible distention and rupture of the alveoli, usually resulting from partial obstruction of a bronchus or bronchiole. The left upper lobe most often is affected and may cause severe respiratory distress in early infancy. Diagnosis is made on roentgenogram, which reveals a radiolucent, overinflated lobe with mediastinal shift. Treatment involves surgical excision of the affected lobe.

Cystic adenomatoid malformation is the second most common congenital anomaly of the lungs. In this lesion there is malformation of the terminal bronchiolar structures leading to cystic enlargement of the affected lobe. The lesion typically causes severe respiratory distress in the neonatal period. Chest roentgenograms reveal a cystic mass and mediastinal shift that may be confused with congenital diaphragmatic hernia. Emergency surgical excision of the affected lobe is life saving.

Other congenital anomalies of the lungs include pulmonary hypoplasia, pulmonary sequestration, and bronchiogenic cysts.

ACQUIRED

Atelectasis

Atelectasis refers to the imperfect expansion or collapse of lung parenchyma. It is a common problem in childhood and may occur with restrictive or obstructive pulmonary disease. Respiratory excursion may be dampened as a result of neuromuscular or musculoskeletal conditions, or secondary to splinting in an effort to moderate pleuritic pain. Air travel through a bronchus may be impeded by anything that reduces the diameter of the bronchus. Extrinsic causes include enlarged lymph nodes, tumors, or cardiac enlargement. Intrinsic causes include foreign bodies, mucous plugs, edema, and granulomas.

Small areas of atelectasis are likely to be asymptomatic and well tolerated. When large areas of the lung are affected, *clinical manifestations* include dyspnea, shallow respirations, tachypnea, and cyanosis. Complications of atelectasis include pneumonias secondary to decreased ciliary clearance of mucus.

Diagnosis usually is made on roentgenograms, with areas of pulmonary consolidation being found.

Treatment decisions are based on the underlying cause. Mucous plugs often are liberated by chest physiotherapy and postural drainage. Foreign bodies usually require bronchoscopic removal. Splinting, especially in the postoperative period, should be treated with analgesics and incentive spirometry. β-Adrenergic drugs may be helpful in patients with asthma who have atelectasis. Prognosis is good.

Emphysema

Pulmonary emphysema is a condition of the lungs in which there is irreversible distention and rupture of the alveoli. It may be congenital or caused by acquired obstructive processes that interfere primarily with expiration. Emphysema may be localized or generalized, with symptoms varying with the amount of lung involved.

Localized emphysema typically results from a ball–valve obstruction of a primary or secondary bronchus. This type of emphysema commonly is seen with foreign bodies, intrabronchial tuberculosis, or tumors. During inspiration, the lumen of the bronchus increases slightly, allowing air to pass by. During expiration, however, the lumen of the bronchus narrows, with trapping of the air distal to the obstruction. *Manifestations* may be mild and include tachypnea and shallow breathing. Chest examination reveals decreased breath sounds in the affected lobe with hyper-resonance on percussion. On chest roentgenograms, hyperlucency of the affected lobe may be seen, which is especially apparent on expiratory films. There also may be shift of the mediastinal contents to the contralateral side.

Generalized emphysema typically is seen with chronic pulmonary disease such as asthma, cystic fibrosis, and chronic aspiration pneumonia. It also may be seen as a complication of severe acute pulmonary disease. With generalized emphysema, the patient experiences expiratory dyspnea. Respirations typically are shallow and rapid. Retractions of the accessory muscles of respiration commonly are seen. Chest roentgenograms reveal generalized hypolucency of the lung parenchyma with flattening of the diaphragm. Decreased diaphragmatic excursion may be seen on fluoroscopy.

Pulmonary Edema

Pulmonary edema results from the transudation of fluid from the pulmonary capillaries into the lung parenchyma. It may be the result of cardiogenic or noncardiogenic causes. The most common cardiogenic cause is left ventricular failure, in which pulmonary venous congestion leads to increased hydrostatic pressure in the pulmonary capillaries and subsequent leakage of fluid into the tissues. Noncardiogenic causes include hypervolemia, infections, drugs, or toxins.

Clinical manifestations of pulmonary edema include cough with production of frothy pink sputum, tachypnea, and tachycardia. Physical examination may reveal moist rales heard best at the lower portions of the chest with dullness to percussion. Chest roentgenograms reveal dense perihilar infiltrate in a butterfly distribution.

Treatment of pulmonary edema should attempt to correct its underlying cause. Morphine commonly is used to relieve dyspnea. Diuretics often are used in an effort to decrease hydrostatic pressure and volume overload. Oxygen commonly is used to moderate hypoxemia.

Adult Respiratory Distress Syndrome

Adult respiratory distress syndrome (ARDS) is a severe form of noncardiogenic pulmonary edema that can be precipitated by a number of alveolar insults, including shock, trauma, toxic inhalations, disseminated intravascular coagulation, and drug overdose. The exact pathogenesis of ARDS is not well understood, but there is widespread injury of the vascular epithelium that leads to progressive pulmonary edema.

Clinical manifestations may be mild immediately after the acute injury but progress to severe tachypnea and dyspnea 8–48 hr following the initial insult. Respiratory failure is common. Pathologic changes begin with pulmonary edema and progress to pulmonary fibrosis.

Treatment of ARDS includes mechanical ventilation utilizing high positive end-expiratory pressure (PEEP) settings in an effort to maintain functional residual volume in the increasingly noncompliant lung. Diuretics may be a helpful adjunct to care. Corticosteroids do not appear to be effective in the treatment of this disease. ARDS is a grave diagnosis that carries a mortality of greater than 50%.

Pulmonary Embolism and Infarction

Pulmonary embolism is an uncommon diagnosis in infants and children. It is most commonly seen following periods of prolonged inactivity. Recent abortion, intravenous drug abuse with right-sided bacterial endocarditis, sickle cell anemia, and fat emboli may also lead to pulmonary embolism.

Clinical manifestations include pain that may be substernal, pleuritic, or radiate to the shoulder. Large emboli can cause symptoms of acute right heart failure. Auscultation may reveal distant breath sounds or moist rales. Percussion may reveal impaired resonance. Chest roentgenograms often are normal.

Although pulmonary angiography is *diagnostic*, decisions to perform this test should be weighed against the risks of empiric therapy.

Treatment consists of anticoagulation with intravenous heparin followed by 3–6 mo of oral coumarin therapy.

Pulmonary Suppuration

Suppurative conditions of the lung include pulmonary abscesses and bronchiectasis.

Pulmonary abscesses commonly are associated with infections caused by *S. aureus, Klebsiella,* or oral anaerobes. Manifestations include fever, malaise, cough, hemoptysis, and production of copious amounts of foul-smelling, purulent sputum. Treatment of pulmonary abscesses includes a prolonged course (4–6 wk) of antibiotics against the offending bacteria. Symptoms typically improve within 1 wk of the institution of therapy. The disease has an excellent prognosis.

Bronchiectasis refers to the permanent dilation of the smaller airways with inflammatory destruction of their surrounding tissue and abscess formation. Bronchiectasis may be congenital or acquired. The former may be due to an arrest in the embryonic bronchial development with subsequent cyst formation. The majority of cases are acquired after birth, usually as a result of chronic pulmonary infection. Associated conditions include sinusitis, ciliary dyskinesia, agammaglobulinemia, tuberculosis, asthma, and cystic fibrosis. Manifestations include a chronic, recurrent cough with production of copious mucopurulent sputum during periods of acute infection. Clubbing of the fingers may be present. Treatment includes systemic antibiotic therapy with postural drainage and chest physiotherapy. In severe cases unresponsive to medical management, segmental or lobar resection should be considered.

CYSTIC FIBROSIS
(*NELSON TEXTBOOK*, SEC. 14.89)

Cystic fibrosis (CF) is the most common life-threatening genetic trait found in Caucasian populations. CF is most prevalent in populations of Northern and Central European origin, with an incidence as high as $1:625$ live births. Incidence varies in other populations, being much less common among blacks and Asians.

The abnormal gene that is responsible for CF is carried on the long arm of chromosome 7. The gene codes for the CF transmembrane regulator protein (CFTR), a 1,480–amino acid protein that seems to alter the apical membrane permeability to chloride ion, causing secretions that are viscous and salt rich. Although there is a great deal of ill-understood heterogeneity in the symptoms and signs of patients with CF, the organs most commonly affected by these viscous secretions are the lungs and the gastrointestinal tract.

CLINICAL MANIFESTATIONS

Cough is the most common symptom of disease in the *respiratory tract*. Initially dry and hacking, the cough typically becomes productive of copious purulent sputum. Wheezing is another common symptom of CF, resulting from inspissated secretions and bronchiolitis. Other respiratory manifestations include shortness of breath, dyspnea, and exercise intolerance. Physical examination may reveal any or all of the following: increased anterior–posterior diameter of the chest, hyper-resonance of the lungs, rales, wheezing, cyanosis, or digital clubbing.

Gastrointestinal manifestations of CF are common and may present in the newborn period. *Meconium ileus* is found in 10% of patients with CF. Diagnosis is made after the failure to pass meconium in the first days of life. Associated signs include vomiting and abdominal distention. Abdominal roentgenograms reveal evidence of ileus with air–fluid levels and distended bowel loops in the proximal areas of the bowel.

Insufficiency of the exocrine pancreas is common in CF. The most prominent manifestation is a protuberant abdomen with bulky, malodorous stools secondary to fat malabsorption. Symptoms and signs related to fat-soluble vitamin (A, D, E, K) deficiencies may be apparent and include night blindness (vitamin A), decreased bone density (vitamin D), hemolytic anemia and neurologic dysfunction (vitamin E), or bleeding (vitamin K). Patients often also are noted to be glucose intolerant and sometimes require insulin therapy, although ketoacidosis is rare.

Biliary cirrhosis is an uncommon problem in patients with CF. Manifestations include jaundice, ascites, and hematemesis due to esophageal varices.

Other affected organs include the *reproductive tract* and the *sweat glands*. Decreased fertility is common among women with CF, in part as a result of thickened cervical secretions. About 95% of men with CF are azoospermic. Excessive salt loss in the sweat may lead to a salty taste of the skin or hypochloremic alkalosis and prostration if severe.

DIAGNOSIS

The diagnosis of CF should be suspected in any patient with chronic lower respiratory tract disease or pneumonia caused by *Staphylococcus* or *Pseudomonas* species. Suspicious gastrointestinal symptoms include meconium ileus, malabsorption, steatorrhea, rectal prolapse, and biliary cirrhosis. Nonspecific findings suspicious for CF include failure to thrive, sinusitis, azoospermia, nasal polyps, or salty taste when kissed.

The gold standard of postnatal diagnosis remains the *sweat chloride test*. In this test, pilocarpine iontophoresis is used to collect sweat for analysis. A sweat chloride concentration of >60 mEq/L is diagnostic for CF when clinical symptoms are present. Other conditions associated with a high sweat chloride concentration include adrenal insufficiency, ectodermal dysplasia, glucose-6-phosphatase deficiency, and hypothyroidism.

Prenatal diagnosis can be performed with specific gene probes for CF mutations or by linkage analysis, which requires chromosome samples from both parents and at least one affected sibling. Neonatal diagnosis using an assay for immunoreactive trypsinogen in the blood has been advocated for patients at risk, but this test lacks the sensitivity and specificity to be useful in widespread screening programs.

TREATMENT

Largely because of improvements in respiratory care, the life expectancy of patients with CF has increased dramatically over the past 30–40 yr. The median life expectancy of a patient with CF is now almost 30 yr. Therapy is primarily aimed at optimizing respiratory function through judicious use of antibiotics, bronchodilators, and chest physiotherapy, while minimizing pancreatic dysfunction with enzyme, hormone, and vitamin supplements.

The major objectives of pulmonary therapy are twofold: clear the airways and treat infections. Aerosol therapy with normal saline is used to increase the moisture of respiratory secretions. Bronchodilators or antibiotics may be added to the saline in an effort to treat airway hyper-reactivity or infection if present. Chest physiotherapy involves sequential vibration and percussion with postural drainage to each of the lobes of the lung in an effort to liberate mucous plugs and secretions.

S. aureus and *Pseudomonas* species commonly colonize the lungs. Antibiotics against these bacteria should be given in high doses in an effort to prevent antibiotic resistance by oral, intravenous, or inhalational methods. Infection with *Pseudomonas cepacia* may be especially difficult to treat.

Pulmonary complications include atelectasis, hemoptysis, pneumothorax, ABPA, and respiratory failure. *Atelectasis* is caused by inspissation of secretions. Chest physiotherapy, antibiotics, and bronchoscopy in severe cases are the treatments of choice for atelectasis. *Hemoptysis* usually is due to rupture of one of the dilated bronchial arteries and/or coagulopathy. Treatment consists of vitamin K and temporary cessation of chest physiotherapy. *Pneumothorax* typically occurs secondary to bronchiectasis and the rupture of a lung bleb. It may resolve with 100% oxygen or chest tube drainage but more commonly requires invasive pleural stripping or sclerosis. *ABPA* usually is treated with corticosteroids, but may require aerosolized amphotericin B or systemic 5-fluorocytosine in refractory cases.

Respiratory failure in patients with CF may be acute or chronic. Acute respiratory failure usually is the result of intercurrent infection. Therapy consists of pulmonary toilet and antibiotics; prognosis is good. Chronic respiratory failure results from progressive respiratory deterioration in which chronic hypoxemia leads to increases in the pulmonary vascular resistance and cor pulmonale. Treatment consists of supplemental oxygen and diuretics. Digoxin is of limited value for cor pulmonale. Heart–lung transplantation has been effective in severe cases.

Nutritional support consists of a high-calorie, high-protein diet in an effort to meet the increased metabolic demands resulting from the increased work of breathing. Fat-soluble vitamins should be provided. A number of pancreatic enzyme supplements are available and should be used. The dose of these enzymes should be titrated to prevent steatorrhea.

Gastrointestinal complications include constipation, gastroesophageal reflux, and rectal prolapse. Constipation may resolve with stool softeners or increased liquid intake. More severe cases require enemas. Gastroesophageal reflux is not uncommon and should be treated with Nissen fundoplication if severe. Rectal prolapse is common in infants with CF and should be treated with manual replacement. Taping the buttocks closed will prevent immediate recurrence.

Treatment of pancreatic and hepatic complications is discussed in Chapter 11.

DISEASES OF THE PLEURA
(*NELSON TEXTBOOK*, SECS. 14.90–14.95)

The two pleural surfaces, the parietal and the visceral, are normally separated only by a thin layer of fluid that bathes them and reduces friction associated with breathing. Any accumulation that interrupts the proximity of these surfaces may cause pain with respiration and may progress to florid respiratory distress. Examples of such accumulations include air (pneumothorax), exudates, transudates, pus (empyema), blood (hemothorax), or chyle (chylothorax).

On physical examination, breath sounds are distant on the affected side. If air has accumulated in the intrapleural space, percussion is tympanitic on the affected side. If fluid has accumulated in the intrapleural space, percussion is dull. Diagnosis is confirmed by roentgenogram and aspiration of the offending substance. Therapy includes treatment of underlying disease and removal of the offending accumulation. Relief of pain with nonsteroidal anti-inflammatory drugs or opiates should be provided.

Pneumothorax typically accompanies underlying destructive lung disease. Small pneumothoraces may resolve spontaneously. Moderate pneumothoraces may resolve with nitrogen washout utilizing inspiration of 100% oxygen. Large pneumothoraces require thoracentesis with closed vacuum-assisted drainage. Persistent pneumothoraces require evacuation and surgical or chemical adhesion of the pleural surfaces.

Transudates are most commonly found with associated pulmonary infection. They also may be associated with congestive heart failure, renal disease, malignancy, or collagen vascular disease. They are differentiated from exudates (which also are typically seen with infection) by laboratory assay: exudates have a specific gravity of >1.015, a protein level >3 g/dL, and a lactate dehydrogenase level of >200 IU/L. Treatment of both includes vacuum-assisted thoracentesis.

Empyema typically complicates pneumonia caused by *S. aureus*, *H. influenzae*, and *S. pneumococcus* (especially types 1 and 3). Purulent secretions must be drained and appropriate IV antibiotics given.

Hemothorax is uncommon in children. Drainage and treatment of underlying vascular disease or coagulopathy is essential.

Chylothorax occurs as a result of interruption of the thoracic duct. Treatment consists of a low-fat diet with surgical ligation of the thoracic duct in severe cases.

13

THE CARDIOVASCULAR SYSTEM

Disorders of the cardiovascular system may be due to anatomic variations in the heart or the blood vessels. Although these variations may be acquired in various disease states, such as rheumatic fever or Kawasaki syndrome, most heart disease of childhood is congenital.

EVALUATION OF THE CARDIOVASCULAR SYSTEM
(*NELSON TEXTBOOK*, SECS. 15.1–15.9)

HISTORY

Whereas older children may show the more classic signs and symptoms of cardiac disease, symptoms of heart disease in young children often are subtle and nonspecific. Symptoms include:

poor feeding and vomiting
easy fatigability
increased perspiration
tachypnea, shortness of breath, or dyspnea
failure to thrive
cyanosis

PHYSICAL EXAMINATION

A thorough physical examination is essential when evaluating a patient with confirmed or suspected heart disease. Before auscultating the heart, a thorough examination should include assessments of:

skin color: cyanosis, pallor, cutis marmorata (mottling)
quality of peripheral pulses and capillary refill
work of breathing: tachypnea, dyspnea
presence of hepatomegaly, edema, jugular venous distention, or rales consistent with right or left heart failure
assessment of the blood pressure in four extremities to rule out coarctation of the aorta
assessment of the precordium and cardiac impulse: its location, its intensity, and the presence or absence of a thrill

The heart should then be auscultated in a systematic fashion.

Cardiac Auscultation

QUALITY AND TIMING OF THE HEART SOUNDS.
The *1st heart sound* is due to the closure of the atrioventricular (A-V) valves. It typically is single, muffled, and heard best at the apex. A sharp ejection click resulting from valvular pulmonic or aortic stenosis may be heard at the left sternal border and often is confused as a split 1st heart sound.

The *2nd heart sound* has two components: the closure of the aortic valve followed by the closure of the pulmonic valve. The relationship of these sounds normally varies with respiration: during inspiration, the blood flow to the right side of the heart increases, causing elongation of the right ventricular emptying time and delay of the pulmonic component of the 2nd heart sound. The 2nd heart sound is widely split in cases in which there is a fixed increase in blood return to the right side, such as with atrial septal defects (ASDs) and anomalous pulmonary venous return. The pulmonic component also is delayed with pulmonic stenosis and right bundle-branch block. The pulmonary component of the 2nd heart sound moves closer to the aortic component in conditions in which pulmonary artery diastolic pressure is high, such as pulmonary hypertension. The 2nd heart sound may be single with severe pulmonary hypertension or with semilunar valvular atresia. Delay of the aortic component of the 2nd heart sound may occur with aortic stenosis or left bundle branch block.

The *3rd heart sound* is low pitched and is heard best at the apex in mid-diastole. Although it may be heard in adolescents, it typically is heard in patients with congestive heart failure as a gallop rhythm. The *4th heart sound* is heard late in diastole and is due to atrial contraction.

MURMURS. The examination should focus next on the presence or absence of any heart murmurs caused by turbulent flow. Murmurs most commonly are innocent and not the result of cardiac pathology. Murmurs usually are described by their pitch, intensity, duration, timing, and location. Intensity typically is graded on a six-point scale:

I—barely audible
II—of medium intensity
III—loud
IV—loud and associated with a thrill
V—may be heard with the stethoscope only partly on the chest
and VI—may be heard with the stethoscope near the chest

Systolic murmurs generally are classified as ejection murmurs, pansystolic murmurs, or continuous murmurs. Ejection murmurs generally are due to turbulent flow across the semilunar valves. They may be due to increased flow or valvular anomalies. They typically are high pitched, crescendo–decrescendo murmurs that are strongly related to the heart sounds. Pansystolic murmurs typically are due to septal defects or regurgitant A-V valves. They begin almost simultaneously with the 1st heart sound and may gradually decrescendo. Continuous murmurs spill over from systole into diastole and typically are due to shunt vessels such as patent ductus arteriosus (PDA), arteriovenous malformations, aorticopulmonary collateral vessels, and surgically placed shunts connecting the right and left circulations.

Diastolic murmurs are due to regurgitant semilunar valves or turbulent blood flow across one of the A-V valves. This latter situation arises with stenosis of the mitral or tricuspid valves or when there is high blood flow across a normal valve, such as with a large ventricular septal defect (VSD) or ASD. Regurgitant semilunar valves commonly cause early diastolic, decrescendo murmurs heard best at the left sternal border. Murmurs associated with the A-V valves typically are mid-diastolic rumbles.

Benign or *innocent murmurs* also may be heard at any time during childhood. They are normal variants and usually are early systolic, soft, nonradiating murmurs. Examples of innocent murmurs include the vibratory or Still murmur, the pulmonic ejection murmur, the carotid bruit, the mammary souffle, and the venous hum.

CHEST ROENTGENOGRAM

The chest roentgenogram is helpful in the diagnosis of cardiovascular disease. Cardiac enlargement is diagnosed when the posterio–anterior projection of the cardiac diameter exceeds 55% of the thoracic diameter in infants less than 1 yr of age and 50% of the thoracic diameter in older children. Specific chamber enlargement may be inferred in this projection, although the sensitivity and specificity of this method is poor.

Assessment of the pulmonary vascularity may be helpful in diagnosis. Cardiac lesions associated with left-to-right shunts, such as ASD, VSD, and PDA, cause pulmonary arterial engorgement. Conversely, lesions associated with right-to-left shunts or pulmonary stenosis decrease the prominence of these vessels. Lesions associated with obstructed pulmonary venous return, such as anomalous pulmonary veins, cor triatriatum, or mitral stenosis, cause pulmonary venous engorgement.

ELECTROCARDIOGRAM

Analysis of the electrocardiogram (ECG) may be helpful in diagnosis of myriad cardiac conditions. Chamber hypertrophy may be diagnosed by a combination of voltage criteria and morphology of the P wave or QRS complex. Metabolic conditions, such as hyperkalemia, may be diagnosed by changes in the wave morphology. Inflammation of the heart, such as that due to myocarditis and pericarditis, may be inferred from the ECG. Complete analysis of the ECG includes assessment of the rate, rhythm, P wave, P-R interval, QRS complex, Q-T interval, ST segment, and T wave.

The *P wave* represents atrial depolarization. Its morphology is best assessed in lead II, because the vector of this lead is most closely related to the direction of atrial depolarization. The P wave is peaked with right atrial hypertrophy and biphasic with left atrial hypertrophy.

The *P-R interval* represents the time it takes for electrical current to travel from the right atrium to the ventricles. The P-R interval is shortened in conditions in which the conduction velocity is increased, such as Wolff-Parkinson-White syndrome or glycogen storage disease. P-R interval lengthening usually is indicative of drug effect or disease in the A-V node, although it also may be due to disease in the atrial myocardium, the bundle of His, or the Purkinje system.

The *QRS complex* represents ventricular depolarization. The Q wave represents septal depolarization, the R wave represents depolarization of most of the ventricular myocardium, and the S wave represents the unbalanced depolarization of the remaining (posterior and superior) left ventricular myocardium. Assessment of the axis of the QRS complex is helpful in diagnosing right or left ventricular hypertrophy. Assessment of its morphology and duration is helpful in diagnosing hypertrophy and conduction problems.

The *Q-T interval* is measured from the beginning of the QRS complex to the end of the T wave. It is prolonged in metabolic conditions such as hypocalcemia and hypokalemia. It also is prolonged in the *prolonged Q-T syndrome* or as a result of drugs such as quinidine.

ST segment elevations or depressions are nonspecific markers of cardiac abnormality. ST segment changes may be due to ischemia, infarction, and drugs such as digoxin.

The *T wave* represents ventricular repolarization. Changes in the orientation of the T wave may be due to right ventricular hypertrophy.

ECHOCARDIOGRAPHY

Echocardiography and color flow Doppler ultrasonography are the most important noninvasive tools used in the diagnosis of cardiac lesions. They may provide enough anatomic and hemodynamic information that more invasive testing with cardiac catheterization and angiography may not be warranted.

OTHER NONINVASIVE TESTS

Magnetic resonance imaging has emerged as an important tool in the diagnosis of cardiac disease. It may provide excellent images of cardiac anatomy and metabolism and obviate the need for catheterization. *Radionuclide studies* are helpful in demonstrating cardiac perfusion. *Exercise testing* may be helpful in assessing the heart's ability to meet metabolic demands in various physiologic states.

CARDIAC CATHETERIZATION AND ANGIOGRAPHY

These tests are indicated when the information obtained from less invasive tests is insufficient for making optimal treatment decisions. Indications include diagnosis and presurgical evaluation of complex cardiac lesions, periodic monitoring of lesions at risk for progressive deterioration, and invasive procedures such as balloon dilation of stenotic valves, closure of ASDs and PDAs, or myocardial biopsy.

Cardiac catheterization yields especially good hemodynamic data. Injection of radiographic contrast material enables the cardiologist to diagnose and quantify shunts through the use of saturation and pressure measurements.

CONGENITAL HEART DISEASE
(*NELSON TEXTBOOK*, SECS. 15.11–15.61)

Congenital heart disease occurs in 8:1,000 live births. The incidence is significantly higher in stillborns (2%) and abortuses (10–25%). Ninety percent of congenital heart disease is not associated with teratogens or identifiable gene defects, and the recurrence risk varies from 1 to 4% for subsequent siblings. Parents with congenital heart disease have a risk of 4–5% of having a child with a congenital heart disease.

Of the congenitally acquired lesions, VSDs comprise 25–30%. ASD and PDA each comprise 6–8% of cardiac lesions, Coarctation of the aorta, tetralogy of Fallot, and pulmonary and aortic valve stenosis each account for 5–7% of cardiac lesions. d-Transposition of the great arteries is the second most common cyanotic lesion, acounting for 3–5% of all cardiac lesions. Other lesions are less common.

CONGENITAL CARDIAC DISEASE WITH CYANOSIS
(*NELSON TEXTBOOK*, SECS. 15.11–15.30)

Tetralogy of Fallot

The four components that comprise tetralogy of Fallot are (1) obstruction to right ventricular output, (2) VSD, (3) aorta overriding the VSD, and (4) right ventricular hypertrophy. The VSD always is large and nonrestrictive; the obstruction to right ventricular outflow may vary from mild to complete. When mild, blood flow may pass from the right ventricle to the pulmonary arteries relatively easily. Cyanosis therefore is mild, and these children sometimes are referred to as "pink tets." When the obstruction to right ventricular outflow is complete, all of the deoxygenated right ventricular flow passes across the VSD and into the systemic circulation. Cyanosis in these cases is severe and presents early in life.

CLINICAL MANIFESTATIONS. The main symptoms of tetralogy of Fallot are cyanosis, dyspnea, and paroxysmal hypercyanotic attacks ("tet spells") that generally worsen during the 1st yr of life. Tet spells are caused by increased shunting of deoxygenated blood across the VSD as a result of either increased pulmonary vascular resistance or decreased systemic vascular resistance, or a combination of the two.

Attacks typically are short, and children generally cope with hypercyanotic spells by squatting, which increases systemic vascular resistance, thereby decreasing right-to-left flow. Prolonged attacks may be treated by (1) placing the child on the abdomen in a knee–chest position, (2) administration of oxygen, (3) morphine, and (4) drugs that increase systemic vascular resistance, such as methoxamine or phenylephrine.

Typically found on cardiac examination are normal pulse, normal blood pressure, harsh systolic ejection murmur resulting from pulmonic stenosis, and a single 2nd heart sound if complete obstruction of the right ventricle is present. The ECG reveals right ventricular hypertrophy and right axis deviation. Chest roentgenograms typically show decreased pulmonary blood flow and a heart that is "boot shaped" (coeur en sabot) as a result of decreased pulmonary artery shadow and right ventricular hypertrophy.

Complications of tetralogy of Fallot include cerebral thromboses and ischemia resulting from hemoconcentration and hypoxemia, brain abscesses, bacterial endocarditis, and congestive heart failure.

TREATMENT. Immediate stabilization in the neonatal period includes the use of prostaglandin E_1 (PGE_1) to maintain the patency of the ductus arteriosus and prevention of hemoconcentration. Hypercyanotic spells should be treated as detailed above.

Correction includes surgical closure of the VSD and widening of the pulmonic outflow tract. This corrective repair may be attempted early in life or may be performed after a palliative systemic-to-pulmonary shunt is placed. Although any of a number of shunts may be used, a classic or modified Blalock–Taussig shunt connecting the subclavian artery to the ipsilateral pulmonary artery is performed most commonly because it best approximates normal pulmonary blood flow.

Complications of surgical correction include surgically induced pulmonary valvular incompetence, which typically is without hemodynamic significance. Conduction disturbances involving the A-V node or the bundle of His also are common because those structures typically are close to the VSD and are injured during closure.

Pulmonary Atresia with VSD

This lesion essentially is an extreme form of tetralogy of Fallot, and is complicated by bizarre anatomic distortions of the distal pulmonary arteries. Depending on the distortion of these vessels, blood flow may be entirely ductal dependent or via bronchial collateral vessels.

Presentation typically is early in life, with cyanosis and dyspnea. A systolic murmur usually is soft or absent; the 2nd heart sound is single. Chest roentgenogram and ECG findings are similar to findings when there is a tetralogy of Fallot.

Treatment in the newborn period involves the use of PGE_1 to maintain the patency of the ductus arteriosus until the pulmonary artery anatomy can be delineated. A palliative systemic-to-pulmonary shunt typically is placed. If the distal pulmonary arteries are relatively normal, repair involves closure of the VSD and use of a homograft between the right ventricles and the distal pulmonary arteries, with ligation of any bronchial collateral vessels. More complicated anatomy requires heart–lung transplantation.

Pulmonary Atresia with Intact Ventricular Septum

With this lesion, right-sided blood flow exits via the only route it can: a patent foramen ovale. Pulmonary blood flow is via a PDA. Because the deoxygenated blood returning from the body completely mixes with that returning from the lungs, the child typically is cyanotic and dyspneic from birth. Cardiac examination reveals a single 2nd heart sound, often with no murmur. An ECG is helpful because the axis always is between 0 and 90 degrees, characteristic of unbalanced left ventricular forces. A peaked P wave also is seen. Chest roentgenograms reveal a variably sized heart and decreased pulmonary vascularity.

Palliative treatment includes the use of PGE_1 and surgical creation of a systemic-to-pulmonary shunt in the newborn period. Definitive correction involves either the creation of a right ventricle–to–pulmonary artery conduit wherever possible or a Fontan procedure, in which systemic venous blood return is routed directly to the pulmonary arteries.

Tricuspid Atresia

In tricuspid atresia, there is no outlet from the right atrium; systemic venous return therefore must cross a patent foramen ovale and mix with oxygenated blood. Blood flow to the lungs is via a PDA, or, if a VSD is present, via the pulmonary artery. Patients present with cyanosis and dyspnea at birth. The majority of children have pansystolic murmur at the left sternal border and a single 2nd heart sound. The ECG reveals left axis deviation and peaked or biphasic P waves. Chest roentgenograms reveal pulmonary undercirculation.

Palliative *treatment* includes PGE_1 and the creation of a systemic-to-pulmonary shunt. Rashkind balloon atrial septostomy, in which a balloon catheter is used to rip the intra-atrial septum, may be beneficial in some patients. Correction is via a Fontan procedure in which the systemic venous return is routed directly to the lungs either through the right atrium or via extracardiac shunts. The Fontan procedure depends on enough central venous pressure to overcome pulmonary vascular resistance; the procedure therefore is contraindicated in young infants or in children with elevated pulmonary vascular resistance or pulmonary artery hypoplasia. Good outcome depends on a sinus rhythm and the absence of mitral regurgitation or elevated left ventricular end-diastolic pressure (LVEDP).

D-Transposition of the Great Arteries

In d-transposition of the great arteries (TGA) the aorta arises from the right ventricle, pumping deoxygenated blood to the body, while the pulmonary artery arises from the left ventricle, pumping already oxygenated blood back to the lungs. Oxygenation of the systemic blood may occur by mixing at any or all of three levels: a patent foramen ovale, a VSD, or a PDA.

CLINICAL MANIFESTATIONS. In situations in which the ventricular septum is intact, cyanosis and tachypnea are recognized in the first hours or days of life. Cardiac examination often is subtle. The ECG reveals normal neonatal right-sided dominance. Chest roentgenograms reveal normal pulmonary vascular markings with a narrow cardiac waist and a globular heart ("egg on a string" appearance).

In situations in which there is an associated large VSD, the patient presents with symptoms of congestive heart failure and cyanosis may be subtle. Cardiac examination is remarkable for a pansystolic VSD-type murmur. The ECG typically shows peaked P waves and either right ventricular or biventricular hypertrophy. Chest roentgenograms reveal cardiomegaly with a narrow cardiac waist and significant pulmonary vascular markings.

TREATMENT. Palliative treatment of these lesions consists of PGE_1 and Rashkind balloon atrial septostomy in an effort to increase mixing, and, in cases associated with VSD, help decompress the left atrium. Whereas atrial baffle (Mustard, Senning) procedures once were the corrective procedure of choice for cases of TGA with an intact ventricular septum, the corrective procedure of choice for infants less than 2 wk of age now is the arterial switch (Jatene) procedure. In this procedure, the great arteries are reanastomosed to their correct ventricles and the coronary arteries are reimplanted. The survival rate in most centers is 80–90%. The cases of older infants are complicated by the physiologic fall in pulmonary vascular resistance, which leaves the left ventricle without the muscle mass necessary to assume systemic function. In an effort to prepare the left ventricle for the systemic load it will have to assume after corrective repair, the Jatene procedure typically is performed only after pulmonary arterial banding. In cases associated with a large VSD, the left ventricle continues to face systemic vascular resistance; repair therefore is more elective.

Total Anomalous Pulmonary Venous Return

In total anomalous pulmonary venous return (TAPVR), the return of oxygenated blood is to the right side of the circulation, rather than the left atrium. The anomaly may be supracardiac (return to the superior vena cava, innominate vein, or azygous system); intracardiac (return to a coronary sinus or directly to the right ventricle); or subdiaphragmatic (return to the portal vein, ductus venosus, or inferior vena cava). An associated ASD or patent foramen ovale always is present, aiding in the decompression of the right atrium and filling the left side of the circulation with mixed blood.

CLINICAL MANIFESTATIONS. Three types of clinical patterns are seen. When there is obstruction of pulmonary venous return, as is common in the infradiaphragmatic type, cyanosis and tachypnea are seen in the newborn period. Cardiac examination frequently reveals no murmurs. In patients in whom the pulmonary return is only mildly obstructed, there is a large left-to-right shunt in the presence of pulmonary hypertension, with the result being severe congestive heart failure. Cardiac examination may reveal a murmur or a gallop rhythm, and cyanosis is mild. In the third group of patients there is no obstruction to pulmonary venous return and no pulmonary hypertension. Although this variant is rare and more common with intracardiac lesions, patients may be asymptomatic. In all three variants, the ECG typically shows peaked P waves and right ventricular hypertrophy. Chest roentgenograms of the supracardiac variant may reveal cardiomegaly with the typical "figure 8" or "snowman" appearance, and those of the infracardiac variant typically show marked pulmonary venous congestion with a small heart.

TREATMENT. After stabilization with PGE$_1$ and possible balloon atrial septostomy, the defect should be anatomically repaired and the ASD closed in the newborn period. Prognosis is excellent.

Ebstein Anomaly

In this lesion, there is "atrialization of the right ventricle": the tricuspid valve usually is incompetent and inferiorly displaced in the right ventricle. Symptoms depend on the degree of displacement and incompetence of the tricuspid valve. A right-to-left shunt through the foramen ovale is responsible for cyanosis and polycythemia. Cardiac dysrhythmias are common. The ECG usually shows a right bundle branch block, large, peaked P waves, and occasionally a prolonged P-R interval. On chest roentgenograms, heart size varies from normal to grossly enlarged. Treatment includes control of arrhythmias and repair of the tricuspid valve with closure of the ASD.

Truncus Arteriosus

In this lesion there is a single trunk arising from the two ventricular chambers, which are typically connected via a VSD. There are three anatomic variants of the truncus arteriosus:

> *type I,* in which a pulmonary artery trunk arises off the truncus, later dividing into right and left pulmonary arteries
>
> *type II,* in which the right and left pulmonary arteries arise separately from the posterior of the truncus
>
> *type III,* in which the right and left pulmonary arteries arise separately from the lateral aspects of the truncus

Truncus arteriosus may be an isolated condition or may occur as part of another complex disorder such as occurs in DiGeorge syndrome.

CLINICAL MANIFESTATIONS. Symptoms vary, depending on the degree of pulmonary obstruction or vascular resistance. Typically, there is no obstruction to pulmonary blood flow and the lungs are flooded. Symptoms include tachypnea, dyspnea, and congestive heart failure. Cyanosis is minimal or mild. Cardiac examination reveals a hyperdynamic precordium, a systolic ejection murmur, and a loud, single 2nd heart sound. The ECG is variable but may show ventricular hypertrophy. Chest roentgenograms usually show cardiomegaly and increased pulmonary vascular markings.

TREATMENT. Surgical treatment usually involves closure of the VSD and creation of a right ventricle–to–pulmonary artery homograft.

Single Ventricle

In this condition, both atria empty into a common ventricle from which two great arteries arise. Cyanosis is due to mixing and may be exacerbated by pulmonic stenosis if present. In situations without obstruction to pulmonary blood flow, such flow may be torrential and congestive heart failure the predominant feature of disease. The ECG and chest roentgenograms are nonspecific, showing ventricular hypertrophy and cardiomegaly. Surgical correction is staged: in the first procedure, blood flow to the lungs is optimized with either a pulmonary artery band or a systemic-to-pulmonary shunt. The second procedure is a Fontan.

Eisenmenger Syndrome

Eisenmenger syndrome refers to the reversal of blood flow (as a result of pulmonary hypertension) through a shunt that typically is left to right (VSD, ASD, PDA, A-V canal, etc.). This condition is due to increased pulmonary vascular resistance secondary to changes in the intimal and medial layers of the pulmonary arteries. Such changes typically arise after prolonged exposure to elevated pulmonary artery pressure, and become apparent in the 2nd or 3rd decade of life.

Cardiac examination reveals a right ventricular heave and a loud, narrowly split 2nd heart sound. The ECG reveals peaked P waves and evidence of right ventricular hypertrophy. Chest roentgenograms may show a normal or enlarged heart.

Hypoplastic Left Heart Syndrome

Hypoplastic left heart syndrome (HLHS) includes a number of cardiac lesions in which underdevelopment of the left ventricle and the ascending aorta is common. Pulmonary venous blood returns to the left atrium and passes through an obligatory atrial communication, either an ASD or a PDA into the right side of the heart and the pulmonary artery. Systemic blood flow almost exclusively is the result of retrograde blood flow through a patent foramen ovale.

CLINICAL MANIFESTATIONS. Infants with HLHS typically are full term and vigorous in the nursery; they may be discharged without suspicion of cardiac disease. Symptoms begin as the ductus arteriosus begins to close: the child appears grey and limp, with poor perfusion to the body, while being tachypneic and dyspneic as a result of pulmonary overcirculation. The ECG may reveal right axis deviation and evidence of right atrial and ventricular hypertrophy. Chest roentgenograms may reveal cardiomegaly and pulmonary overcirculation.

TREATMENT. Medical palliation of HLHS includes PGE_1 infusion in an effort to maintain systemic blood flow through a PDA. Surgical correction involves the multistaged Norwood procedure. In the first stage of the Norwood procedure, the coarcted segment of the aorta is repaired and an anastomosis with the pulmonary artery is formed, essentially creating a truncus arteriosus–like lesion. In the second (and perhaps third) stages of the Norwood procedure, a modified Fontan procedure is performed in which the systemic veins are connected to the pulmonary arteries directly, and the right heart becomes the systemic pump exclusively. Because mortality with this procedure is high, cardiac transplantation is considered the treatment of choice in some centers.

CONGENITAL HEART DISEASE WITH LITTLE OR NO CYANOSIS
(*NELSON TEXTBOOK*, SECS. 15.30–15.61)

Ventricular Septal Defect

VSD is the most common congenital heart disease. It accounts for 25% of all congenital heart disease, with the defect most commonly found in the membranous portion of the intraventricular septum.

CLINICAL MANIFESTATIONS.   VSD typically is not diagnosed in the newborn period. Because pulmonary vascular resistance is high, there may be little or no shunting across the defect in this period. As pulmonary vascular resistance falls, left-to-right shunting of blood occurs and a pansystolic murmur is audible at the left sternal border.

Clinical symptoms depend on the degree of shunting, which in turn depends on the pulmonary vascular resistance and the size of the VSD. If the defect is small, the VSD is said to be "restrictive." Hemodynamics are relatively normal and clinical symptoms are mild or inapparent. Diagnosis typically is suspected by detection of the characteristic murmur on physical examination. The ECG typically is normal, as is the chest roentgenogram.

If the VSD is large and pulmonary vascular resistance is low, the ratio of left ventricular output that goes to the lungs is far greater than that which goes to the body ($\dot{Q}_p/\dot{Q}_s$ is high). This torrential blood flow to the lungs (and subsequently back to the left ventricle) causes left ventricular hypertrophy and heart failure. Symptoms include dyspnea, tachypnea, poor feeding and growth, and diaphoresis. Cardiac examination reveals a pansystolic murmur that may have an associated thrill. A low-pitched, mid-diastolic murmur resulting from turbulent flow across the mitral valve may be audible. The ECG typically reveals left ventricular hypertrophy and may reveal left atrial enlargement. Chest roentgenograms usually show cardiac enlargement and pulmonary overcirculation.

COMPLICATIONS.   Although the VSD closes in the majority of cases, complications of VSD include the small risk (<2%) of infective endocarditis and sequelae of persistent pulmonary overcirculation, including recurrent bouts of respiratory distress, congestive heart failure, and Eisenmenger syndrome.

TREATMENT. Parents should be reassured in most cases, with antibiotic prophylaxis prior to dental and genitourinary manipulations being the only treatment necessary. If the defect is large and the child symptomatic, the symptoms of congestive heart failure are treated with diuretics and digoxin. Surgical correction may be performed in patients with unrestrictive defects in the 1st yr of life with good outcome.

Double Outlet Right Ventricle Without Pulmonary Stenosis

In this anomaly, the left and right ventricles are connected by a VSD, but both great arteries arise from the right ventricle. If the great arteries are normally related, the patient presents as with a large, unrestrictive VSD. The ECG typically reveals a left superior axis deviation and evidence of biventricular hypertrophy. Correction is accomplished by closure of the VSD and funneling blood to the aorta.

If the great vessels both arise from the right ventricle but are transposed, the patient has the Taussig–Bing anomaly. In this lesion, the VSD is doubly committed and shunts blood to both the aorta (which is itself commonly obstructed) and the pulmonary artery. Patients typically present with cyanosis and congestive heart failure. The ECG may show superior axis deviation and ventricular hypertrophy. Chest roentgenograms show pulmonary overcirculation and cardiomegaly. Treatment typically involves palliative pulmonary banding in an effort to reduce pulmonary blood flow, and subsequently a Rastelli procedure in which the VSD is closed and a right ventricle–to–pulmonary artery conduit is placed.

Atrial Septal Defect (ASD)

ASD is a classic example of a high-flow, low-pressure left-to-right shunt. In this lesion there is an intra-atrial communication through which blood flows down the path of least resistance (i.e., from the high-resistance systemic side of the heart to the low-resistance pulmonary side of the heart). The ratio of pulmonary to systemic flow (Q_P/Q_s) may be very elevated, resulting in torrential pulmonary blood flow. Although this lesion may be quite well tolerated in childhood, pulmonary vascular changes and Eisenmenger syndrome may result if it is not corrected.

The same physiology may be found with other lesions. Partial anamolous pulmonary venous return causes a large, fixed, left-to-right shunt, as do ostium primum defects and A-V canals. With all of these lesions, a pulmonic ejection murmur may be audible at the left upper sternal border as a result of pulmonary overcirculation. The pulmonary component of the 2nd heart sound is delayed, resulting in a fixed, widely split 2nd heart sound. A soft, mid-diastolic rumble may be heard as a result of blood flow across the tricuspid valve.

Ostium secundum defects are the most common variety of ASD. A child with an ostium secundum defect most commonly is asymptomatic, although exercise intolerance may be noted in older children. Diagnosis typically is made by auscultation of the heart. The ECG may show increased right atrial and ventricular forces as well as an rsR' configuration in the right precordial leads consistent with right ventricular conduction delay. Chest roentgenograms may reveal increased heart size with increased pulmonary arterial markings. Although these defects may be well tolerated until the 3rd decade of life, they should be repaired electively. Closure usually is done prior to school entry. In some centers, closure may be performed with occlusional devices in the catheterization laboratory. Left unrepaired, ostium secundum defects produce complications that include atrial dysrhythmias, tricuspid regurgitation, and pulmonary hypertension. Infective endocarditis is rare.

Ostium primum defects and *A-V canals* are embryologically related. In both, there is interatrial communication through which blood shunts from left to right and associated irregularities in the A-V valves. A-V canals, common among patients with Down syndrome, also are associated with interventricular communication and shunting. Ostium primum defects typically are well tolerated in childhood, whereas children with A-V canal typically present with congestive heart failure in infancy. Chest roentgenograms typically show cardiomegaly and increased pulmonary arterial markings. The ECG findings are distinctive and include left superior axis deviation, biventricular hypertrophy, and right ventricular conduction delay. Surgical repair includes plastic repair of the A-V valves and closure of the interchamber communications. This may be done primarily or after protective pulmonary artery banding.

Patent Ductus Arteriosus

PDA is the most common of the "aortic runoff" syndromes, in which aortic blood flow is shunted left to right. Other examples include aorticopulmonary septal defects, coronary artery fistulae, and ruptured sinus of Valsalva. In all of these syndromes, there is aortic communication with the low-resistance right-side circulation, causing increased pulmonary blood flow, widened pulse pressure, and bounding arterial pulsations. Symptoms vary with the degree of blood flow across the communication. Large lesions lead to pulmonary congestion, dyspnea, and congestive heart failure. The ECG may show left ventricular or biventricular hypertrophy. Chest roentgenograms may reveal prominent pulmonary arterial markings. Small lesions typically are asymptomatic, without ECG or roentgenographic changes.

The ductus arteriosus typically closes shortly after birth. The precise mechanisms leading to closure are incompletely understood, but arterial oxygenation is known to play a role. In premature infants, PDA is a common finding that is related to hypoxemia. In term infants, PDA is uncommon and relates to deficiencies in the medial muscular layer of the vessel that pre-empt its closure. Because the long-term risk associated with PDA far outweighs the risks of closure, closure typically is performed before the 2nd yr of life. Surgical therapy consists of ligation and separation; closure also may be done in the catheterization laboratory, using arterial occlusion devices.

Pulmonary Stenosis with Intact Ventricular Septum

Obstructions of the right ventricular outflow tract are common and may vary in severity. All cause a pulmonic outflow murmur most audible at the left upper sternal border and radiating to the lung fields. They may occur as isolated lesions or as part of more complex anatomy. They may be progressive or static, symptomatic or asymptomatic.

Valvular pulmonic stenosis is the most common form of outlet obstruction. Symptoms vary with the degree of stenosis. Mildly stenotic lesions may be asymptomatic and are diagnosed on routine cardiac examination. They typically do not progress, and no therapy except antibiotic prophylaxis is warranted. More severely stenotic valves may lead to cyanosis and symptoms of right congestive heart failure. Cardiac examination reveals a pulmonic ejection murmur and a single 2nd heart sound. The ECG findings may include right atrial and ventricular hypertrophy. Chest roentgenograms may reveal right-sided cardiac enlargement and decreased peripheral pulmonary vascular markings. The main pulmonary artery frequently appears normal on chest roentgenograms as a result of poststenotic dilation. Therapy consists of valvuloplasty, which may be performed surgically or in the catheterization laboratory.

Infundibular pulmonic stenosis is a fairly common finding that may occur as an isolated lesion or in conjunction with valvular stenosis. Infundibular stenosis is due to subvalvular muscular hypertrophy and fibrosis. The severity of symptoms depends on the degree of obstruction. Repair is surgical myotomy.

Peripheral pulmonic stenosis is common and may occur as an isolated finding or in conjunction with more severe cardiac disease. Isolated peripheral pulmonic stenosis typically is mild and the diagnosis is made by auscultation. Usually no therapy is necessary.

Pulmonary Insufficiency

Pulmonary insufficiency typically occurs as part of more complex cardiac disease or following correction of right ventricular outflow tract obstruction. Incompetence usually is mild and is diagnosed by the presence of a soft, low-pitched diastolic murmur at the left mid- and upper sternal border. Treatment consists of therapy directed at associated cardiac lesions, with valvular replacement if necessary.

Coarctation of The Aorta

The *symptoms* of coarctation of the aorta vary with the location and degree of obstruction. When there is obstruction of the aortic isthmus and flow to the dependent parts of the body primarily occurs via a PDA, the lesion is said to be of the infantile type. Congestive heart failure, cyanosis, poor feeding, and failure to thrive are common presentations. Most coarctations are juxtaductal, with more insidious symptoms and presentations. Coarctations may be isolated cardiac lesions, or part of more complex cardiac disease. Coarctation of the aorta usually is associated with hypertension resulting from poor renal perfusion and increased renin secretion.

Diagnosis usually is made after measurement of blood pressures in all four extremities. With coarctation of the aorta, the blood pressure is decreased in those extremities distal to the coarctation. Associated findings include a systolic murmur heard best at the left sternal border and radiating to the back, and faint femoral pulses that may be delayed relative to those palpated in the upper extremities. The ECG findings depend on the degree and location of the obstruction: in the infantile variant right ventricular hypertrophy is seen, whereas in older patients left ventricular changes resulting from persistent hypertension are present. Chest roentgenograms may reveal cardiomegaly.

Coarctation of the aorta *should be surgically repaired*, because hypertensive cardiac disease invariably will result. Repair may be done emergently, as in newborns, or electively. Elective repair usually is done at 2–4 yr, at which time the risks of surgery are minimal. Surgical repair frequently is complicated by postoperative hypertension, requiring medical management.

Congenital Aortic Stenosis

Congenital obstruction of the left ventricular outlet accounts for 5% of congenital heart disease. Stenosis typically is mild and may not present until adulthood, but may be severe and present in the newborn period with associated endocardial fibroelastosis. Stenosis typically is valvular in origin, but also may be subvalvular or supravalvular, as is seen most commonly in Williams syndrome.

Clinical manifestations of stenosis vary with degree of obstruction, and may include left heart failure, fatigability, angina, or syncope. Cardiac examination reveals a harsh ejection murmur at the right upper sternal border that may radiate to the neck. If the lesion is valvular in origin, an opening click may be heard. In severe lesions, the 2nd heart sound may be paradoxically split. The ECG may be normal or reveal left ventricular hypertrophy. Evidence of ventricular strain may be present on resting ECG or elicitable on graded exercise testing. Chest roentgenograms frequently reveal cardiomegaly.

Treatment of aortic stenosis may include surgical excision of the stenotic area, valvuloplasty, or balloon dilation of the stenotic valve in the catheterization lab. Treatment may carry a high risk; therefore, interventions should be limited to patients with symptomatic disease or demonstrating a high pressure gradient across the stenotic area. Antibiotic prophylaxis of dental or genitourinary manipulations is required.

Congenital Mitral Stenosis

This is a relatively rare lesion in which there is obstruction of left atrial flow. Symptoms are those of left heart failure, with poor growth, poor feeding, and easy fatigability. Cardiac examination reveals a rumbling diastolic murmur at the apex. An opening click or loud 1st heart sound also may be heard. The ECG reveals a normal or bifid P wave consistent with left atrial enlargement. Right ventricular hypertrophy may be seen in extreme cases. Prognosis is poor, and surgical results have been variable.

Congenital Mitral Insufficiency and Mitral Valve Prolapse

Both of these lesions cause regurgitation of left ventricular blood across an incompetent mitral valve and are associated with a systolic ejection murmur heard best at the apex. Mitral valve prolapse may have an associated mid-systolic click. Patients generally are asymptomatic, although severe lesions may be associated with left heart failure. The ECG may show left atrial enlargement, and right ventricular enlargement in severe cases. Treatment generally is symptomatic, although valve replacement may be warranted in severe cases.

DISTURBANCES OF THE RATE AND RHYTHM OF THE HEART
(NELSON TEXTBOOK, SECS. 15.62–15.65)

Disturbances of the rate and rhythm of the heart are a fairly common problem in pediatrics. They may occur in the normal or diseased heart; they may be transient or permanent; they may be minor or severe. The major risk associated with rhythm disturbances is that of a severe tachycardia or bradycardia, which greatly compromises cardiac output, leading to syncopy, shock, or death.

Normal rhythm disturbances include sinus arrhythmia, sinus bradycardia, and extrasystoles. Pathologic disturbances of rate and rhythm are best divided into those that cause rapid heart rates (tachyarrhythmias) and those that produce slow heart rates (bradyarrhythmias).

Sinus arrhythmia refers to the normal variation in sinus heart rate found with respiration. In all individuals there is a normal slowing of the heart rate during expiration and acceleration during inspiration. Although this variation may be quite pronounced in children, it should not be confused with a significant rhythm disorder. The diagnosis of sinus arrhythmia is made when normal P waves are followed by a normal P-R interval and a normal QRS complex on a rhythm strip; the only variation seen is the lengthening and shortening of the interval between systoles.

Sinus bradycardia is a bradyarrhythmia in which there is slowing of the impulses originating from the sinus node. Although it is commonly found in healthy individuals and athletes, it also may be a symptom of disease states such as hypothyroidism. A diagnosis of sinus bradycardia is made when the heart rate is less than two standard deviations below the mean for a given age. P waves, P-R intervals, and QRS complexes all are normal on the rhythm strip.

Extrasystoles are common phenomena that are produced by electrical discharge from an ectopic focus anywhere in the myocardium. They typically are of no clinical or prognostic significance and usually are categorized as premature atrial complexes or premature ventricular complexes.

Premature atrial complexes may occur in the normal or diseased myocardium. They are diagnosed on rhythm strip by the appearance of an abnormally located P wave that has a morphology that is different from the regularly recurring sinus P wave.

Premature ventricular complexes (PVCs) are common in children and adolescents. They are characterized by premature, wide, bizarre QRS complexes that are not preceded by a P wave. They are infrequent and disappear with exercise or tachycardia. PVCs should be investigated further under the following circumstances:

sequential ventricular depolarizations occur without intervening sinus beats

PVCs are multifocal in origin

the frequency of PVCs increases with exercise

the PVCs interfere with normal repolarization (R on T phenomenon)

in the presence of underlying heart disease

if the patient feels marked anxiety from the awareness of PVCs

TACHYARRHYTHMIAS

The tachyarrhythmias must be divided into those that are supraventricular in origin and those that are ventricular in origin. Most of the time this is accomplished easily by inspection of the QRS complex. If the heart rate is fast and the QRS complex is normal and narrow, the tachyarrhythmia is supraventricular in origin. If the QRS complex is wide and bizarre in appearance, the tachyarrhythmia may be ventricular in origin, or supraventricular in origin in cases in which there is aberrant conduction through the ventricular system. The tachyarrhythmias include sinus tachycardia, atrial tachycardia, atrial fibrillation, atrial flutter, ventricular tachycardia and ventricular fibrillation.

Sinus Tachycardia

This may occur in the normal or diseased myocardium and commonly is seen with fever, dehydration, and pain or secondary to drug effects, especially those of the sympathomimetics. It usually is diagnosed when the heart rate is less than 225/min and varies with respiration. On a rhythm strip, the P waves always are present and have a normal axis, QRS complexes always follow the P waves, and the P-R interval is normal.

Treatment involves treating the underlying cause.

Atrial Tachycardia or Supraventricular Tachycardia

Supraventricular tachycardia (SVT) typically is caused by a re-entry circuit through the A-V node. SVT may occur in the normal or diseased myocardium, and attacks are characterized by their abrupt onset and cessation. Heart rate typically is 180–320/min and does not vary with respiration. On a rhythm strip, P waves may be present 50% of the time, although their morphology and axis may be abnormal. QRS complexes may be normal or abnormal in cases in which aberrant conduction is present. In these cases, differentiation from ventricular tachycardia is difficult but essential. The complete absence of P waves and the presence of wide QRS complexes that are dissimilar to the QRS complexes found during sinus rhythm are diagnostic of ventricular tachycardia.

Treatment depends on the symptoms of the child. In urgent situations the patient should be electrically cardioverted with 1–2 watt-sec/kg of electrical current. Asymptomatic patients may be treated with various vagal maneuvers, such as placement of iced saline on the face, breath holding, or a Valsalva maneuver, or pharmacologic therapy may be used. Digoxin is the mainstay of therapy for patients with supraventricular tachycardia. Other drugs that have been used include quinidine, propranolol, and verapamil.

Atrial Flutter

This most commonly is found in children with diseased myocardium. It frequently is seen in children with large stretched atria resulting from diseases or surgical repairs, such as Ebstein anomaly, mitral regurgitation, or following the Fontan procedure. Atrial flutter is a regular or regularly irregular tachycardia in which the atrial rate is found to be 250–400/min, with variable conduction of the ventricular impulse at a rate of 100–320/min. On a rhythm strip, atrial flutter shows a characteristic saw-toothed pattern, with QRS complexes that may be either normal or prolonged in those cases with aberrant conduction.

Treatment usually begins with digitalis in an effort to slow the ventricular response to atrial flutter by prolonging conduction through the A-V node. After full digitalization, quinidine or procainamide may be added to convert the patient back to sinus rhythm. In symptomatic patients with congestive heart failure, electrical cardioversion is the treatment of choice.

Atrial Fibrillation

This most commonly is found in diseased myocardium and is associated with diseases in which the atria are large and stretched. In atrial fibrillation, the atrial excitation is irregularly irregular, with an atrial rate of 300–500/min and a ventricular rate of 120–180/min. On a rhythm strip the P waves are abnormal and variable and the QRS complexes may be normal or prolonged in cases with aberrant conduction.

Digitalis is the *treatment* of choice because it slows the ventricular rate. After full digitalization, normal sinus rhythm may be restored with quinidine, procainamide, or electrical cardioversion.

Ventricular Tachycardia

This is diagnosed by the appearance of three or more consecutive premature ventricular beats at a rate of greater than 120/min. Although ventricular tachycardia may occur in the normal myocardium, it is seen more commonly in patients with cardiac disease, in postoperative patients, or with sympathomimetic drug use.

Ventricular tachycardia should be treated promptly because it may be associated with hypotension or progress to ventricular fibrillation. Lidocaine, bretylium, and electrical cardioversion commonly are used in the treatment of this arrhythmia.

Ventricular Fibrillation

This is diagnosed by the appearance of completely irregular tracings on the rhythm strip without identifiable P waves or QRS complexes. Invariably accompanied by hypotension, this arrhythmia is fatal unless promptly treated. Defibrillation is the treatment of choice.

BRADYARRHYTHMIAS

Various parts of the heart have their own inherent automaticity. Because the impulses arising from the sinus node have a faster inherent rate than the impulses arising from the A-V node (which has a faster rate than that of the ventricles), sinus rhythm usually results. Bradyarrhythmias result from slowing of the normal sinus impulse or because of various degrees of A-V block.

Sinus pause results when the ventricle does not conduct a sinus impulse. Sinus pauses are rare in childhood, but may be the result of digoxin or previous surgery.

There are three degrees of **A-V block.** With *1st-degree A-V block,* there is prolongation of the P-R interval but all P waves are followed by QRS complexes. *Second-degree A-V* block is subdivided into two types, Mobitz type I (Wenckebach) and Mobitz type II. In Wenckebach, the P-R interval progressively elongates until a QRS complex is skipped, after which the P-R interval shortens again. In Mobitz II, occasional atrial contractions are not followed by QRS complexes, without the regular cycles of prolongation of the P-R interval seen in Wenckebach. *Third-degree A-V block* is diagnosed when no atrial impulses are conducted to the ventricles, which must rely on their own automaticity for contraction. Patients with 1st-degree heart block often are asymptomatic and require no therapy except for periodic monitoring. Patients with 3rd-degree heart block may require a pacemaker.

INFECTIVE ENDOCARDITIS
(*NELSON TEXTBOOK*, SEC. 15.66)

ETIOLOGY AND EPIDEMIOLOGY

Infections of the endocardium may be caused by bacteria, viruses, fungi, and other agents. *Streptococcus viridans* is responsible for approximately 50% of cases of infective endo-carditis and staphylococcal infections are responsible for another 30%. Infective endocarditis caused by group D enterococcus is common after lower bowel or genitourinary manipulation, and *Pseudomonas aeruginosa* and *Serratia marcescens* are common causes among IV drug users.

Although the endocardium of normal hearts may become infected, infections most commonly occur in areas of extremely turbulent flow. Some lesions that commonly are complicated by infective endocarditis include VSD, aortic stenosis, PDA, TGA, and tetralogy of Fallot.

CLINICAL MANIFESTATIONS

The early signs and symptoms of infective endocarditis usually are mild, especially when *S. viridans* is the infecting organism. Symptoms include fever, chills, chest pain, dyspnea, malaise, night sweats, weight loss, arthralgias, and myalgias. Signs include fever, tachycardia, arrhythmias, heart failure, and new or changing murmurs. Embolic phenomena may be manifested as Roth spots, petechiae, splinter nail bed hemorrhages, Osler nodes, or ocular lessions. Additionally, small, painless, erythematous or hemorrhagic lessions on the palms and soles, known as Janeway lesions, may be present.

Complications occur in 50–60% of children with documented infective endocarditis. Complications include congestive heart failure resulting from vegetations involving the aortic or mitral valve, myocardial abscesses, pulmonary emboli, and aneurysm formation.

LABORATORY FINDINGS

Attempts should be made to identify the causative agent. Blood cultures must be obtained as promptly as possible in each child in whom infective endocarditis is suspected. Three to five blood cultures typically are recommended, although two blood cultures will identify the bacteria in 90% of the cases. The laboratory should be notified that endocarditis is suspected in case specially enriched media or prolonged growth periods are required for adequate growth.

A number of acute-phase reactants may be elevated in infective endocarditis, including erythrocyte sedimentation rate, C-reactive protein, and leukocytosis. Additionally, hypergammaglobulinemia, hypocomplementemia, cryoglobulinemia, and an elevated rheumatoid factor may be found.

TREATMENT

Antibiotic therapy is the mainstay of treatment for infective endocarditis. Antibiotics chosen should be broad-spectrum initially and then subsequently tailored to the organism identified. High serum bacteriocidal levels must be established and maintained, with a total duration of therapy of 4–6 wk. Complications of infective endocarditis, especially congestive heart failure, should be treated with digoxin, fluid restriction, and diuretic therapy.

PREVENTION

Susceptible patients should receive antibiotic prophylaxis prior to some medical procedures associated with bacteremia, including dental procedures and genitourinary manipulation. Recommended agents and their doses are given in Table 13–1.

TABLE 13–1. RECOMMENDATIONS FOR PREVENTION OF BACTERIAL ENDOCARDITIS*,†

Dental Procedures and Surgery of Upper Respiratory Tract

(1) For most patients: Oral amoxicillin	*Adults:* 3 g 1 hr before a procedure and 1.5 g 6 hr after the initial dose *Children:* 50 mg/kg 1 hr before a procedure and 25 mg/kg 6 hr after the initial dose‡
(2) Penicillin allergy: Oral erythromycin	*Adults:* 1 g 2 hr before a procedure and 500 mg 6 hr after the initial dose *Children:* 20 mg/kg 2 hr before a procedure and 10 mg/kg 6 hr after the initial dose‡
or Oral clindamycin	*Adults:* 300 mg 1 hr before a procedure and 150 mg 6 hr after the initial dose *Children:* 10 mg/kg 1 hr before a procedure and 5 mg/kg 6 hr after the initial dose‡
(3) High-risk patients§: Parenteral ampicillin plus gentamicin (IV or IM)	*Adults:* Ampicillin 2 g 30 min before a procedure‖ Gentamicin 1.5 mg/kg 30 min before a procedure‖ *Children:* Ampicillin 50 mg/kg 30 min before a procedure‖ Gentamicin 2 mg/kg 30 min before a procedure‖
(4) High-risk penicillin-allergic patients: Vancomycin (IV)	*Adults:* 1 g infused slowly in 1 hr, initiated 1 hr before a procedure; no repeat dose needed *Children:* 20 mg/kg infused as adults; no repeat dose needed‡

Gastrointestinal and Genitourinary Tract Surgery and Instrumentation

(1) For most patients: Parenteral ampicillin plus gentamicin (IV or IM)	*Adults:* Ampicillin 2 g 30 min before a procedure‖ Gentamicin 1.5 mg/kg 30 min before a procedure‖ *Children:* Ampicillin 50 mg/kg 30 min before a procedure‖ Gentamicin 2 mg/kg 30 min before a procedure

(continued)

TABLE 13–1. RECOMMENDATIONS FOR PREVENTION OF BACTERIAL ENDOCARDITIS*,†
Continued

(2) Penicillin allergy: Parenteral vancomycin plus gentamicin	*Adults:* Vancomycin 1 g infused slowly over 1 hr before a procedure¶ 　Gentamicin 1.5 mg/kg 30 min before a procedure¶ *Children:* Vancomycin 20 mg/kg infused slowly over 1 hr before a procedure‡ 　Gentamicin 2 mg/kg 30 min before a procedure¶
(3) Oral regimen for low-risk patients: Amoxicillin	*Adults:* 3 g 1 hr before a procedure and 1.5 g 6 hr later *Children:* 50 mg/kg 1 hr before a procedure and 25 mg 6 hr later‡

* From Behrman RE (ed): Nelson Textbook of Pediatrics, 14th ed. Philadelphia, WB Saunders Company, 1992, p 1203. (Adapted from JAMA 264:2919, 1990, American Medical Association, and from Med Lett Drug Ther 31:112, 1989.) Oral regimens are less expensive, more convenient, and safer than parenteral routes. Amoxicillin is recommended because of excellent bioavailability and good activity against streptococcus and enterococci. Parenteral routes are more effective and are recommended by some authorities for high-risk patients.

† Prophylaxis is recommended for patients with previous endocarditis, valvular heart disease, prosthetic heart devices, indiopathic hypertrophic subaortic stenosis, mitral valve prolapse with regurgitation, cardiac transplantation (possibly), and congenital heart disease except for an isolated secundum atrial septal defect and for patients who have recovered at least 6 mo from surgery for a patent ductus arteriosus or simple atrial septal defect without a patch.

‡ Maximal doses for children should not exceed adult doses.

§ High risk includes prostetic valves, previous endocarditis, continuous penicillin prophylaxis for rheumatic fever, and surgically constructed systemic–pulmonary shunts or conduits.

¶ Additional parenteral (ampicillin and gentamicin), or more often oral (amoxicillin), dose should be given 6–8 hr after the initial dose in high-risk patients. The dose of gentamicin should not exceed 80 mg.

¶ Additional dose may be repeated 8 hr after the initial dose.

RHEUMATIC HEART DISEASE
(*NELSON TEXTBOOK*, SEC. 15.67)

Rheumatic heart disease may result after pharyngeal infection with some strains of group A streptococci (see Chap. 9). Rheumatic disease begins weeks to months following acute infection. Rheumatic fever may recur, so lifelong antibiotic prophylaxis may be necessary. The endocardium, myocardium, or pericardium may be affected in rheumatic fever, but valvular lesions are the most prognostically important. The mitral valve is affected most frequently, with the aortic valve affected next most in frequency.

MITRAL INSUFFICIENCY

This results from the loss of valvular substance and the shortening and thickening of the chordae tendineae. With mitral insufficiency, the patient typically experiences left ventricular enlargement with subsequent dilation of the left atrium as a result of regurgitation of ventricular blood. Ultimately, the patient goes on to develop left-sided heart failure with dyspnea, orthopnea, and other symptoms related to pulmonary edema. Cardiac examination is remarkable for a pansystolic murmur heard best at the apex. A systolic thrill or a mid-diastolic rumble suggestive of severe insufficiency also may be found on examination. The ECG reveals bifid P waves suggestive of left atrial enlargement with QRS complexes suggestive of left ventricular hypertrophy. On chest roentgenograms, there typically is cardiomegaly with prominence of the left atrium and ventricle. Lung fields may reveal fluffy infiltrates suggestive of pulmonary venous congestion.

Mitral insufficiency generally is well tolerated by patients. In most cases, the insufficiency regresses and therapy is limited to antimicrobial prophylaxis. If mitral insufficiency is complicated by congestive heart failure, arrhythmias, or infective endocarditis, they should be treated as described elsewhere in this chapter.

MITRAL STENOSIS

Mitral stenosis of rheumatic origin is a chronic problem that usually develops many years after acute rheumatic fever. It results from fibrosis of the mitral ring with fibrosis and thickening of the valve leaflets and their attachments. Symptoms include orthopnea, dyspnea, and overt pulmonary edema, with the ECG revealing prominent bifid P waves. In severe cases, evidence of right ventricular hypertrophy resulting from pulmonary arterial hypertension may be seen. Chest roentgenograms may reveal pulmonary vascular congestion in severe cases. Cardiac examination reveals a loud 1st heart sound with a loud opening snap of the mitral valve. A long, low-pitched, rumbling mitral distolic murmur may be audible.

Treatment of mitral stenosis includes maneuvers aimed at opening the stenotic valve. Where possible, the valve may be opened with balloon catheterization. If this is unsuccessful, surgical commisurotomy or valve replacement must be undertaken.

AORTIC INSUFFICIENCY

This results from sclerosis of the aortic valves with distortion and retraction of the cusps. Long-standing aortic insufficiency results in left ventricular enlargement and hypertrophy, with ultimate left heart failure. Symptoms include dyspnea, orthopnea and chest pain, with the cardiac examination typically revealing a blowing, high-pitched diastolic murmur most audible at the upper and middle left sternal border. The ECG reveals left ventricular enlargement and a notched P wave consistent with left atrial enlargement. Chest roentgenograms may reveal enlargement of the left ventricle and aorta.

Unlike mitral incompetence, aortic insufficiency does not regress. *Treatment* in most cases consists of antimicrobial prophylaxis against recurrences of rheumatic fever and infective endocarditis, with valve replacement when necessary.

DISEASES OF THE MYOCARDIUM
(*NELSON TEXTBOOK*, SECS. 15.68–15.74)

Myocardial damage may result from myriad medical conditions. Common hereditary causes include Duchenne muscular dystrophy, hypertrophic cardiomyopathy, mitochondrial myopathy syndromes, and the storage diseases. Infectious causes include coxsackievirus B infections; bacterial infections, including diphtheria and Lyme disease; and parasitic infections, most notably Chagas disease. Thyroid disease, pheochromocytoma, hypercholesterolemia, and beriberi all are known to cause myocardial disease. Collagen vascular diseases, including systemic lupus erythematosus, rheumatoid arthritis, scleroderma, and dermatomyositis, may cause cardiac disease. Drugs and toxins, most notably adriamycin, also may cause myocardial disease.

Myocarditis refers to inflammation of the heart resulting from any cause. Symptoms may be overt, including congestive heart failure, shock, or sudden death, or mild, including arrhythmia, gallop rhythm, or ECG changes. Tests helpful in diagnosis include elevation of the erythrocyte sedimentation rate, creatine phosphokinase, and lactic dehydrogenase. Poor cardiac function may be demonstrated on echocardiograms. Myocardial biopsy may confirm the diagnosis. *Treatment* consists of treating arrhythmias and congestive heart failure as described elsewhere in this chapter.

Cardiomyopathy may be primary or secondary to congenital anomalies, hypertension, or other acquired disease. Primary cardiomyopathy typically is classified as hypertrophic, dilated, or restrictive. All three are manifested clinically by heart failure, chest pain, dyspnea, arrhythmias, or sudden death.

Hypertrophic cardiomyopathy also is known as idiopathic hypertrophic subaortic stenosis and is marked by hypertrophy of the ventricles, especially the septum. In this disease there is decreased ventricular filling as a result of poor compliance, which in turn leads to poor cardiac output. Because the gradient across the subaortic obstruction may be increased during the Valsalva maneuver, competitive sports and strenuous physical activity should be discouraged. *Treatment* may include β-blockers, calcium channel blockers, or septal myotomy in severe cases.

Restrictive cardiomyopathy also is marked by poor ventricular compliance and poor diastolic filling. *Dilated cardiomyopathy* is characterized by dilation of the ventricles. In this disease, the ventricles are too compliant: filling is increased but contraction is poor. Prognosis of both of these diseases is invariably poor, and cardiac transplantation ultimately is necessary for survival.

CONGESTIVE HEART FAILURE

"Heart failure" is the term used to describe a state in which cardiac output is insufficient in meeting the metabolic de-

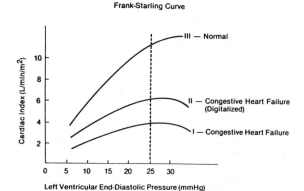

Figure 13–1. As the left ventricular end-diastolic pressure (LVEDP) increases, cardiac index increases, even in the presence of congestive heart failure, until a critical level of LVEDP is reached. Adding an inotropic agent (digoxin) shifts the curve from I to II. (From Gersony WM, Steep CN: *In* Dickerman JD, Lucey JF [eds]: Smith's The Critically Ill Child: Diagnosis and Medical Management, 3rd ed. Philadelphia, WB Saunders Company, 1984.)

mands of the body. Cardiac output is measured by the product of stroke volume and rate (CO = SV × rate), and cardiac output may be increased by increasing either of these variables. The body typically regulates its own heart rate, with tachycardia often being the first symptom of congestive heart failure. Various chronotropic drugs, such as isoproterenol, also may be used to increased heart rate and thereby increase cardiac output.

Physicians also may increase cardiac output by increasing stroke volume. The relationship of cardiac muscle resting length (LVEDP) and the cardiac index is shown in the Frank–Starling curve (Figure 13–1). Note that the cardiac index increases with LVEDP up to a point, after which there is a decline in the cardiac index. This curve demonstrates that one may manipulate preload (or LVEDP) with either fluid boluses or diuretics in an effort to maximize cardiac output on a given Frank–Starling curve. If judicious fluid management does not sufficiently increase cardiac output, heart failure must be treated with drugs that increase cardiac contractility, such as digoxin, dopamine, and dobutamine, or decrease the resistance (afterload) against which the heart is pumping. Afterload reducers are vasodilators and include nitroprusside, hydralazine, and captopril.

DISEASE OF THE PERICARDIUM
(*NELSON TEXTBOOK*, SEC. 15.75)

The pericardium is the tissue surrounding the heart and lining the mediastinum. Within this enclosed sac is a small amount of transudative fluid that bathes and lubricates the external surface of the heart. Although the heart is able to tolerate small increases in the fluid surrounding the heart without adverse effects on cardiac output, larger accumulations of fluid interfere with ventricular filling and ultimately with cardiac output.

Pericarditis may result from many disease processes. It may be the only manifestation of cardiac disease or be one component of a complex of cardiac manifestations. It also may be associated with more widespread systemic illness. Infectious diseases that are a major cause of pericarditis include viruses (coxsackie B, Epstein–Barr virus), bacteria (*S. aureus, Pneumococcus, Haemophilus influenzae,* tuberculosis), fungi, and parasites. Other common causes include collagen vascular diseases (rheumatoid arthritis, systemic lupus erythematosus), rheumatic fever, uremia, and postpericardotomy syndrome.

All of these diseases may share the same cardiac symptoms, including tachycardia, chest pain, congestive heart failure, pulsus paradoxicus, and ultimately tamponade. A friction rub may be heard on cardiac examination, and heart sounds may be distant. The ECG typically shows nonspecific low voltages, ST segment changes, and T wave inversions. Chest roentgenograms may reveal a typical "water bottle" configuration in the upright film as a result of settling of the pericardial fluid in the mediastinum.

Treatment typically consists of steroids or nonsteroidal anti-inflammatory drugs in an effort to reduce inflammation and antibiotics where indicated. Although pericardiocentesis commonly is done for diagnostic and therapeutic purposes, decisions to place a pericardial drain must be made carefully. They typically are based on the rapidness of the accumulation of fluid and the potential for tamponade. Open pericardial drainage often is necessary for purulent pericarditis because this readily may progress to tamponade.

SYSTEMIC HYPERTENSION
(*NELSON TEXTBOOK*, SEC. 15.80)

Hypertension is diagnosed when blood pressure is found to be greater than the 95th percentile for age on three different measurements. Hypertension typically is classified as primary (essential) or secondary. In pediatrics, the majority of cases of hypertension are secondary.

ETIOLOGY

A renal etiology is found in 75% of patients with secondary hypertension. Renal causes include infection, glomerulonephritis, renovascular disease, obstructive uropathy, and hemolytic uremic syndrome. The most common cardiac cause is coarctation of the aorta. Endocrine causes include hyperaldosteronism, Cushing syndrome, pheochromocytoma, and congenital adrenal hyperplasia. Drugs, especially corticosteroids, birth control pills, and sympathomimetics, commonly

TABLE 13–2. ANTIHYPERTENSIVE DRUGS*

Drug	Mechanism of Action	Dosage Range	Route	Duration	Side Effects
Vasodilators					
Hydralazine	Relax arteriolar smooth muscle	0.4–0.8 mg/kg/dose 0.5–2 mg/kg and increase to max 200 mg/24 hr	IV PO	2–4 hr 6–8 hr	Tachycardia, nausea Drug-induced lupus
Diazoxide	Relax smooth muscle	2–5 mg/kg/dose, max 100 mg	IV	6–24 hr	Tachycardia, hypotension, hyperglycemia
Nitroprusside	Dilatation of arterioles and venules	0.5–8.0 μg/kg/min	IV	With infusion	Thiocyanate production, rarely hypothyroidism
Minoxidil	Arteriolar dilatation	0.2–1.0 mg/kg/24 hr, max 50 mg/24 hr	PO	12–24 hr	Hypertrichosis, fluid retention
Adrenergic blockade					
Phentolamine	α-Receptor blockade	0.1 mg/kg/dose, max 5 mg	IV	1 hr	Reflex tachycardia
Phenoxybenzamine	α-Receptor blockade	2–5 mg/24 hr	PO	6–12 hr	Tachycardia may progress to arrhythmia
Prazosin	α-Receptor blockade	1-mg initial dose, may increase to 15 mg/24 hr	PO	8–12 hr	First dose orthostatic hypotension
Propranolol	β-Receptor blockade Reduces renin release	0.025–0.1 mg/kg/dose 0.25–1.0 mg/kg/dose	IV PO	6–8 hr	Bronchospasm bradycardia, vivid dreams
Labetalol	α-β Blockade	titrate 0.2–2 mg/kg/hr (based on adult dose) 100–400 mg (adult)	IV PO	With infusion 12 hr	Orthostasis, dizziness, bronchospasm

Sympatholytic agents					
α-Methyldopa	Decrease sympathetic tone	10 mg/kg/24 hr and increase	PO	6–8 hr	Sedation, hepatic dysfunction, positive Coombs reaction
Clonidine	2-α Agonist in CNS	3–5 µg/kg/dose	PO	6–8 hr	Sedation, constipation rebound withdrawal hypertension
Renin–angiotension					
Captopril	Converting-enzyme inhibition of angiotensin II synthesis	0.1–0.3 mg/kg/dose and increase to max 2 mg/kg/dose	PO	8 hr	Proteinuria, neutropenia, rash, dysgeusia
Enalaprilat	Same as captopril	0.005–0.010 mg/kg/dose	IV	8–12 hr	Transient hypotension
Calcium channel					
Nifedipine	Calcium channel blocker	0.2–0.5 mg/kg, max 10–20 mg	PO Sub†	Repeat q 30–60 min	Facial flushing, tachycardia
Verapamil	Calcium channel blocker	120–240 mg (adults)	PO	12–24 hr	Limited pediatric experience
Diuretic agents					
Hydrochlorothiazide	Diuresis	1–2 mg/kg/24 hr	PO	12–24 hr	Hypokalemia, hyperuricemia, hypercalcemia
Furosemide	Diuresis	1 mg/kg/dose	IV	4–6 hr	Hypokalemia, alkalosis
		2 mg/kg/dose	PO	4–6 hr	

* From Behrman RE (ed): Nelson Textbook of Pediatrics, 14th ed. Philadelphia, WB Saunders Company, 1992, p 1226. (Adapted from Med Lett Drugs Ther 1:25, 1989; 31:31, 1989.)
† Sublingual.

may be associated with hypertension. Other causes include hypercalcemia, seizures, neuroblastoma, and lead poisoning.

CLINICAL MANIFESTATIONS

Symptoms of hypertension are nonspecific. Infants may present with respiratory distress, vomiting, irritability, failure to thrive, or congestive heart failure. Children may present with the above symptoms or with headaches, visual symptoms, easy fatigability, or epistaxis.

DIAGNOSIS

Diagnostic tests include complete blood count, urinalysis, serum electrolytes, blood urea nitrogen creatinine, and uric acid. Blood pressures should be measured in all four extremities to rule out coarctation. Specific renal tests, including ultrasound, radionuclide scan, and angiography, should be considered.

TREATMENT

This includes pharmacologic and nonpharmacologic approaches. Weight loss and sodium restriction may be helpful in treatment of hypertension. Pharmacologic therapies are varied and should be tailored to the individual patient based on the patient's underlying physiology. Antihypertensive drug therapies are summarized in Table 13–2.

14

DISEASES OF THE BLOOD

DEVELOPMENT OF THE HEMATOPOIETIC SYSTEM
(*NELSON TEXTBOOK*, SECS. 16.1–16.3)

Blood formation starts by the 3rd wk after conception in mesodermal tissues. By birth, most blood formation takes place in the bone marrow.

RED BLOOD CELLS

Production of red blood cells is regulated by erythropoietin hormone produced in kidneys. Hemoglobin is the major protein of red blood cells.

HEMOGLOBIN

Hemoglobin is an oxygen-carrying protein that consists of an iron-containing heme group and a protein moiety, globin. The hemoglobin molecule is a tetramer of two pairs of globin proteins, each containing a heme group.

- Fetal hemoglobin (Hb F)

    is composed of two alpha and two gamma globin chains $(\alpha_2\gamma_2)$.

    represents 70% of total hemoglobin at birth but decreases rapidly postnatally to 2% in older children and adults

- Major adult hemoglobin (Hb A)

    is composed of two alpha and two beta globin chains $(\alpha_2\beta_2)$

    represents 30% of total hemoglobin at birth but increases thereafter

- Minor adult hemoglobin (Hb A_2)

    is composed of two alpha and two delta chains $(\alpha_2\delta_2)$ comprises 2–3.4% of total hemoglobin at 1 yr of age

METABOLISM OF THE RED BLOOD CELL

The red blood cell extrudes its nucleus during maturation. Red blood cells contain more than 40 enzymes, but no mitochondria, and generate adenosine triphosphate (ATP) from glucose, mostly by anaerobic glycolysis.

The functions of ATP include maintenance of electrolyte gradients, maintenance of red blood cell membrane and shape, maintenance of heme iron in reduced form, and maintenance of levels of organic phosphates.

The pentose phosphate pathway accounts for 10% of glucose metabolism.

THE ANEMIAS
(NELSON TEXTBOOK, SEC. 16.4–16.32)

Anemia is defined as reduction of red blood cell volume or hemoglobin concentration below the range of values occurring in healthy persons (Table 14–1). Black children have hemoglobin levels 0.5 g/dL lower than white or Oriental children.

Physiologic disturbances occur when hemoglobin falls below 7–8 g/dL. Signs and symptoms of anemia include pallor in skin and mucous membranes, weakness, tachypnea, tachycardia, shortness of breath, and congestive heart failure. Physiologic adjustments include tachycardia, increased cardiac output, rightward shift in the hemoglobin dissociation curve, and deviation of blood flow to vital organs. Few symptoms are evident initially if anemia develops slowly.

The anemias can be divided into two large groups (Table 14–2): (1) those resulting from decreased production of red blood cells or hemoglobin, and (2) those resulting from increased destruction or loss of red blood cells. In addition, a morphologic classification is possible based on mean corpuscular volume (MCV):

microcytic: MCV <75 fL
normocytic: MCV 75–100 fL
macrocytic: MCV >100 fL

TABLE 14–1. NORMAL HEMOGLOBIN LEVELS*

Age	Hemoglobin (g/dL)		Hematocrit (%)	
	Mean	Range	Mean	Range
Cord blood	16.8	13.7–20.1	55	45–65
2 wk	16.5	13.0–20.0	50	42–66
3 mo	12.0	9.5–14.5	36	31–41
6 mo–6 yr	12.0	10.5–14.0	37	33–42
7–12 yr	13.0	11.0–16.0	38	34–40
Adult				
Female	14	12.0–16.0	42	37–47
Male	16	14.0–18.0	47	42–52

* Adapted from Behrman RE (ed): Nelson Textbook of Pediatrics, 14th ed. Philadelphia, WB Saunders Company, 1992, p 1232.

TABLE 14–2. CLASSIFICATION OF THE ANEMIAS*,†

Anemias resulting primarily from inadequate production of red blood cells or hemoglobin
Decreased numbers of red blood cell precursors in the marrow
  "Pure red blood cell" anemias
    Congenital pure red blood cell anemia
    Acquired pure red blood cell anemias (e.g., TEC‡)
Inadequate production despite normal numbers of red blood cell precursors
  Anemia of infection, inflammation, and cancer
  Anemia of chronic renal disease
  Congenital dyserythropoietic anemias
Deficiency of specific factors
  Megaloblastic anemias
    Folic acid deficiency or malabsorption
    Vitamin B_{12} deficiency, malabsorption, or transport
    Orotic aciduria
  Microcytic anemias
    Iron deficiency
    Pyridoxine-responsive and X-linked hypochromic anemias
    Lead poisoning
    Copper deficiency
    Thalassemia trait

Hemolytic anemias
Intrinsic abnormalities of the red blood cell
  "Structural" defects
    Hereditary spherocytosis
    Hemolytic elliptocytosis
    Paroxysmal nocturnal hemoglobinuria
    Pyropyknocytosis
  Enzymatic defects (nonspherocytic hemolytic anemias)
    Enzymes of glycolytic pathway—pyruvate kinase, hexokinase, and others
    Enzymes of the pentose phosphate pathway and glutathione complex
  Defects in synthesis of hemoglobin
    Hb S, C, D, E, etc., alone and in combination
    Thalassemia

Extrinsic (extracellular) abnormalities
Immunologic disorders
  Passively acquired antibodies (hemolytic disease of the newborn)
    Rh isoimmunization
    A or B isoimmunization
    Other blood group families
  Active antibody formation
    Idiopathic autoimmune hemolytic anemia; cold agglutinin diseases
    Symptomatic—lupus, lymphoma
    Drug induced

Nonimmunologic disorders
Toxic from drugs, chemicals
Infections—malarial, clostridial

* From Behrman RE (ed): Nelson Textbook of Pediatrics, 14th ed. Philadelphia, WB Saunders Company, 1992, p 1233.
† See also anemia in pancytopenias and leukemia.
‡ TEC = transient erythropenia of childhood.

ANEMIA RESULTING FROM INADEQUATE PRODUCTION OF RED BLOOD CELLS

Congenital Pure Red Cell Anemia (Diamond-Blackfan Syndrome)

This anemia results from a deficiency of red blood cell precursors in bone marrow and reticulocytopenia. Serum erythropoietin levels are increased, and red blood cells have increased hemoglobin F and increased adenosine deaminase. Patients usually become symptomatic in early infancy (2–6 mo). Congenital pure red cell anemia frequently is associated with congenital anomalies, including triphalangeal thumbs.

Corticosteroid therapy frequently is beneficial, and many responsive patients ultimately outgrow the dependence on steroid therapy. Patients who do not respond to corticosteroids (10–15%) are transfusion dependent.

Acquired Pure Red Cell Anemias

These occur infrequently. Etiologies may include thymoma, antibody to erythropoietin or erythroblasts, chloramphenicol, or viral infections.

Transient erythroblastopenia of childhood occurs in children 6 mo to 5 yr of age. There is reticulocytopenia with decreased red blood cell precursors in bone marrow. It is a normochromic normocytic anemia with normal adenosine deaminase and hemoglobin F, and thus can be distinguished from Diamond-Blackfan anemia. Spontaneous remission occurs occasionally. Transfusions occasionally may be necessary until recovery occurs.

Anemias of Chronic Disease

Anemia complicates a number of chronic systemic diseases associated with infection, inflammation, and renal disease. Hemoglobin concentration usually is in the range of 6–9 g/dL, with most symptoms attributable to underlying disease, not anemia. Laboratory findings include low serum iron levels, normal total iron-binding capacity, and elevated serum ferritin (acute-phase reactant).

Anemia resulting from chronic disease does not respond to iron therapy, and transfusions rarely are indicated. Erythropoietin treatment can increase the hemoglobin level in patients with anemia secondary to end-stage renal failure.

Congenital Dyserythropoietic Anemias

These rare normocytic or macrocytic anemias display multinuclearity in marrow red blood cell precursors. Laboratory findings include ineffective erythropoiesis and chronic hemolysis. There is no treatment other than blood transfusions.

Physiologic Anemia of Infancy

In this type of anemia there is a progressive decline in hemoglobin levels after which hemoglobin reaches a nadir, rarely falling below 9 g/dL. The "anemia" is a physiologic adaptation to extrauterine life secondary to a decrease in erythropoietin as arterial oxygenation increases at birth, shortened survival of fetal red blood cells, and expansion of blood volume with growth. Premature infants have an exaggerated response with earlier onset (3–6 wk) and lower hemoglobin nadir (7–9 g/dL). Iron deficiency is not a cause, but in premature infants vitamin E deficiency may cause hemolytic anemia.

Physiologic anemia usually requires no therapy; transfusions may be required in symptomatic cases or if frequent blood drawing is necessary. Use of recombinant erythropoietin is under evaluation in preterm infants.

Megaloblastic Anemias

In these anemias red blood cells are larger than normal, and the marrow shows asynchrony between maturation of nucleus and cytoplasm. Almost all cases in children result from deficiency of folic acid, vitamin B_{12}, or both. These anemias are uncommon in the United States.

FOLIC ACID DEFICIENCIES

Megaloblastic Anemia of Infancy. This is caused by deficient intake or absorption of folic acid. Human and cow milks provide adequate amounts of folic acid but goat milk is deficient. The peak incidence is at 4–7 mo of age. The anemia is progressive, with MCV >100. Hypersegmented neutrophils are seen, and red blood cell folate levels are low. Treatment is with folic acid; low doses have no effect on primary vitamin B_{12} deficiencies.

Folic Acid Deficiency of Malabsorption Syndromes. Folic acid is absorbed through the small intestine. Celiac disease, chronic infectious enteritis, and enteroenteric fistulas may impair folic acid absorption markedly.

Folic Acid Deficiency Complicating Hemolytic Anemia. Chronic hemolytic processes may increase the requirement for folic acid. This may lead to more severe anemia.

Folic Acid Deficiency Associated with Drugs. Anticonvulsant drugs may cause low serum levels of folate but megaloblastic anemia is rare. Methotrexate, trimethoprim–sulfamethoxazole, and other drugs also may cause megaloblastic anemia.

VITAMIN B_{12} DEFICIENCIES. Dietary deficiency is rare but may be seen in cases of extreme dietary restriction (strict vegetarians).

Juvenile Pernicious Anemia (Congenital Pernicious Anemia). This rare disease results from inability to secrete gastric intrinsic factor, which is required for absorption of dietary vitamin B_{12}. Symptoms become prominent at 9 mo to 10 yr of age and include anemia and neurologic manifestations. Absorption of vitamin B_{12} is assessed by Schilling test. Treatment is IM injections of vitamin B_{12}.

Transcobalamin Deficiency. This is a congenital deficiency in transcobalamin II, a vitamin B_{12} transport protein.

Vitamin B_{12} Deficiency in Older Children. Some cases have atrophy of gastric mucosa, antibody to intrinsic factor, or structurally abnormal intrinsic factor.

Vitamin B$_{12}$ Malabsorption of Intestinal Causes. These include familial occurrence of specific intestinal defect in absorption, surgical resection, inflammatory diseases, overgrowth of intestinal bacteria, or infestation with fish tapeworm.

Microcytic Anemias

IRON-DEFICIENCY ANEMIA. This is the most common hematologic disease of infancy and childhood. Iron is absorbed more efficiently from human milk than from cow's milk, so the diets of formula-fed infants should include iron-fortified cereals or formula to prevent iron deficiency. The newborn has iron stores for blood formation for the first 6–9 mo of life; therefore, dietary iron deficiency is uncommon until 9–24 mo of age. The usual dietary pattern observed in infants with iron-deficiency anemia is the consumption of large amounts of cow's milk and carbohydrates unsupplemented with iron. However, blood loss also must be considered:

occult gastrointestinal bleeding may be caused by lesion such as peptic ulcer, Meckel diverticulum, or polyp
chronic intestinal blood loss may be induced by whole cow's milk

Clinical manifestations include pallor, tachycardia, cardiac dilation, systolic murmurs, irritability, and anorexia; pica is sometimes prominent. Laboratory findings include:

decreased serum iron and increased total iron-binding capacity, with percentage saturation falling below 15
red blood cells become smaller (microcytic) and their hemoglobin content decreases (hypochromic) (Table 14–3)
decreased ferritin
increased free erythrocyte protoporphyrin
thrombocytosis

Differential diagnosis includes lead poisoning and thalassemia trait.

Treatment includes oral iron preparations, which should

TABLE 14–3. MEAN CORPUSCULAR VOLUME IN CHILDREN*

Age	MCV (fL) Mean (Range)
Birth	119 (110–128)
6–24 mo	77 (70–85)
2–6 yr	81 (75–90)
6–12 yr	85 (78–95)
Adult	90 (80–100)

* From Behrmann RE (ed): Nelson Textbook of Pediatrics, 14th ed. Philadelphia, WB Saunders Company, 1992, p 1240. (Modified from Koerper MA, Mentzer WC, Brecher G, et al: J Pediatr 89:580, 1976.)

be continued for 4–6 wk after blood values are normal. Response to iron therapy (increased reticulocyte count) is noted within 72–96 hr. Blood transfusion is indicated only for severe anemia. If hemoglobin is under 4 g/dL, packed red blood cells should be given slowly in small amounts.

HEMOLYTIC ANEMIA

In hemolytic anemias, there is shortened survival time of red blood cells (normal red blood cell survival is 100–120 days). The reticulocyte count is increased and exceeds 2%, and hyperplasia of erythropoietic marrow elements occurs. Indirect bilirubin may be elevated, but jaundice is rare. Aplastic crises characterized by reticulocytopenia can cause life-threatening anemia.

Hemolytic Anemias Caused by Intrinsic Abnormalities of the Red Blood Cell

HEREDITARY SPHEROCYTOSIS. This is the most common hereditary hemolytic state next to glucose-6-phosphate dehydrogenase deficiency; it usually is autosomal dominant, with 25% of cases being sporadic. Affected cells have a characteristic spherocytic shape and are sequestered and destroyed in the spleen.

Clinical Manifestations. The onset is in infancy, and it may present in the neonatal period with anemia and hyperbilirubinemia severe enough to require phototherapy or exchange transfusions. The spleen generally is enlarged, and 50% of patients form gallstones in late childhood or adolescence. Aplastic crises associated with parvovirus infections are the most serious complications during childhood.

Laboratory Findings. Evidence of hemolysis includes anemia, reticulocytosis, and hyperbilirubinemia. The characteristic spherocytic cell is smaller than the normal red cell and lacks central pallor. Red blood cell membrane abnormality can be demonstrated by increased osmotic fragility.

Differential Diagnosis. Acquired spherocytosis is seen in autoimmune hemolytic anemia; Coombs test is usually positive.

Treatment. Splenectomy produces clinical cure, but it should be delayed until the child is 5–6 yr of age or older. Splenectomy prevents gallstones and eliminates the threat of aplastic crises. Pneumococcal vaccine should be given prior to splenectomy, and prophylactic penicillin is given afterward.

HEREDITARY ELLIPTOCYTOSIS. This is similar to hereditary spherocytosis but the red blood cells have an oval or elliptic shape. It usually is benign, but a less common variant is associated with hemolysis.

OTHER STRUCTURAL DEFECTS. *Paroxysmal nocturnal hemoglobinuria* is a rare chronic anemia with prominent intravascular hemolysis.

Hereditary stomatocytosis is a rare abnormality in which red blood cells are swollen and display a mouth-like slit; hemolytic anemia may be present.

In *acanthocytosis,* distorted red blood cells have sharp projections as a result of abetalipoproteinemia.

Pyropoikilocytosis is a rare hemolytic anemia characterized by bizarre fragmented cells with reduced thermal stability.

Hemolytic Anemias Caused by Enzymatic Defects of the Red Blood Cells

PYRUVATE KINASE DEFICIENCY. This type of congenital hemolytic anemia is due to a homozygous autosomal recessive gene that causes marked reduction in pyruvate kinase activity. Clinical manifestations may include jaundice and anemia in the neonatal period; most patients have pallor, jaundice, and splenomegaly. Exchange transfusions may be indicated for hyperbilirubinemia in the newborn period. Transfusion of red cells may be necessary for severe anemia. Splenectomy after 5–6 yr of age may lead to higher hemoglobin and reticulocyte counts.

DEFICIENCIES OF OTHER ENZYMES. Congenital anemias may stem from defects in other enzymes, including hexokinase, glucose phosphate isomerase, and phosphofructokinase.

DEFICIENCIES OF ENZYMES OF THE PENTOSE PHOSPHATE PATHWAY. The pentose phosphate pathway produces NADPH, which is necessary for conversion of oxidized to reduced glutathione. If glutathione is decreased, hemoglobin may become denatured and precipitate into inclusions called Heinz bodies. Red blood cells with Heinz bodies are rapidly removed from the circulation.

GLUCOSE-6-PHOSPHATE DEHYDROGENASE (G-6-PD) DEFICIENCY. The most important disease in this group, G-6-PD is responsible for two clinical syndromes: (1) episodic hemolytic anemia induced by infections and certain drugs (common), and (2) spontaneous chronic nonspherocytic hemolytic anemia (rare). Because synthesis of G-6-PD is determined by an X-chromosome–linked gene, *drug-induced hemolytic anemia* occurs more frequently in males. There is considerable variation in the defect among racial groups; the defect in affected blacks is less severe than that in affected whites. Hemolysis becomes apparent 48–96 hr after patient has ingested a substance with oxidant properties. Drugs that have these properties include antipyretics, sulfonamides, antimalarials, and naphthaquinolones. Favism is an acute and severe hemolytic syndrome caused by fava beans. Death may occur as consequence of severe anemia.

Laboratory findings include anemia and hemoglobinuria and red blood cells with Heinz bodies. *Diagnosis* depends on demonstration of reduced G-6-PD activity in red blood cells.

Treatment involves prevention of oxidant exposure and blood transfusions; spontaneous recovery is the rule.

Hemoglobin Disorders

Clinical disorders result from abnormalities of the globin genes. These disorders can be subdivided into three major groups:

1. Hemoglobinopathies resulting from changes in the amino acid sequences of the globin chains.
2. Hereditary persistence of fetal hemoglobin syndromes that are characterized by elevated levels of Hg F.
3. Thalassemias that are due to decreased synthesis of one or more of the normal globin genes.

HEMOGLOBIN STRUCTURAL ABNORMALITIES (Hemoglobinopathies)

Sickle Cell Hemoglobinopathies. Sickle hemoglobin (Hb S) differs from normal adult hemoglobin by substitution of valine for glutamic acid at the sixth position of the β chains. Sickling occurs when this hemoglobin is deoxygenated. Erythrocytes from heterozygous individuals (sickle cell trait) are more resistant to malarial parasites. Mutation is found in high frequency in regions where *P. falciparum* has been endemic. Hb S is readily identified by electrophoresis and molecular techniques.

Sickle Cell Anemia. This is the homozygous expression of sickle hemoglobin gene (Hb SS). It is characterized by severe chronic hemolytic disease resulting from destruction of poorly deformable erythrocytes and painful crises from vascular occlusion.

- Clinical manifestations

    Hemolytic anemia develops over the first 2–4 mo of life, paralleling the replacement of fetal hemoglobin by Hb S.

    Dactylitis, the hand–foot syndrome, with painful symmetric swelling of the hands and feet, frequently is the first evidence of sickle cell disease.

    Painful vaso-occlusive episodes occur intermittently and may be precipitated by intercurrent illnesses accompanied by fever, hypoxia, and acidosis.

    Acute splenic sequestration occurs when large amounts of blood become acutely pooled in the spleen.

    Splenic infarcts eventually lead to loss of splenic function ("autosplenectomy").

    Patients have increased susceptibility to meningitis, sepsis, and other serious infections caused by pneumococci and *Haemophilus influenzae* as a result of reduced splenic function.

    Pulmonary infarction may lead to acute chest syndrome.

    Other sequelae include cerebrovascular occlusion and damage to myocardium, liver, and kidneys.

    Plastic episodes may occur in association with parvovirus infection.

    Hemolytic crises may occur with concomitant G-6-PD deficiency.

- Laboratory findings

    Hemoglobin concentrations usually range from 5 to 9 g/dL; reticulocyte counts are 5–15%.

    Peripheral smear shows irreversibly sickled cells.

    Nucleated red blood cells and Howell–Jolly bodies often are present.

Total white blood cell count is elevated to 12,000–20,000/mm^3.

Hyperbilirubinemia is present as a result of red blood cell destruction.

Diagnosis is established by hemoglobin electrophoresis.

- Treatment

Measures are directed toward prevention of serious complications.

Immunizations with *H. influenzae,* and hepatitis B vaccines are indicated.

Prophylactic penicillin against pneumococcal infections is highly efficacious.

Parenteral antibiotics are given to patients with acute onset of high fever.

Painful episodes are managed with oral acetaminophen alone or with codeine; more severe episodes may require hospitalization and parenteral narcotics and fluids for correction of dehydration or acidosis.

Blood transfusions are useful for patients with ischemic organ damage, stroke, splenic sequestration, or aplastic crises, or in preparation for major surgery.

Sickle Cell Trait. This is the heterozygous expression of sickle hemoglobin gene (Hb AS). Eight percent of American blacks have sickle cell trait. The clinical course usually is benign but, under conditions of severe hypoxia, vaso-oclusive complications may occur in Hb AS individuals. Hyposthenuria usually is present in older children and adults.

Other Hemoglobinopathies.
- Hemoglobin C

Lysine at position 6 of the β globin gene occurs in about 2% of American blacks.

In the heterozygous state (Hb AC), no anemia or disease is present.

In the homozygous state (Hb CC), moderately severe hemolytic anemia with hemoglobin levels from 8–11 g/dL is observed.

Hb SC disease, resulting from the concurrence of Hb S and Hb C genes, is less severe than Hb SS but more severe than Hb CC.

- Hemoglobin E

Lysine at position 26 of the β chain is prevalent in populations from Southeast Asia.

Homozygous Hb E is characterized by hemolytic anemia, target cells, microcytosis, and moderate to severe splenomegaly.

The syndrome Hb E–B^0-thalassemia may be expressed as a severe anemia.

Unstable Hemoglobin Disorders. Abnormal hemoglobins may denature and precipitate within red blood cells and form Heinz bodies. The disorder may range from mild to severe, becoming more pronounced with infection or following exposure to oxidant drugs.

Abnormal Hemoglobins with Increased Oxygen Affinity. Rare abnormal hemoglobins that have increased oxygen affinity (e.g., Hb Chesapeake) release oxygen poorly to tissues. Affected individuals have elevated hemoglobin levels (16–19 g/dL).

Abnormal Hemoglobins Causing Cyanosis. Rare hemoglobin variants with markedly decreased oxygen affinity (e.g., Hb Kansas) may produce benign cyanosis. Other abnormal hemoglobins (Hb M syndrome) are characterized by benign cyanosis and a brown color of the blood.

HEREDITARY PERSISTENCE OF FETAL HEMOGLOBIN. This is characterized by production of elevated levels of Hb F beyond the neonatal period. Various molecular abnormalities have been identified. Hemoglobin F inhibits the sickling of Hb S.

THALASSEMIA SYNDROMES. The thalassemias are a heterogeneous group of hypochromic anemias. Numerous underlying genetic defects decrease production of α or β globin chain synthesis. Thalassemia genes are remarkably widespread and are believed to be the most prevalent of all human genetic diseases. These genes may increase resistance to lethal malarial infections.

Homozygous β^0-Thalassemia. This becomes symptomatic as a severe hypochromic microcytic and hemolytic anemia during the second 6 mo of life. Regular blood transfusions (every 4–5 wk) are necessary to support life and maintain hemoglobin levels above 10 g/dL. Untreated or infrequently treated patients may develop:

Compensatory hypertrophy of erythropoietic tissues in medullary and extramedullary spaces; the spleen and liver become enlarged

Massive expansion of the marrow of the face and skull that produces characteristic facies

Thin bones and pathologic fractures

Growth is impaired in older children.

Hemosiderosis (deposition of iron in tissues) is an inevitable consequence of prolonged transfusion therapy and may involve the myocardium, liver, pancreas, and other organs. It can be decreased with the iron-chelating drug desferoxamine. Cardiac complications caused by myocardial hemosiderosis are common terminal events. Bone marrow transplantation is curative.

Heterozygous β-Thalassemia. Most forms are associated with mild hypochromic microcytic anemia. Heterozygotes often are misdiagnosed as having iron-deficiency anemia and inappropriately treated with iron. Most β-thalassemia trait individuals have elevated levels of Hb A_2 (3.4–7%).

α-Thalassemia. This is due to deficient synthesis of α globin chains. Four α globin chain genes are present in normal individuals, and four distinct forms of α-thalassemia have been identified, corresponding to deletions of one, two, three, or all four of these genes.

Deletion of one gene produces silent carrier phenotype with mild microcytosis.

Deletion of two genes produces α-thalassemia trait with microcytic anemia.

Deletion of three genes produces a thalassemia intermedia–like syndrome with moderately severe anemia in which Hb H (β₄ tetramers) can be identified by electrophoresis.

Deletion of all four genes is accompanied by total absence of α chain synthesis

- Affected individuals usually are stillborn or die shortly after birth (hydrops fetalis)
- Hb Barts (γ₄ tetramers) are present

Hemolytic Anemia Resulting from Extrinsic Factors

AUTOIMMUNE HEMOLYTIC ANEMIAS ASSOCIATED WITH "WARM ANTIBODIES". In this type of anemia, abnormal antibodies of the immunoglobulin G (IgG) class (active at 37°C) directed against red blood cells are produced. Most are idiopathic, but they may be associated with drugs or, more rarely, with lymphoma, lupus erythematosus, or immunodeficiency.

Clinical Manifestations. There are two general types:

acute transient type—occurs in infants and young children; it frequently responds to steroid therapy and full recovery within 3 mo is characteristic

chronic type—has a prolonged course over many months or years and often is attributable to an underlying systemic disease; mortality is about 10%

Diagnosis. The anemia may be profound, and the direct Coombs test is strongly positive.

Treatment. Transfusions usually are of only transient benefit but may be required by the severity of the anemia. Prednisone is used to reduce the rate of hemolysis; intravenous gamma globulin, immunosuppressive agents, or splenectomy also may be of benefit.

AUTOIMMUNE HEMOLYTIC ANEMIAS ASSOCIATED WITH "COLD ANTIBODIES". In this type of anemia, antibodies are of the IgM class, are more active at low body temperature, and need complement for activity. These antibodies often are found after viral or mycoplasma infections. When very high titers are present, severe episodes of intravascular hemolysis may occur following exposure to cold.

POLYCYTHEMIA
(*NELSON TEXTBOOK*, SEC. 16.33)

Polycythemia exists when the red blood cell count and the hemoglobin and hematocrit levels exceed the upper limits of normal. *Secondary polycythemia* may be associated with chronic arterial oxygen desaturation secondary to cardiovascular or pulmonary diseases. Polycythemia also may be associated with hemoglobins that have altered oxygen affinity, renal tumors or cysts, and vascular tumors of the cerebellum.

Polycythemia rubra vera, characterized by polycythemia, leukocytosis, thrombocytosis, and hyperplasia of the bone marrow, has been reported in a few children.

THE PANCYTOPENIAS
(*NELSON TEXTBOOK,* SECS. 16.34–16.36)

Bone marrow aplasia may lead to anemia, thrombocytopenia, and neutropenia. Pancytopenia may be constitutional or acquired. Bone marrow examination is essential to diagnosis.

CONSTITUTIONAL APLASTIC PANCYTOPENIA
(Fanconi Syndrome)

This is a familial disorder, inherited as an autosomal recessive condition. About two thirds of affected children have congenital anomalies, especially microcephaly, microphthalmia, absence of the radii and thumbs, abnormalities of the heart and kidney, hyperpigmentation, and short stature.

Laboratory studies reveal severe pancytopenia with macrocytic red blood cells. The bone marrow is strikingly hypocellular, with decreased numbers of precursors. Chromosomal studies reveal an abnormally high percentage of chromatid breaks, gaps, and rearrangements.

Therapy is supportive, with blood transfusions and antibiotics. Androgenic steroids and corticosteroids are beneficial and extend the lifespan. Androgens produce signs and symptoms of masculinization and may lead to hemorrhagic cysts of the liver and hepatoma.

ACQUIRED APLASTIC PANCYTOPENIAS

Marrow depressants include ionizing radiation and chemotherapeutic drugs. A small number of patients develop pancytopenia as an idiosyncratic reaction to drug exposure (i.e., chloramphenicol). It also may follow infection with hepatitis or parvovirus.

Hemorrhage secondary to thrombocytopenia is the first clinical manifestation. Chromosome studies are normal, unlike in Fanconi anemia.

The prognosis in severe aplastic pancytopenia is grave. Immunosuppressive therapy with antithymocyte globulin, steroids, or cyclosporin may be of benefit. Bone marrow transplantation is effective when a suitable donor is available.

PANCYTOPENIA CAUSED BY MARROW REPLACEMENT

Bone marrow replacement by tumor cells (such as neuroblastoma), osteopetrosis, or myelofibrosis can lead to pancytopenia.

TRANSFUSIONS
(*NELSON TEXTBOOK*, SECS. 16.37–16.39)

INDICATIONS FOR TRANSFUSION

Acute Hemorrhage

Tachycardia, hypotension, and shock may accompany severe and rapid blood loss (15–20% of the circulating blood volume). Anemia of acute blood loss is normochromic and normocytic. *Treatment* includes measures to control hemorrhage and replace of blood volume with whole blood or packed cells if necessary.

Chronic Anemias

Patients may have few symptoms if anemia develops slowly. Transfusion is indicated if anemia is profound or complications are present. In chronic anemia complicated by congestive heart failure, small amounts of blood should be administered slowly or exchange transfusion performed. Administration of 5 mL/kg of packed cells usually increases hematocrit by 5%.

USE OF BLOOD FRACTIONS

Platelet Transfusions

The life span of transfused platelets is 9–10 days. They may be used to obtain temporary hemostasis in thrombocytopenia of inadequate production but are not useful in states characterized by peripheral hyperdestruction. Repeated transfusion may lead to formation of antibodies to platelet antigens.

Granulocyte Transfusions

These lower mortality in profoundly leukopenic patients with gram-negative sepsis. They also have been recommended for treatment of septic newborns who have neutropenia and depletion of granulocyte reserves.

SPECIAL CONSIDERATIONS

Blood for transfusion should be of the same blood group as the recipient's. Blood for chronically transfused children should be as fresh as possible.

Risks involved in blood transfusions include clerical errors, isoimmunization, hepatitis, acquired immunodeficiency syndrome (AIDS), cytomegalovirus infection, circulatory overload, and iron overload.

Reactions to blood transfusions include allergic reactions, febrile reactions, hemolytic transfusion reactions (blood transfusion should be terminated immediately when this is suspected), and graft-versus-host disease.

DISORDERS OF THE LEUKOCYTES
(NELSON TEXTBOOK, SECS. 16.41–16.62)

TYPES OF LEUKOCYTES

Neutrophils (Polymorphonuclear Leukocytes)

These are the most important phagocytic cells that defend the host against acute bacterial infection. Neutrophils are attracted to pathogens by chemotactic factors, and their granules contain proteins vital for killing of bacteria.

Disorders associated with impaired neutrophil function are characterized by recurrent infections. Infection, corticosteroids, and epinephrine can increase the number of circulating neutrophils. Neutrophil production in the bone marrow is regulated by colony-stimulating factors (GM-CSF and G-CSF).

Patients with severe neutropenia (less than 500/mm³) have an increased susceptibility to infections, including cellulitis, abscesses, and life-threatening septicemia. The organisms most commonly isolated from neutropenic patients are *Staphylococcus aureus* and gram-negative organisms.

Eosinophils

These have large, coarse granules with prominent red color and a nucleus with 1 or 2 segments. They normally account for fewer than 5% of circulating leukocytes. Eosinophil counts are increased in parasitic infections, allergic phenomena, and dermatologic conditions.

Basophils

These contain coarse, deep blue granules that fill the cytoplasm and obscure the nucleus. They are increased in certain diseases, including chronic myelogenous leukemia and ulcerative colitis.

Lymphocytes

These constitute 30–60% of blood leukocytes. They are characterized as T or B lymphocytes. Lymphocytosis can be seen in certain infections, including pertussis and infectious mononucleosis.

Monocytes

After leaving the bloodstream, these large phagocytic cells differentiate into tissue histiocytes and may remain for as long as 2 yr. Increased monocyte counts may be seen in the recovery period after chemotherapy and with disease, including tuberculosis and systemic mycosis.

QUANTITATIVE DISORDERS OF THE NEUTROPHILS

The normal absolute number of neutrophils is 1,500–2,500/mm³. Levels below this range are designated neutropenia, and levels above this are designated neutrophilia.

Neutrophilia

Acute neutrophilia accompanies physical exercise, panic response, epinephrine, and glucocorticoids. *Chronic neutrophilia* may be associated with glucocorticoids, chronic inflammatory reactions, or chronic anxiety.

Disorders of Proliferation of Committed Stem Cells

BENIGN NEUTROPENIA. This may be associated with familial inheritance or immunologic disorders. There are few serious sequelae. Bone marrow aspiration may reveal normal myeloid maturation or an arrest at any earlier stage, including the promyelocyte level.

SEVERE CONGENITAL NEUTROPENIA (Kostmann Disease). The onset of this disorder is in early infancy. Children have recurrent severe pyogenic infections, which are often fatal. Administration of G-CSF can lead to a marked decrease in infections.

CYCLIC NEUTROPENIA. This consists of profound neutropenia with periodic episodes of fever and oral ulcerations. Neutropenia persists for 3–6 days, with cycles of 21 days. Administration of G-CSF may shorten the duration of the low neutrophil count.

Phenotypic Abnormalities

SCHWACHMAN SYNDROME. This is a chronic moderate neutropenia and pancreatic insufficiency with occasional thrombocytopenia and anemia. Malabsorption and growth failure are prominent.

Disorders of Neutrophil Survival

INFECTION. The most common cause of transient neutropenia in childhood is viral infections (e.g., hepatitis A and B, respiratory syncytial virus, influenza A and B). Neutropenia corresponds to the period of acute viremia and may persist for 3–6 days. Sepsis is one of the more serious causes of neutropenia.

ISOIMMUNE NEONATAL NEUTROPENIA. This is analogous to Rh hemolytic anemia; during gestation, maternal sensitization to fetal neutrophil antigen inherited from the father produces antibody that crosses the placenta and destroys the infant's neutrophils. It occurs in 3% of live births. Cutaneous infections predominate during neutropenia. The neutrophil count returns to normal by a median age of 7 wk.

AUTOIMMUNE NEUTROPENIA. This is due to autoimmune antineutrophil antibodies. It occurs in infants from 5 to 24 mo of age and may persist for 6–24 mo prior to spontaneous remission. Corticosteroids may be effective.

RETICULOENDOTHELIAL SEQUESTRATION. Splenic enlargement can lead to neutropenia.

ACQUIRED NEUTROPENIA. This can result from malignancies such as leukemia or lymphoma, myelofibrosis, and nutritional deficiencies of vitamin B_{12} or folic acid.

DRUG-INDUCED NEUTROPENIA. Drugs can induce neutropenia by idiosyncratic or hypersensitivity reaction.

The most important therapeutic measure is the withdrawal of the offending drug. Duration of neutropenia varies from a few days to months or years.

Inherited Leukocyte Abnormalities

In these abnormalities, 90% of neutrophils have two to four segments, 5% have no segmentation (bands), and 5% have more than four segments.

Hereditary hypersegmentation (large neutrophils with 6–10 lobes) and *hereditary hyposegmentation* with 1–2 lobes (Pelger–Huet anomaly) usually are not associated with any other abnormality.

In *Alder–Reilly anomaly*, neutrophil granules are larger and stain more prominently.

May–Hegglin anomaly is associated with mild neutropenia, inclusions similar to Dohle bodies, and thrombocytopenia with bizarre giant platelets. Most individuals are in good health.

QUALITATIVE ABNORMALITIES OF THE NEUTROPHILS

Disorders of Cell Motility and Chemotaxis

Migration of neutrophils to inflammatory sites leads to accumulation of exudate responsible for the clinical signs of inflammation and infection. Patients with chemotactic disorders have an increased susceptibility to various microorganisms, including gram-positive and gram-negative bacteria and fungi.

Disorders of Neutrophil Ingestion

Leukocyte adherence deficiency is due to absence of C3bi receptor in neutrophils and monocytes. This deficiency results in substantial defect in particle ingestion. Patients have recurrent pyogenic infections.

Disorders of Degranulation

CHEDIAK-HIGASHI SYNDROME. This is an autosomal recessive disorder in which the leukocytes contain giant cytoplasmic granules. Patients have partial albinism, moderate neutropenia, and increased susceptibility to infection. There is a propensity for lymphohistiocytic proliferation (known as the accelerated phase), which aggravates the neutropenia.

Disorders of Oxidative Microbicidal Activity

CHRONIC GRANULOMATOUS DISEASE. Phagocytic cells ingest but do not kill catalase-positive micro-organisms because the cells fail to generate hydrogen peroxide and other oxygen metabolites that normally kill these microbes. In the X-linked form of the disease, there is a defect in the cytochrome b gene.

Diagnosis is based on the nitroblue tetrazolium (NBT) test (see Chap. 9).

DIAGNOSTIC EVALUATION OF THE PATIENT WITH RECURRENT INFECTIONS

This initially includes history, examination, and complete blood count. Secondary studies may include immunoglobulin and complement work-up along with analysis of phagocyte function.

HEMORRHAGIC AND THROMBOTIC DISEASES
(*NELSON TEXTBOOK*, SECS. 16.63–16.89)

SCHEMA OF HEMOSTASIS

Platelet plug formation (the primary hemostatic mechanism) requires platelets and von Willebrand factor. Formation of a stable fibrin clot (the secondary hemostatic mechanism) requires the coagulation factors (Table 14–4).

EVALUATION OF THE PATIENT WITH A SUSPECTED HEMOSTATIC DEFECT

The first step is to obtain a bleeding history and physical examination. Next screening laboratory studies should be

TABLE 14–4. THE COAGULATION FACTORS*

International Numbers	Synonyms	Comment
I	Fibrinogen	Number rarely used—congenital deficiency known (afibrinogenemia)
II	Prothrombin	Number rarely used—congenital deficiency known
III	Thromboplastin	No specific factor identified
IV	Calcium	Number rarely used
V	Labile factor, proaccelerin	Congenital deficiency known (parahemophilia, Owren disease)
VI	Activated labile factor, accelerin	No longer differentiated from factor V
VII	Stable factor, SPCA, proconvertin	Congenital deficiency known
VIII	Antihemophilic factor (AHF) or globulin (AHG)	Hemophilia A (classic hemophilia)—results from congenital deficiency
IX	Christmas factor, plasma thromboplastin component (PTC)	Hemophilia B—results from congenital deficiency
X	Stuart-Prower factor	Congenital deficiency known
XI	Plasma thromboplastin antecedent (PTA)	Congenital deficiency known
XII	Hageman factor	No clinical symptoms associated with congenital deficiency
XIII	Fibrin-stabilizing factor	Congenital deficiency known

* From Behrman RE (ed): Nelson Textbook of Pediatrics, 14th ed. Philadelphia, WB Saunders Company, 1992, p 1272.

obtained—platelet count, bleeding time, prothrombin time, and activated partial thromboplastin time. Further studies to assess platelet function and factor levels can be obtained as necessary.

CONGENITAL AND INHERITED COAGULATION DISORDERS

Factor VIII Deficiency (Classic Hemophilia, Hemophilia A)

This accounts for 80% of all hemophilia cases. It is caused by a defective X chromosome gene (the expression of this defect occurs almost exclusively in males). Eighty percent of patients have a positive family history. Patients have reduced factor VIII activity levels, and clinical severity depends on level of factor VIII activity (severe, less than 1%; moderate, 1–5%; mild, 6–30%).

The hallmark of hemophilia is hemarthrosis with spontaneous bleeding into joints, which may produce degenerative changes. Laboratory findings reveal prolonged partial thromboplastin time and decreased factor VIII.

Treatment is with factor VIII concentrates. Some patients develop inhibitors of factor VIII (these are IgG globulins); factor IX concentrates with a factor VIII bypassing activity or porcine factor VIII may be useful in these patients.

Factor IX Deficiency (Christmas Disease, Hemophilia B).

This accounts for about 12–15% of hemophilias. It is transmitted as an X-linked recessive.

Factor IX deficiency is clinically indistinguishable from factor VIII deficiency. Laboratory findings show prolonged partial thromboplastin time and low levels of factor IX.

Treatment involves replacement with factor IX concentrates.

Factor XI Deficiency (Hemophilia C)

This is the least common type of hemophilia. Postoperative and post-traumatic hemorrhage is characteristic; spontaneous bleeding is rare.

Treatment is with fresh frozen plasma.

Factor XII Deficiency (Hageman Factor Deficiency)

In this coagulation disorder, partial thromboplastin time is prolonged but there is no clinical abnormality.

Von Willebrand Disease

This is inherited as an autosomal dominant trait that leads to decreased levels of von Willebrand factor. There are at least three major varieties of von Willebrand disease. Von Willebrand protein functions as a carrier for factor VIII and is needed for platelet aggregation.

Clinical manifestations include bleeding from the gums and increased bleeding after trauma or surgery. Laboratory findings include prolonged bleeding time.

Therapy is with fresh frozen plasma or cryoprecipitate. DDAVP is useful in patients with mild disease.

ACQUIRED COAGULATION DISORDERS

Hemorrhagic Disease of the Newborn

(See Chapter 7)

Postneonatal Vitamin K Deficiency

Vitamin K deficiency rarely occurs after the neonatal period but may be associated with malabsorption of fats, prolonged administration of broad-spectrum antibiotics, cystic fibrosis, and biliary atresia. Vitamin K is necessary for carboxylation and therefore activity of factors II, VII, IX, and X.

Liver Disease

Coagulation abnormalities are common in patients with liver disease (all coagulation factors are produced in the liver, although factor VIII can be produced in other organs) because of decreased production of factors.

Inhibitors

These inhibit coagulation of normal blood (usually immunoglobulins) and are rare in normal children. Patients with inhibitors against specific coagulation factors may have bleeding problems and need to be treated similarly to a hemophiliac with an inhibitor. Other types of inhibitors, such as those found in patients with systemic lupus erythematosus, do not cause bleeding and do not need treatment.

Consumption Coagulopathy (Disseminated Intravascular Coagulation)

In disseminated intravascular coagulation (DIC) widespread intravascular deposition of fibrin may lead to tissue ischemia and necrosis as well as a generalized hemorrhagic state. DIC most frequently accompanies severe systemic disease.

Laboratory findings include prolongations of prothrombin and partial thromboplastin time as a result of consumption of certain coagulation factors (II, V, VIII, fibrinogen), and thrombocytopenia resulting from platelet consumption.

Treatment involves control or reversal of the process that initiated DIC (i.e., infection, shock, hypoxia, etc). Supportive care is with blood products (red blood cells, platelets, and cryoprecipitate; occasionally, heparin therapy may be useful).

PLATELET AND BLOOD VESSEL DISORDERS

Congenital and Inherited Disorders

WISKOTT–ALDRICH SYNDROME. This is characterized by eczema, thrombocytopenia, and increased susceptibility to infection resulting from an underlying immunologic defect. It is transmitted as an X-linked recessive trait. A few cases may develop lymphoreticular malignancy.

THROMBOCYTOPENIA WITH CAVERNOUS HEMANGIOMA (Kasabach–Merritt Syndrome).   This is a large cavernous hemangioma associated with severe thrombocytopenia, red cell fragments, and evidence of intravascular coagulation. Spontaneous thrombosis may lead to obliteration of vascular channels and recovery. When feasible, external compression should be attempted. Surgery may be associated with uncontrollable hemorrhage.

Treatment modalities include radiation therapy, corticosteroids, and interferon.

THROMBOCYTOPENIA ABSENT RADIUS SYNDROME.   Severe thrombocytopenia is associated with aplasia of the radii and thumbs, and occasionally with cardiac and renal anomalies. There are no other hematologic manifestations.

PLATELET FUNCTION DEFECTS.   Congenital defects in platelet adhesion or aggregation can lead to mucous membrane bleeding. The platelet count is normal or moderately reduced; the defects are identified by platelet function tests. The most common of these disorders are Bernard–Soulier syndrome and Glanzmann thrombasthenia.

Acquired Disorders

IDIOPATHIC THROMBOCYTOPENIC PURPURA (ITP).   This is the most common thrombocytopenic purpura of childhood. It is associated with petechiae and mucocutaneous bleeding. Antecedent viral disease is common; a probable immune mechanism is the basis of the disorder.

Onset frequently is acute, with petechiae and hemorrhage. Platelet count is reduced below 20×10^9/L, and platelets seen on blood smear are large (megathrombocytes). Bone marrow aspiration reveals normal or increased numbers of megakaryocytes.

Treatment is with gamma globulin, corticosteroids, or splenectomy for chronic patients. Ninety percent of affected children have normal platelet counts 9–12 mo after diagnosis, and relapses are unusual.

DRUG-INDUCED THROMBOCYTOPENIA.   Drugs can induce thrombocytopenia by an immunologic mechanism or megakaryocyte injury. These drugs include carbamazepine, phenytoin, and sulfonamides.

HEMOLYTIC–UREMIC SYNDROME (HUS).   This usually follows an episode of acute gastroenteritis. It is associated with hemolytic anemia, thrombocytopenia, and acute renal insufficiency.

THROMBOTIC THROMBOCYTOPENIC PURPURA.   This rare disease is similar to HUS, except for prominent central nervous system signs.

NEONATAL THROMBOCYTOPENIA ASSOCIATED WITH INFECTION.   The associated infection may be viral, protozoal, or bacterial. Infants usually have hemolysis, jaundice, anemia, and enlarged liver and spleen.

IMMUNE NEONATAL THROMBOCYTOPENIA.   Thirty percent of infants born of mothers with active ITP have thrombocytopenia resulting from the transplacental transfer of antiplatelet antibody. The duration of the thrombocytopenia is 2–3 mo. IV gamma globulin may be helpful.

Alloimmunization may occur if the fetus has platelet antigens that the mother does not have; the PLA-1 antigen is most frequently involved. Washed maternal platelets and IV gamma globulin are helpful.

PLATELET FUNCTION DISORDERS. These are caused by toxic metabolic products (uremia, autoantibodies, immune complexes, fibrin split products) and drugs such as aspirin.

VASCULAR DISORDERS. *Schönlein–Henoch syndrome* (anaphylactoid purpura) is a vascular type of nonthrombocytopenic purpura. It is associated with rash on the legs and buttocks, arthritis, nephritis, and gastrointestinal bleeding. Treatment is supportive.

THROMBOCYTOSIS. In this disorder platelet counts are in excess of 750×10^9/L. Thrombocytosis may accompany hemorrhage, iron-deficiency anemia, hemolytic disease, primary myeloproliferative disorders, and inflammatory states, including Kawasaki disease. No specific therapy is necessary.

THROMBOTIC DISORDERS

Occlusion of the blood vessel with platelet plug or fibrin clot may occur in vessels of any size. Clinical manifestations reflect organ or tissue injury resulting from the absence of or a severe reduction in blood perfusion; diagnosis is by angiography.

The formation of fibrin clot is regulated by a complex inhibitor system. *Congenital and inherited thrombotic disorders* result from deficiency in antithrombin III, protein C, or protein S (homozygous deficiency of protein C leads to purpura fulminans neonatalis).

Acquired defects are uncommon in children but may include venous thrombosis and thrombophlebitis, pulmonary embolism, arterial thrombosis, and stroke.

Anticoagulant and Thrombolytic Therapy

HEPARIN. This enhances the rate at which antithrombin III neutralizes the activities of several of the activated clotting proteins. It is contraindicated in certain patients, including those with pre-existing coagulation defects and recent central nervous system hemorrhage or surgery. It is given as an intravenous or subcutaneous injection, in an intermittent bolus or as a continuous infusion. Activated partial thromboplastin time must be maintained at 1.5–2 times pretreatment value.

WARFARIN. This decreases the rate of synthesis of the vitamin K–dependent factors, II, VII, IX, and X. It takes 4–5 days to induce anticoagulation. Warfarin anticoagulation can be assessed with prothrombin time. The most serious side effect is hemorrhage; effects can be reversed by discontinuation of the drug and administration of vitamin K.

THROMBOLYTIC THERAPY. This involves removal of blood clots by enzymatic digestion with tissue plasminogen activator or urokinase.

THE SPLEEN
(*NELSON TEXTBOOK*, SECS. 16.90–16.93)

The spleen is a large mass of lymphoid and phagocytic reticuloendothelial cells. It has numerous functions, including a reservoir function, hematopoiesis (during fetal life), culling (removal of antibody or spherocytic cells), destruction of old red blood cells, and filtering and immunologic functions.

On physical examination, the tip is palpable in 5–10% of normal children. The spleen must be increased to 2 to 3 times its average size before it can be felt regularly. And enlarged spleen must be differentiated from other masses. Important causes of splenic enlargement include hematologic disease, infections, congestive splenomegaly, infiltrations, cysts, and neoplasms.

CONGESTIVE SPLENOMEGALY

Venous outflow from the spleen may be obstructed within the liver or in the portal or splenic veins. Vascular obstruction produces congestion and splenomegaly. Pancytopenia of varying degree is seen.

ANOMALIES AND TRAUMA

Anomalies of the spleen include splenic cysts, accessory spleens, congenital absence of the spleen, and functional hyposplenia. Rupture of the spleen may result from traumatic injury; symptoms may be mild or severe, with shock requiring laparotomy and splenectomy.

SPLENECTOMY

Splenectomy is performed for various indications, including primary surgical indications (rupture, removal of tumors or cysts, shunting procedures, relief of mechanical distress resulting from massive enlargement). Hematologic indications include congenital hemolytic states such as hereditary spherocytosis, autoimmune hemolytic anemia, chronic ITP, and hypersplenism.

Overwhelming sepsis may follow splenectomy. It should be deferred until 5–6 yr of age if possible. Prophylactic use of penicillin has been advocated. Severe infection caused by pneumococci, *H. influenzae,* or meningococci may occur; immunization with capsular antigens of these viruses probably reduces the frequency of postsplenectomy infection. Febrile illness calls for immediate medical evaluation.

THE LYMPHATIC SYSTEM
(*NELSON TEXTBOOK*, SECS. 16.94–16.96)

The lymphatic system includes lymphocytes of the blood and lymph and organized lymphatic structures such as the lymph nodes, spleen, Peyer patches, appendix, and tonsils. Diseases of the *lymph vessels* include acute lymphangitis (inflammation of the lymphatics draining an area of infection) and lymphedema (obstruction of lymph drainage). Diseases of the *lymph nodes* include acute lymphadenitis (inflammation resulting from acute infection) and chronic lymphadenitis (frequently associated with hyperplasia of the lymph nodes).

15

NEOPLASMS AND NEOPLASM-LIKE STRUCTURES

GENERAL CONSIDERATIONS
(*NELSON TEXTBOOK*, SEC. 17.1)

Cancer causes more deaths for children ages 1–15 yr than any other disease in the United States. The incidence of childhood cancer is 14 new cases per 100,000 per year (6.1% increase from 1973–74). However, overall mortality has decreased by 35.6% to 3.6:100,000, mostly as a result of improved treatments.

ENVIRONMENTAL ETIOLOGIES

These include ionizing and solar radiation, asbestos, drugs, diet, and viruses.

GENETIC MECHANISMS

Oncogenes and Malignancy

Oncogenes are DNA sequences that can transform NIH 3T3 (or another cell line) after in vitro transfection. Cellular oncogenes may contribute to childhood cancer development.

Tumor Suppressor Genes

A normal cellular gene that promotes cancer when it loses function as a result of a mutation (instead of gaining excessive or alternate functions, as does an oncogene) is known as an antioncogene. The retinoblastoma gene is the first known example.

OTHER MECHANISMS

Congenital syndromes associated with increased risk of leukemia include Down syndrome, Fanconi anemia, and Bloom syndrome.

The increased incidence of certain tumors (Hodgkin disease, brain tumors, Ewing sarcoma) in siblings with the same tumors suggests there are other genetic factors involved. There are also familial associations with syndromes (hemihypertrophy, neurofibromatosis).

Pediatricians should counsel patients and parents about avoiding carcinogens (sunlight, tobacco, excessive dietary fats) and following routine preventive care (Pap smears for sexually active girls.).

PRINCIPLES OF DIAGNOSIS
(*NELSON TEXTBOOK*, SEC. 17.2)

Cancer is rare (1:10,000 children) but should be suspected when a child presents with:

prolonged (>3–4 wk), unexplained pain or fever
unexplained (esp. growing) masses
weight loss
prolonged ear pain, nasal discharge, retropharyngeal swelling, trismus (nasopharyngeal or ear tumor)
cervical node enlargement (Hodgkin or non-Hodgkin lymphoma), especially nonpainful, persistent, enlarging
localized, persistent bone pain (osteosarcoma, Ewing sarcoma), especially in 2nd decade of life; frequently associated with an episode of trauma
low-grade fever, bone or joint pain (leukemia); there may or may not be changes in the complete blood count (CBC) early on
"blueberry muffin" spots on the skin (congenital leukemia)

WORK-UP OF SUSPECTED MALIGNANCY

The work-up depends on the particular malignancy suspected. Differential diagnosis varies with presenting symptoms, mass location, and age. Work-up generally includes measuring the extent and degree of dissemination ("staging") before surgical biopsy or removal of tumor (accomplished via blood chemistries and CBC, radiologic studies). Bone marrow aspiration and/or biopsy often can lead to a diagnosis without the need for surgical biopsy.

Note: Be sure blood chemistries are determined before computerized tomography (CT) scan, because radiopaque dye can precipitate renal failure in the presence of pre-existing renal compromise resulting from massive tumor burden.

Definitive diagnosis can be made only by histologic examination of the tumor. Often, prognostic variables depend on the results of special stains, immunoreactive tests, or electron microscopic studies of fresh tumor. Local lymph nodes and regional organs should be examined for tumor; clean margins can affect prognosis.

PRINCIPLES OF TREATMENT
(*NELSON TEXTBOOK*, SEC. 17.3)

Treatment includes two aspects: specific antitumor therapy and general supportive care. Specific antitumor therapy involves a combination of three modalities: surgical removal, irradiation, and chemotherapy. Most childhood malignant neoplasms have widespread metastases, even those tumors with only a local detectable mass. Therefore, the majority are treated with more than simply surgery alone.

Prognosis varies with tumor type, extent of disease (stage), and other variables (patient age, sex, etc.). The best chance for cure is with the initial course of treatment (relapsed tumors are more drug resistant), so children with cancer should be referred early to a children's cancer center. Children's cancer protocols have enabled the cure rate to increase to its current level (approximately half of all tumors are curable) and ensure optimal care of the patient (studies show a higher cure rate in children enrolled in such protocols).

Chemotherapy drugs include hormones, antimetabolites, antibiotics, plant alkaloids, and alkylating agents (see *Nelson Textbook*, Table 17.2, for summary). Drugs generally are discovered through tests with tissue cell cultures and animals, and then tested for safety (phase I) and efficacy (phases II and III) in adult studies before use in children.

Bone marrow transplantation (BMT) has proven effective (cure rates approximately 40–60%) for certain leukemias in complete remission and more recently for other neoplasms. *Allogeneic BMT* (bone marrow donated from someone other than the patient or an identical twin) requires that human leukocyte antigen (HLA) type be identical or very similar. Graft-versus-host disease (GVHD) is a potentially fatal complication of allogeneic BMT, involving an immunologic attack of infused bone marrow cells against the body of the recipient. Cyclosporin and other immunosuppressants decrease its incidence. The chance of developing GVHD increases with a patient's age.

Syngeneic BMT (bone marrow donated from an identical twin) does not require immunosuppression. It therefore may have a slightly higher relapse rate. *Autologous BMT* (the patients' own marrow is harvested, frozen, and reinfused after a transplant conditioning procedure, which involves lethal doses of total body irradiation, or chemotherapy) usually is purged of undetectable tumor cells in vitro with monoclonal antibodies or chemotherapy before freezing. It has no risk of GVHD but has a higher risk of recurrence.

Other post-transplant problems include interstitial pneumonitis, veno-occlusive disease of the liver, sterility, cataracts, and relapse.

GENERAL COMPLICATIONS OF CHEMOTHERAPY

Metabolic

With initial treatment of cancer, massive amounts of uric acid, potassium, and phosphate can be released from dying cells. Particularly with leukemia or lymphoma tumors, this can lead to renal failure and fatal hypocalcemia or hyperkalemia. Before treatment, frequent blood chemistry measurements ("lysis labs": potassium, creatinine, blood urea nitrogen, phosphate, calcium, uric acid), allopurinol, and IV hydration (with bicarbonate, no potassium) must be started.

Hematologic

These complications can result from marrow infiltration and also from chemotherapy. *Anemia* can be treated with packed red blood cell transfusions. *Thrombocytopenia* is treated with platelet transfusions. Both blood products should be irradiated to prevent GVHD in an immunosuppressed patient. Cytomegalovirus (CMV)-negative patients should receive CMV-negative products.

Neutropenia, with absolute neutrophil count less than 500/mm^3, can allow life-threatening infections without obvious localizing symptoms. Any fever or other sign of infection in a neutropenic patient is treated with broad-spectrum antibiotics until the granulocyte count begins to rise. Cultures should be taken to identify possible drug-resistant bacterial pathogens.

Immunosuppression

This results from chemotherapy and often from underlying malignancy. Patients should not receive any live virus vaccines, and siblings should not receive live polio vaccine. Nonimmune patients exposed to varicella should receive varicella–zoster immune globulin and, if varicella develops, they should be treated with acyclovir.

Fungal infections may develop, and thrush can be treated with oral or topical antifungals.

Pneumocystis carinii can produce rapidly fatal infection, and patients with leukemia, lymphoma, and other cancers may receive prophylactic treatment with oral trimethoprim–sulfamethoxazole or IV pentamidine.

NUTRITION

Weight loss can result from the tumor or, more often, from treatments. Chemotherapy causes nausea and vomiting; irradiation, particularly to the head and neck and gastrointestinal tract, can prevent normal eating and/or absorption of food. Patients may lose 10% or more of body weight. Parenteral nutrition may be needed.

EMOTIONAL SUPPORT

This is critical for patient well-being. Both parents and patient should understand as much as possible about the disease and about potential complications of therapy (hair loss, possible amputation for solid tumor, etc.). School absence is frequent, and can be minimized by use of tutors or in-hospital teaching.

LATE SEQUELAE

These include limb dysfunction or absence, which requires prosthesis and rehabilitation, and radiation damage to organs such as bones and/or spine (can cause growth deformities later on), thyroid (can become hypoactive), gonads (become sterile), and brain (can develop neurologic and intellectual deficit).

Chemotherapy also can cause irreversible damage, including leukoencephalopathy from high-dose methotrexate, sterility from alkylating drugs, myocardial damage from anthracyclines, pulmonary fibrosis from bleomycin, pancreatitis after asparaginase, and hearing loss and renal damage from cisplatin.

Both radiation and chemotherapy can induce second cancers (overall, 0.5%/yr, to 12% for patients beyond 25 years off therapy), and all cancer survivors should have yearly check-ups.

THE LEUKEMIAS
(*NELSON TEXTBOOK*, SECS. 17.4–17.8)

These are the most common form of childhood cancer (approximately one third of new cases). Three fourths of cases are acute lymphocytic leukemia, with peak incidence at age 4 yr; one fifth are acute nonlymphocytic leukemia, the incidence of which increases with age; and the remainder are chronic myelocytic leukemia.

ACUTE LYMPHOCYTIC LEUKEMIA

Aside from massive radiation exposure, other environmental factors are not known to cause acute lymphocytic leukemia (ALL). Boys have a slightly higher incidence than girls, and there is an increased incidence in people with immunodeficiency, chromosomal abnormalities, and ataxia–telangiectasia.

Pathologic Subclassification

The *French–American–British* (FAB) working group has classified the morphology of bone marrow blasts

L-1: small with little cytoplasm
L-2: larger with more cytoplasm, irregular nuclear membranes, and more prominent nucleoli
L-3: cytoplasmic vacuolization, often associated with surface immunoglobulin (sIg) in B cell ALL.

Cell surface membrane markers are detected by specific antibodies. These are frequently more useful than the FAB classification to determine prognosis. T cells may be positive for CD5 and CD7 antigens. This T+ subtype is more common in older children, especially boys, who typically present with mediastinal mass, and has a worse prognosis. Mature B cells have sIg, (sIg+ subtype), and B cell precursors (preB ALL cells) contain intracellular Ig and not sIg (cIg+ subtype). Early preB cells do not react with any of the above antibodies and antigens (T−, sIg−, cIg− subtype). The common ALL antigen (cALLa+ subtype) is the most common and has the best prognosis. A few leukemias do not express any of these antigens and may be biphenotypic. Many leukemias in infants (<6 mo old) fit this pattern.

Cytogenetics (chromosome structure) also provide prognostic and therapeutic information. Translocations can help determine the cell type. Hyperdiploidy (>46 chromosomes in the leukemic cells) carries an improved prognosis, whereas a normal or decreased number of chromosomes is correlated with earlier relapse or failure to achieve remission. The presence of the Philadelphia chromosome (Ph+) translocation (t9:22) is a predictor of particularly poor response to chemotherapy and usually warrants BMT.

A formal staging generally is not used, because at the time of diagnosis leukemic cells already have spread to essentially all organs and usually are grossly detectable in marrow, lymph nodes, and spleen. However, certain high- and low-risk features (see below) do help dictate therapy.

Clinical Manifestations

Initial symptoms are nonspecific (e.g., viral syndrome, anorexia, irritability, lethargy) and are present for less than 4 wk before diagnosis in the majority of cases. They progress to symptoms of bone marrow failure resulting from tumor infiltration: pallor and fatigue (anemia), bleeding (thrombocytopenia), and fever (neutropenia), and complaints of bone pain or tenderness.

Physical examination shows pallor, petechiae, and mucous membrane bleeding (50% of patients); 25% of patients have fever. Most patients have lymphadenopathy and splenomegaly; hepatomegaly is less frequent. Less commonly, meningismus and headache occur from central nervous system (CNS) involvement.

Diagnosis

The CBC shows anemia (25% of patients as low as 6 g of hemoglobin/dL) and thrombocytopenia (only 25% of patients as high as $100,000/mm^3$). White blood cell count (WBC) can be low, normal, or high. Blasts often can be seen in the peripheral smear (esp. with high WBC), but the definitive test is bone marrow aspirate (BMA). This shows effacement of normal architecture with monotonous infiltrate of blasts. Occasionally, leukemic cells cannot be aspirated ("dry tap") and diagnosis must be made from bone marrow biopsy.

Other routine studies include chest roentgenogram to check for mediastinal mass. Other roentgenograms for bone pain usually are not necessary but, if done, they often show signs of leukemic infiltration of bone marrow. Lumbar puncture is done to check for CNS leukemia (usually done with the first dose of CNS chemotherapy). Serum chemistries (see "Metabolic Complications of Chemotherapy," above) are done to check for tumor lysis syndrome and renal compromise.

Differential diagnosis includes bone marrow infiltration by other malignant cells (neuroblastoma, rhabdomyosarcoma, Ewing sarcoma, retinoblastoma). These usually have a detectable mass elsewhere. It also includes:

  aplastic anemia (can distinguish on bone marrow biopsy)
  myelofibrosis
  infectious mononucleosis (peripheral cells clearly are not
      blasts, and BMA is normal)

Treatment

This varies with risk features. Low-risk features are age >2 yr and <10 yr, WBC <100,000, no mediastinal mass, no CNS involvement, early preB phenotype, hyperdiploidy, and absence of translocations.

Initial treatment (*induction*) is 4–6 wk of prednisone, vincristine, and L-asparaginase and CNS prophylactic injections of methotrexate, cytosine arabinoside (ara-C), and hydrocortisone. Most patients achieve remission (no detectable disease).

Continuation therapy (consolidation and/or *maintenance*) follows for 2.5–3 yr with methotrexate and 6-mercaptopurine, and CNS prophylaxis. Without CNS treatment, >50% of patients will have a relapse (the CNS is a systemic chemotherapy sanctuary site). Early CNS treatment with chemotherapy alone now is used to prevent CNS relapse.

T cell ALL requires more intensive chemotherapy and has a lower cure rate. B cell ALL (L-3 morphology, sIg +) also is more difficult to cure.

Relapse

Relapse occurs in:

- Bone marrow

    presents with manifestations similar to onset
    treat with more intensive chemotherapy, followed by BMT if suitable donor can be found and if remission can be attained

- CNS

    manifestations are due to increased intracranial pressure
    chemical meningitis (due to intrathecal chemotherapy) can also mimic these manifestations
    periodic examination of CSF can detect relapse
    treat with weekly intrathecal methotrexate and systemic chemotherapy, followed by craniospinal radiation

- Testicles (another sanctuary site)

    presents as painless swelling
    treat with local radiation and resumption of systemic and CNS chemotherapy

Prognosis

Null cell (cALLa +): 95% enter remission; 75% still in complete remission at 5 yr
PreB cell ALL (with t1:19): 95% enter complete remission; 60% in first complete remission at 5 yr
T cell ALL: curable in approximately 50%
B cell ALL: rarely curable
Nontypable (majority of patients <1 yr old): poor prognosis

ACUTE NONLYMPHOCYTIC LEUKEMIA

Acute nonlymphocytic leukemia (ANLL) comprises 20% of childhood leukemia. The incidence increases with age or predisposing conditions (Fanconi anemia; Bloom syndrome; previous chemotherapy, esp. with VP-16 or VM-26).

Clinical Manifestations

These are similar to those for ALL: fatigue, recurrent infections, pallor, fever, active bleeding, bone pain, gastrointestinal distress, and infection. Gingival swelling (resulting from local infiltration) is relatively specific for ANLL. Physical findings include hepatosplenomegaly, lymphadenopathy, joint pain, and bleeding (esp. menorrhagia in girls). Patients also can have symptoms from a local mass of tumor cells (chloroma) causing proptosis or CNS signs.

Diagnosis

Anemia, thrombocytopenia, and variable WBC, with peripheral blasts, sometimes are seen. A BMA for morphology and chromosome analysis shows blastic infiltrate. Coagulation parameters should be checked in the M3 subtype (associated with disseminated intravascular coagulation, excessive bleeding).

The *differential diagnosis* is similar to that for ALL. It also includes dysmyelopoiesis induced from folate or vitamin B_{12} deficiency, but examination of the BMA is diagnostic.

"Preleukemia" or *myelodysplastic syndrome* (MDS) has fewer than 30% blast cells in the BMA and can persist for months before becoming leukemia. It is associated with abnormalities of chromosomes 5 and 7 and poor response to standard chemotherapy.

Subtypes of ANLL often are evident from morphology. Monoclonal antibodies also can distinguish markers from the various subtypes.

Treatment

This generally is more myelosuppressive than ALL therapy. *Induction* with ara-C and daunorubicin induces remission in approximately 70% of patients (some require a second course). All but the M3 subtype go through a period of prolonged marrow hypoplasia before normal cells return. The disseminated intravascular coagulation of M3 ANLL can be treated with heparin before and during induction therapy.

Maintenance treatment involves rotating combinations of chemotherapeutics for 8 mo to 2 yr. CNS prophylaxis is used to prevent or treat CNS ANLL. BMT commonly is used to prevent relapse in patients with a first complete remission if there is an HLA-matched sibling. Thirty to 40% of patients treated with chemotherapy can be cured.

CHRONIC MYELOGENOUS LEUKEMIA

In chronic myelogenous leukemia (CML), clonal expansion of all hematopoietic cell types occurs, but this is found mainly in the myeloid (neutrophil) line. Many clonal cells have Philadelphia chromosome translocation (t9:22). Three percent of childhood leukemia is CML, and peak incidence occurs at age 10–12 yr. Blood and marrow show an increased number of myeloid cells with all maturational forms present.

Clinical Manifestations

These include (massive) splenomegaly, increased vitamin B_{12} levels, fetal hemoglobin in red blood cells, and decreased leukocyte alkaline phosphatase (LAP). The presentation may be subtle, with only the complaint of abdominal fullness (splenomegaly) or a routine CBC showing an elevated WBC.

Diagnosis

This is suggested by high WBC (often $>100,000/mm^3$) with all forms, and sometimes by eosinophilia and basophilia. BMA shows hypercellularity, increased myeloids, and increased megakaryocytes. Platelet count is normal or elevated. Variable anemia with nucleated red blood cells may occur.

Treatment

Initial treatment consists of lowering the WBC to $<100,000/mm^3$ (to decrease blood viscosity) with hydroxyurea or busulfan. Painful splenic enlargement responds to local radiation. Allogeneic BMT (in the chronic phase) can cure CML. Some patients may respond to interferon.

Without BMT, the chronic phase of CML accelerates to a blast crisis, with increasing blast forms seen (myeloid or lymphoid), and development of anemia and thrombocytopenia. Treatment then is changed to that for acute leukemia, and generally is unsuccessful. Median survival from diagnosis is 3 yr.

JUVENILE CML

Juvenile CML, which is completely different from CML, is a clonal panmyelopathy. Children <2 yr of age are affected. Increased WBC, prominent monocytes, splenomegaly, and cutaneous involvement occur. The serum vitamin B_{12} is elevated, LAP is low, and the Ph^1 chromosome is absent.

CONGENITAL LEUKEMIA

This is usually myelocytic, and cutaneous infiltrates ("blueberry muffin lesions"), hemorrhage, and high WBC occur. The prognosis is poor. It should be distinguished from relatively benign proliferation of immature myeloid cells in the newborn (more often in 21-trisomy patients), which spontaneously resolves with little or no treatment.

LYMPHOMA
(NELSON TEXTBOOK, SECS. 17.9 AND 17.10)

Lymphoma, the third most common cancer in children, is divided into two types: Hodgkin disease and non-Hodgkin lymphoma.

HODGKIN DISEASE

This rarely occurs before 5 yr, and the incidence peaks at age 15–34 and again after 50 yr. It is more common in boys and in same-sex siblings of Hodgkin patients. The Reed–Sternberg (R-S) cell seen on histology is thought to arise from an antigen-presenting cell. There is a possible etiologic role for Epstein–Barr virus.

There are four subtypes

lymphocytic predominant: occasional R-S cell occurs with mostly mature lymphocytes; this 10–20% of patients has the best prognosis

nodular sclerosing: 50–70% of cases; collagen bands in lymph nodes, R-S cells appear as lacunar cells

mixed cellularity: 40–50% of cases; mixture of lymphocytes, plasma cells, eosinophils, histiocytes, reticular cells, and R-S cells

lymphocytic depletion: <10% of patients; bizarre malignant reticular cells, R-S cells, and few lymphocytes; this type has the poorest prognosis

Hodgkin disease arises in lymph nodes, and usually spreads to local nodes before dissemination to the spleen, liver, lungs, bone, and bone marrow.

Staging

I—single node region or single extranodal site

II—two or more nodes/sites on the same side of the diaphragm

III—localized nodes/sites on both sides of the diaphragm

IV—diffuse spread (e.g., bone marrow)

For all patients, absence (A) or presence (B) of night sweats, fever, and 10% body weight loss also are noted.

Clinical Manifestations

Enlarged nodes are firm and nontender; enlargement may be discrete, involving single or multiple nodes. The cervical or supraclavicular nodes are the most common location. Mediastinal node enlargement can cause chronic cough, or manifestations of tracheal or bronchial compression. Usually it is seen on chest roentgenograms, but nodes may be confused with the thymus in a young child. Systemic signs include night sweats, persistent fever, weight loss, lethargy, fatigability, anorexia, and pruritus.

Extranodal involvement is uncommon at diagnosis. With progression, disease may involve diffuse lung tissue (sufficient for stage IV diagnosis) and can mimic fungal pneumonia on roentgenograms. Liver metastasis causes obstructive jaundice, and later hepatocellular disease. Bone marrow infiltration can cause pancytopenia. Extradural Hodgkin disease can cause nerve compression symptoms.

Immune disorders also can occur, including immunohemolytic anemia, immunothrombocytopenia, or nephrotic syndrome. Immunoincompetence (cellular) is extreme in patients with Hodgkin disease, as a result of chemotherapy and the underlying neoplasm. Varicella should be treated with acyclovir. Opportunistic fungal infections may become disseminated. Splenectomy (routine for staging) puts patients at severe risk for overwhelming encapsulated bacterial sepsis.

Diagnosis

This is made by biopsy of a persistently enlarged node with no local inflammation to explain it. Hodgkin disease is more common in older children (who often have mononucleosis), so a recent history of mononucleosis should not necessarily deter biopsy. A chest roentgenogram should be obtained before biopsy to detect any mediastinal mass and check for airway compromise. The CBC generally is not helpful, but there may be increased erythrocyte sedimentation rate, serum copper, or ferritin.

Staging involves chest roentgenogram and CT scan; occasionally lymphangiography to check for pelvic/abdominal nodes; staging laparotomy; and bone marrow biopsies. Laparotomy involves splenectomy (it is difficult to detect spleen involvement by scans), liver biopsies, multiple node biopsies, and, in girls, repositioning of the ovaries to sites outside potential radiation fields. In one third of cases, the clinical stage will be modified by surgical findings.

Treatment

Radiation and/or chemotherapy are effective. For stage I or IIA (localized) in a fully grown patient, some oncologists use radiation alone; up to 50% of patients will have recurrence and will do well with chemotherapy. Chemotherapy can be used over approximately 6 mo, with or without the addition of low-dose radiation.

Prognosis

Overall, >90% of children with Hodgkin disease will achieve complete remission. Most patients with stage I and II disease will be cured, 75% with stage III disease will be cured if treated with chemotherapy and radiation, and 50% with stage IV disease are likely to be cured if treated with intensive chemotherapy.

NON-HODGKIN LYMPHOMA

Non-Hodgkin lymphoma (NHL) is more common than Hodgkin disease in younger children; boys are affected three times more often than girls. Immunodeficiencies increase the risk of NHL (e.g., acquired immunodeficiency syndrome, X-linked agammaglobulinemia, severe combined immunodeficiency disease, Wiskott–Aldrich syndrome, ataxia–telangiectasia, or iatrogenic post-transplant immunosuppression).

Pathology

NHL is divided into low, intermediate, and high grades; children generally have the latter. Tumors of T cell origin often have a mediastinal primary and lymphoblastic histology. Those of B cell origin often have an abdominal primary and "undifferentiated," Burkitt, or "histiocytic" histology. Childhood NHL usually is diffuse and rapidly growing.

Staging

I—single tumor or node anywhere except the mediastinum or abdomen

II—single tumor/node with regional node involved; or two nodes/sites on same side of the diaphragm; or primary gastrointestinal tumor, with or without mesenteric nodes

III—tumors on both sides of the diaphragm; or any primary intrathoracic tumor; or any extensive primary intra-abdominal tumor

IV—any of the above with CNS or bone marrow involvement

Clinical Manifestations

These depend on the primary site of tumor. NHL often present as painless, unexplained swelling of cervical, supraclavicular, or other lymph nodes. Nodes are nontender, firm, and discrete early and confluent later, with rapid growth and occasional periods of regression.

Anterior mediastinal (thymic, T cell) lymphoma can present with cough, progressive dyspnea, pleural effusion, or superior vena cava syndrome. Abdominal lymphoma (most frequent in the ileocecal area) can present with mass, intestinal obstruction, and intussusception, with or without ascites. Lymphoma of bone presents with local or diffuse bone pain.

Meningeal extension causes manifestations of increased intracranial pressure, whereas focal intracranial lymphoma (frequently in an immunocompromised host) also may have mass lesion signs. In cases of bone marrow involvement, if more than 25% of BMA cells are blasts, it is classified as leukemia.

With extensive lymphoma, patients may develop systemic signs (fever, weight loss).

Treatment

Surgery is limited to initial diagnosis and to resection of small, localized gastrointestinal tumors. All patients require systemic chemotherapy, because all will have micrometastasis.

NHL cells can grow and die rapidly (especially in Burkitt lymphoma), so there must be a laboratory follow-up for lysis to anticipate possible renal failure. With a mediastinal mass, the physician must prepare for airway compromise and avoid sedation (which can precipitate loss of airway). Also, steroids must be avoided for airway edema, because they often start tumor lysis prematurely.

For localized lymphoma, ALL-type drugs are used but for a shorter period (6 mo). Burkitt lymphoma is treated with high-dose methotrexate and cyclophosphamide. Therapy is intense, but lasts <1 yr, because relapses occur early or not at all. Mediastinal lymphoma (usually T cell) is treated with intensive combinations of 10 or more drugs, given over 1–2 yr. CNS prophylaxis is standard.

Prognosis

With stages I and II NHL, 90% of patients will be cured; with stages III and IV, there is a 50% cure rate. Spread to bone marrow with "leukemia conversion" has a worse prognosis. Relapsed disease often responds well to BMT.

NERVOUS TISSUE TUMORS
(*NELSON TEXTBOOK*, SEC. 17.12)

NEUROBLASTOMA

The incidence is 1:100,000 per year in children <15 yr. It is slightly more common in whites than blacks and in boys than girls. Median age at diagnosis is 2 yr; 75% of cases are diagnosed by <5 yr. Clinical disease can spontaneously regress, especially stage IVS or I in children <1 yr.

Pathology

Neuroblastoma is a firm, gray tumor, with bleeding, necrosis, and calcifications. There is variable differentiation into benign ganglioneuroma, but most cells are primitive neural cells without obvious differentiation ("small blue round cells"). Tumor can arise anywhere neural crest cells migrate:

> 70% arise in the abdomen; one half of these are in the adrenal gland
>
> 20% arise in the thorax, usually the posterior mediastinum
>
> 10% arise elsewhere, or from an unknown site as a result of widespread metastasis

Tumor disseminates by local invasion or by hematogenous or lymphatic spread; metastases are common in the liver, bone marrow, and skeleton. A normal DNA content of tumor cells compared with normal cells (DNA index) or N-*myc* amplification in the tumor carries a worse prognosis.

Clinical Manifestations

The primary tumor is a firm, irregular, nontender mass, often in the upper abdomen. Bleeding into the tumor is common and may cause pallor or hypotension. Liver metastasis may cause enlargement and ascites, and bony metastasis may cause pain and tenderness (irritability in a young child).

Thoracic tumors may be found on chest roentgenograms; large masses may cause respiratory distress. Tumors in the head/neck may be palpated or may cause Horner syndrome. Pelvic tumors may prevent normal defecation or urination. Intra- or extraspinous tumor, or both (dumbell shaped), may cause cord compression, back tenderness, sphincter dysfunction, or gait disturbance. Primary nasopharynx tumors (esthesioneuroblastoma) may cause unilateral epistaxis or nasal obstruction.

Paraneoplastic signs of neuroblastoma include opsoclonus–myoclonus, ataxia, titubation of the head, myoclonic jerks, chaotic eye movements, or progressive dementia. Flushing and sweating can occur regardless of tumor extent and can occur even in a mother with an in utero fetus with neuroblastoma.

Diagnosis

Plain film, ultrasound, and intravenous pyelogram may help with diagnosis. CT scan with oral and IV contrast is indicated for abdominal tumors; 80% have calcifications seen on CT. Liver or skeleton metastasis also may be seen on CT, and a chest roentgenogram can show primary thoracic or paraspinous tumors.

Bone scan (with technetium diphosphonate) is highly sensitive for tumor and metastasis in 60% of patients. Tumor may be difficult to distinguish from trauma and growth plates in children, however. A miBG scan (detects uptake of radiolabeled *meta*-iodobenzylguanidine) can be a very specific/sensitive detector of disease.

BMA and biopsy should be done to detect tumor clumps or marrow effacement by infiltration (advanced infiltration causes pancytopenia). Urine should be checked for elevated catechol metabolites from the tumor (dopa, dopamine, norepinephrine, homovanillic acid, or vanillylmandelic acid, which are found in 90% of patients).

Treatment

Surgical excision is best for localized disease and probably not helpful for widely disseminated disease. Biopsy of surrounding lymph nodes to check for metastasis is helpful.

Chemotherapy (with cyclophosphamide and doxorubicin, or cisplatin and VM-26) can induce complete remission in approximately 50% of patients. (Sometimes, it is a complete remission with the exception of the tumor primary, which then becomes amenable to surgical removal with "second-look" surgery.)

Local radiation usually can cause regression of tumor and is used to treat symptoms (e.g., pain, neural compromise).

Patients with ganglioneuroma only do not need therapy. Also, the majority of IVS patients do not need therapy, unless vital functions are blocked. Tumors in most of these patients will spontaneously regress within a few months.

Prognosis

Prognosis is good with young age (<1 yr) and localized tumor; it is much worse for older children with widespread disease. It varies from >95% cure for stage I to <10% cure for stage IV in children >1 yr.

Complete resection improves the prognosis, as does the presence of hyperdiploidy and increased N-*myc* content of tumor. Prognosis also improves with early detection.

Auto-BMT may achieve a cure rate of 25%, but studies are not complete yet.

NEOPLASMS OF THE KIDNEY
(*NELSON TEXTBOOK*, SECS. 17.13–17.14)

WILMS TUMOR

Wilms tumor is the most common kidney tumor of children; the incidence is 7.8/million per year in children <15 yr. It is associated with genitourinary anomalies (4.4%), hemihypertrophy (2.9%), and sporadic aniridia (1.1%).

Wilms tumor is associated with deletions (major or minor) in chromosome 11, the probable location of tumor suppressor gene. The familial form is more likely to be bilateral and to occur at earlier age. A familial patient is more likely to have congenital anomalies, and the offspring of a familial Wilms tumor patient have a 30% chance of developing the tumor.

Pathology

Wilms tumor is a solitary growth in any part of the kidney and distorts the normal kidney. It has sharp demarcation and is variably encapsulated, and there is occasional hemorrhage into the tumor. A "favorable" histology is one of epithelial and stromal cells. "Unfavorable" types (10% of tumors, accounting for 60% of deaths) include:

"anaplastic": nuclear size variation and abnormal mitotic figures; occurs in older patients

"rhabdoid": not true muscle, but fibrillar eosinophilic inclusions; occurs in very young patients

"clear cell sarcoma": a spindle cell pattern; occurs in boys more often than girls, and often has bony metastasis

Staging (National Wilms Tumor Study [NWTS] Group)

I—limited to kidney and resected without rupture of capsule

II—extends beyond capsule but is resected totally

III—residual nonhematogenous extension of tumor (abdomen only) after surgery

IV—hematogenous metastasis, generally to lung

V—bilateral renal disease (5% of patients: survival estimated by prognosis for most severely affected kidney)

Clinical Manifestations

The median age at diagnosis is 3 yr. Patients generally are older and less ill-appearing than neuroblastoma patients. The tumor typically presents as an asymptomatic smooth, firm abdominal mass that does not cross the midline; usually it is found inadvertently by the parents or physician. Patients have abdominal pain and/or vomiting, and 60% have hypertension resulting from pressure on the renal artery; this can be severe enough to cause cardiac failure.

Diagnosis

The physician should suspect Wilms tumor in a young child with an abdominal mass. A urinalysis should be done; 10–25% of patients have hematuria.

Ultrasound can show an intrarenal mass, and CT shows an inhomogeneous mass arising from the kidney; calcifications are less common than in neuroblastoma. CT determines the intra- versus extrarenal source of the tumor, detects multiple masses, determines the extent of tumor, and allows evaluation of the opposite kidney.

The *differential diagnosis* includes hydronephrosis, renal cysts, mesoblastic nephroma, and other renal neoplasms (renal cell carcinoma, sarcoma, lymphoma).

Pulmonary metastases occur in 10–15% of patients.

Treatment

Initially, this involves complete surgical removal of the tumor and kidney (even if lung metastases are present). Also, the surgeon should check the other kidney, liver, retroperitoneal nodes, and renal vein.

Patients require postsurgical adjuvant therapy to prevent recurrence. Pulmonary lesions may be removed surgically or may be treated with chemotherapy and radiation only.

For stage V disease, preoperative chemotherapy may be used to shrink the tumor and allow one of the kidneys to be saved.

Prognosis

Survival varies from 89 to 92% (stage I) to 66 to 72% (stage IV). Prognosis improves for patient age <2 yr and tumor weight <250 g. Histology affects prognosis (see "Pathology" above). Relapse is very difficult to cure.

OTHER RENAL NEOPLASMS

Nephroblastomatosis

This involves independent foci of malformation or benign neoplasia in both kidneys; it is present in >33% of Wilms tumor patients. There is a high risk for developing a second Wilms tumor; patients should be followed by CT scan.

Mesoblastic Nephroma

This is a congenital massive, firm, infiltrative benign tumor; it occurs more often in boys than girls. Surgery usually is adequate treatment, unless histology shows evidence of clear cell sarcoma.

Renal Cell Carcinoma

This tumor occasionally occurs in teenagers, who present with an abdominal mass and hematuria. It may be cured with complete resection, but incomplete resection has a bad prognosis.

SOFT-TISSUE SARCOMAS
(NELSON TEXTBOOK, SECS. 17.15 AND 17.16)

The incidence of these tumors is 8.4/million per year in white children and half that in black children.

RHABDOMYOSARCOMA

This tumor comprises more than 50% of all soft-tissue sarcomas in children. There are two peaks of incidence: ages <5 yr (tumors of neck, head, prostate, bladder, vagina) and

15–19 yr (genitourinary tract, particularly the testes or paratesticular tissue). It may occur with neurofibromatosis, and can occur in any part of the body.

Pathology

The tumor arises from embryonic mesenchyme; it is one of the "small blue round cell" tumors of childhood (others are neuroblastoma, lymphoma, Ewing sarcoma). Histologic subtypes are:

embryonal: 60% of tumors
botryoid (sarcoma botryoides): variant of embryonal form; tumor projects into body cavity (e.g., vagina, uterus, bladder, nasopharynx, and middle ear); 6% of tumors
alveolar: 20% of cases; cells grow in cores with spaces resembling alveoli; usually in older children, in trunk and extremities; has poorest prognosis
pleomorphic: mainly in adults; 1% of childhood cases
Undifferentiated: found in 20% of childhood cases

Staging (Intergroup Rhabdomyosarcoma Study [IRS])

Group I—localized tumor, completely resectable, no microscopic disease
Group II—grossly resected tumor with local nodes positive or residual microscopic disease
Group III—gross residual disease
Group IV—distant metastatic disease

Clinical Manifestations

The tumor presents as a mass, sometimes painful. Additional features depend on tumor location, and include:

nasopharynx: associated with nasal congestion, mouth breathing, epistaxis, and breathing problems
cranial extension: cranial nerve paralysis, blindness, increased intracranial pressure, headache, and vomiting
face or cheek: swelling, pain, trismus, cranial nerve paralysis
neck: initial swelling, later neurologic signs
orbit: proptosis, periorbital edema, ptosis, visual deficit, pain
middle ear: pain, hearing loss, chronic otorrhea, or visible ear canal mass; can lead to cranial nerve paralysis and intracranial mass effect
larynx: chronic croupy cough, progressive stridor
trunk or extremity: presents as a mass, often after trauma; usually thought to be hematoma but does not resolve with time
genitourinary system: hematuria, recurrent urinary tract infection, incontinence, mass on abdominal or rectal examination
paratesticular: rapidly growing scrotal mass
vaginal: grape-like mass protruding from vaginal orifice, can cause urinary problems, vaginal bleeding, or urethral or rectal obstruction; uterine tumors can cause similar symptoms

The tumor can metastasize early, with lung and/or bony lesions. Metastases may present with pulmonary insufficiency, bony pain, or symptomatic hypercalcemia.

Diagnosis

This often is delayed several months because of the tumor's rarity and failure to consider the diagnosis. Work-up involves plain roentgenograms and CT scan of the primary tumor. For abdominal tumors, ultrasound and oral and IV dye with CT may be included; for genitourinary tumors, cystourethrograms should be included.

Skeletal survey (roentgenograms) and bone scan roentgenogram and CT of chest, and BMA and biopsy are necessary to check for metastatic disease. The tumor must be biopsied and/or resected for tissue diagnosis.

Treatment

The best therapy is complete surgical excision, but this rarely is possible. Tumor margins should be carefully defined. Chemotherapy may be indicated to shrink tumor before resection is attempted. In general:

Group I: resection is followed by chemotherapy to prevent recurrence

Groups II and III: surgery is followed by local radiation and systemic chemotherapy

Group IV: primarily treated with systemic chemotherapy

Prognosis

There is an 80–90% cure rate with complete resection. Unresectable tumors at certain sites (e.g., orbit) have good prognoses. Two thirds of patients with incompletely resected local tumor (only) have long-term survival, whereas with disseminated disease, one half achieve complete remission and less survive long term.

Older patients have a worse prognosis: they are more likely to have an alveolar histology and tumors of the extremities.

OTHER SOFT-TISSUE SARCOMAS
(SEE *NELSON TEXTBOOK*, TABLE 17–11)

NEOPLASMS OF BONE
(*NELSON TEXTBOOK*, SECS. 17.17–17.21)

The annual incidence of bone tumors ranges from 5.6/million (whites) to 4.8/million (blacks). Osteosarcoma is twice as common as Ewing sarcoma in whites.

OSTEOSARCOMA

The onset of this tumor coincides with periods of increased bone growth; mean age at diagnosis is 15 yr (during growth spurt). The tumor most frequently arises in long bones at the metaphyseal ends (where growth occurs). The most common sites are the distal femur, proximal humerus, and proximal tibia, but osteosarcoma can arise in any bone.

There is a high incidence in survivors of familial retinoblastoma and as second tumor following Ewing sarcoma (latency 4–20 yr). Other predisposing diseases include Ollier disease, Maffucci syndrome, multiple hereditary exostoses, osteogenesis imperfecta, and Paget disease.

Pathology

This tumor is one of malignant osteoblasts (produce osteoid). It starts within the medullary canal of the shaft; tumor may break through to cause a big soft-tissue mass or can extend along the cavity. There may be osteosarcomatous, chondrosarcomatous, and fibrosarcomatous features in the same tumor.

Clinical Manifestations

Local pain occurs early, and usually is attributed to trauma. There is a progressive limitation of motion and an obvious mass. Limping, change in gait, tenderness, local erythema, and hyperthermia also may be seen.

The earliest metastases are to the lungs (either asymptomatic or with respiratory distress, effusion, and pneumothorax); later metastases are to other bones, lymph nodes, and the CNS.

Diagnosis

Persistent unexplained bone pain should be evaluated roentgenographically; osteosarcoma shows sclerosis and new bone formation. The tumor should be staged before surgery using bone scan, chest roentgenograms, and CT. CT (with contrast) of the involved extremity should be obtained to define the extent of tumor.

Treatment

Surgical (complete) resection for local disease is indicated. The question of using presurgical chemotherapy to reduce tumor and treat micrometastasis still is being evaluated. All patients should receive adjuvant chemotherapy.

Patients with pulmonary metastases should have surgical removal of those as well as chemotherapy.

Post-treatment rehabilitation includes limb prosthesis; phantom limb pain may be a problem.

Prognosis

This is best with low-grade tumors (parosteal). The cure rate for surgery alone is approximately 20%; it improves to >50% with addition of chemotherapy.

Some patients with few large resectable pulmonary metastases have long-term survival, but diffuse pulmonary disease or bony metastases make survival unlikely.

CHONDROSARCOMA

This tumor is rare in children, and usually occurs in the 2nd decade. There is an equal frequency in boys and girls. It is associated with Ollier disease and Maffucci syndrome.

Histology shows malignant formation of cartilage. Chondrosarcoma is most common in the pelvis but may occur in any bone (flat bones of the trunk, long bones of the extremities). There is metastasis to the lungs and bone, and frequent local extension and recurrence after surgery.

The tumor presents with pain and mass, and roentgenograms suggest the *diagnosis*, which is made by biopsy.

Treatment involves resection or amputation. Tumor does not respond to radiation or chemotherapy.

EWING SARCOMA

Pathology

On histology, there are small, blue, round cells with little cytoplasm or stroma. PAS- (glycogen)-positive tissue helps distinguish it from neuroblastoma. The bone most commonly involved is the femur; the most commonly involved flat bone is the pelvis.

"*Extraosseous Ewing sarcoma* is a histologically similar tumor that arises in soft tissue (of the legs or paravertebral region).

Metastases to the lungs, bone, bone marrow, and CNS are present in one third of children at diagnosis.

Clinical Manifestations

There is pain, fever, and tenderness, and the patient may have a massive soft tissue component. Differential diagnosis includes eosinophilic granuloma and osteomyelitis.

Ewing sarcoma may improve transiently with antibiotics, delaying diagnosis; it should always be considered in culture-negative osteomyelitis.

Diagnosis

Ewing sarcoma is suspected from history and roentgenograms but may be difficult to differentiate from infection unless there is pulmonary metastasis. Diagnosis is by biopsy. Lung roentgenograms and CT, bone scan, and bone marrow biopsy should be obtained, as well as CT of the primary tumor to follow disease.

Treatment

The tumor is sensitive to radiation and chemotherapy. Pathologic fractures may occur through the bone tumor, with poor healing, so patients must be warned against weight bearing on the tumor-containing leg. Radiation usually is high dose and may have side effects of poor bone growth, fibrosis, or secondary osteosarcoma.

Prognosis

This is poor in the presence of metastasis or with a proximal primary tumor; tumors of the pelvis, humerus, or ribs have worse prognoses than tumors of long limb bones. Forty to 60% of children without metastatic disease are free of disease at 3 yr, but late relapses occur.

PRIMITIVE NEUROECTODERMAL TUMORS

These are small, round-cell tumors in peripheral sites (soft tissue and bone) and in the CNS. The cell type is unclear, but it may be a midpoint of development between Ewing sarcoma and neuroblastoma. These tumors usually have more evidence of neural differentiation (neuron-specific enolase, dense core granules) than Ewing sarcoma. The presentation and treatment are similar to those of Ewing sarcoma, but there is a worse prognosis.

RETINOBLASTOMA

The incidence of retinoblastoma is 3.4/million per year; there is an equal frequency in blacks and whites. The average age at diagnosis is 8 mo for bilateral and 26 mo for unilateral cases. Thirty percent are bilateral, and all have a dominantly inherited predisposition; 10–20% of unilateral disease patients also have this predisposition. The genetic defect is a deletion in the chromosome 13q arm (RB locus).

One percent of hereditary retinoblastoma survivors will develop osteosarcomas by age 10 yr. These occur in the radiation port or at other loci, and they can be multifocal. By the age of 30 yr, 30% of patients develop some other second malignancy.

Pathology

Retinoblastoma usually develops in the posterior portion of the retina. It consists of small, closely packed, round cells with little cytosol and an occasional rosette. It often arises in multiple foci.

Endophytic tumor growth from internal layers of the retina into the vitreous cavity is seen by ophthalmoscope. *Exophytic* tumors grow into the subretinal space, causing retinal detachment. Endophytic tumors can seed other parts of the retina and are associated with large tumors (>5 disk diameters [dd]) and a poorer prognosis.

Massive tumors may invade the choroid and may indicate a likelihood of hematogenous spread. Tumor extension through the lamina cribrosa and down the optic nerve to the CNS also occurs. Most tumors have not metastasized by diagnosis, so an attempt to save vision is made.

Staging

    I—one or more tumors <4 dd in size, at or behind the
      equator
    II—same as I, but size 4–10 dd
    III—any tumor anterior to the equator or solitary tumors
      >10 dd behind the equator
    IV—multiple tumors, some >10 dd; or lesion anterior to
      the ora serrata
    V—tumor involving >½ of the retina; vitreous seeding

Clinical Manifestations

There is leukocoria (yellowish white reflex in pupil) of the involved eye. Patients may have visual loss, eye squint, ocular pain, pupillary irregularity, or hyphema. With advanced tumor, proptosis, increased intracranial pressure, and bone pain from metastasis occur.

Over 80% of children with the hereditary form have bilateral disease at diagnosis. Many familial cases are discovered by routine funduscopic examination.

Diagnosis

Leukocoria should be evaluated carefully in children (using funduscopy under anesthesia) to look for retinoblastoma. Roentgenograms show calcifications 75% of the time. CT scan of the orbits is used to check tumor extent in the orbits, optic nerve, and bones.

Differential diagnosis of leukocoria includes retinal detachment, persistent hyperplastic primary vitreous, nematode endophthalmitis, cataract, coloboma of the choroid, and retinopathy of prematurity.

Other useful studies include a skeletal survey, bone scan, CT of the head with contrast, BMA/biopsy, and lumbar puncture. Tumor is frequently associated with increased carcinoembryonic antigen and α-fetoprotein; the latter can be followed after treatment to check for recurrence.

Treatment

Unilateral disease with a small tumor (stages I–III) requires local irradiation; that with a large tumor requires enucleation. With bilateral disease, there should be an attempt to save vision in at least one eye. One or both eyes can be irradiated, but for severe painful glaucoma or blindness, enucleation should be done. The surgeon also should remove as much optic nerve as possible with enucleation.

Postsurgical radiation is used if extraorbital extension is found. Chemotherapy is not used for a totally resected tumor, but it may help with control of residual disease (cyclophosphamide and doxorubicin). Widespread disease responds to chemotherapy but is unlikely to be cured.

Prognosis

With tumors of stages I–IV, there is a 100% survival rate; with stage V tumors, there is an 85% survival rate. Fewer than 10% of patients have extraglobal disease at diagnosis. There is a 0% cure rate with massive or extensive optic nerve disease, and a 30% cure rate if micrometastases are found in periglobal tissues of the optic nerve.

The above numbers do not take into account the high likelihood of a second malignancy later in life as a result of retinoblastoma mutation.

GASTROINTESTINAL NEOPLASMS
(*NELSON TEXTBOOK*, SEC. 17.22)

These are much rarer in children than in adults. A malignant lesion in the mouth in a very young child is likely to be a sarcoma.

SALIVARY GLAND TUMORS

Most enlarged glands are benign (the result of inflammation or mucoceles). Also, most tumors are benign (hemangiomas, hamartomas, mixed tumor of salivary gland–pleomorphic adenoma).

Mixed tumor occurs in the 2nd decade, with an equal frequency in boys and girls. The parotid is the gland most frequently involved; the patient presents with a hard, movable, nontender mass, and can have facial nerve paralysis. *Treatment* is by surgical excision. The tumor has a good prognosis, although it may recur locally.

Mucoepidermoid carcinoma is malignant, usually is found in the 2nd decade, and most often occurs in the parotid gland. Rarely, this tumor metastasizes to local nodes; if it does, the prognosis is poor. Complete excision leads to an excellent prognosis, but this tumor also may recur locally.

NASOPHARYNGEAL CARCINOMA
(Lymphoepithelioma)

This tumor is common in adults in North Africa and the Far East; it occurs in family clusters and is associated with Epstein–Barr virus. In the United States, it occurs mostly in the 2nd decade; blacks are affected 4–7 times more often than whites. The histology is that of undifferentiated carcinoma.

The patient presents with unilateral, tender, cervical adenopathy, trismus, epistaxis, sore throat, and dysphagia (leading to weight loss).

Diagnosis is by biopsy of the cervical node or of the nasopharyngeal primary. Tumor can extend to the base of the skull and to soft tissues of the nasopharynx. Regional node metastasis is common; hematogenous spread to bone and lung also occur.

Radiation of the involved nasopharynx results in a 50% cure rate. Chemotherapy (with cyclophosphamide, doxorubicin, and continuous infusion cisplatin/5-fluorouracil) is being studied.

CARCINOMA OF THE STOMACH

This form is rare in children. The patient presents with mass, bleeding, and obstruction. It is best treated with complete resection.

PANCREATIC CARCINOMA

This lesion also is rare in children. It usually arises in the head of pancreas, and the patient presents with an upper abdominal mass, weight loss, and pain. Patients may present with jaundice if the tumor obstructs the common bile duct. *Treatment* is resection; the prognosis is poor.

Pancreatoblastoma

This is a benign exocrine tumor in the head of the pancreas; it is encapsulated, and distinct from the ducts. The patient presents with an abdominal mass. *Treatment* is resection; this does not interfere with pancreatic function.

Nesidioblastosis (β Cell Endocrine Benign Hyperplasia)

Diagnosis is by hypoglycemia with high serum insulin. *Treatment* is by pancreatectomy.

COLONIC POLYPS

The juvenile (retention) polyp represents 85% of all lower gastrointestinal tract polyps in children. The patient presents with bright red rectal bleeding. Polyps occur mainly in 3–5-yr-olds. They can be removed by sigmoidoscopy; 25% will recur but are not premalignant.

Multiple juvenile polyposis may be premalignant.

ADENOCARCINOMA OF THE COLON AND RECTUM

This tumor is rare in children (<1% of childhood malignancies) but has been reported in a child 9 mo old. The patient presents with bloody stools, melena, abdominal pain, anorexia, and weight loss. An abdominal mass may be found, and the patient may have hepatomegaly as a result of metastasis.

Diagnosis is evident from barium enema or endoscopy. Predisposing conditions are familial multiple polyposis, ulcerative colitis, regional enteritis, and Peutz–Jeghers syndrome.

NEOPLASMS OF THE LIVER
(*NELSON TEXTBOOK*, SEC. 17.23)

There are two types of primary liver cancer: hepatoblastoma and hepatocellular carcinoma (hepatoma).

EPIDEMIOLOGY

Hepatoblastoma is more common than hepatocellular carcinoma, and usually occurs in patients <3 yr old; boys are affected more often than girls (ratio 1.5:1). Hepatocellular carcinoma incidence peaks at age <4 yr and 12–15 yr; boys are affected slightly more often than girls (ratio 1.3:1). These tumors are associated with congenital hemihypertrophy and extensive hemangiomas. Hepatocellular carcinoma with cirrhosis is much rarer in children than in adults, but cirrhosis of malnutrition and biliary cirrhosis resulting from biliary atresia are associated with an increased incidence of malignant liver tumors.

PATHOLOGY

Hepatoblastoma may appear epithelial or gland-like or may have mesenchymal components with primitive osteoid tissue. Cells are poorly differentiated. Hepatocellular carcinoma has well-differentiated, large polygonal cells and eosinophilic cytoplasm. Cells form rudimentary hepatic cords with sinusoids. Frequently, these tumors metastasize to the lungs or extend locally in the abdomen.

CLINICAL MANIFESTATIONS

The patient usually presents with an upper abdominal mass, and less commonly with pain, anorexia, and weight loss. Less common findings are vomiting, jaundice, and virilization in boys as a result of tumor production of gonadotropin.

DIAGNOSIS

The *differential diagnosis* of hepatic enlargement includes neuroblastoma, infantile hemangioendotheliomas, cavernous hemangiomas, and metabolic storage disease. The physician should search for evidence of other metastatic disease or of hemangiomas.

Usually liver function tests are normal, but 20% of patients with these tumors have increased bilirubin or transaminases. Most patients have increased α-fetoprotein. Abdominal roentgenograms show a big liver; 30% have calcifications. Chest roentgenograms and CT may show metastasis (present in 10% of cases). Hepatic angiography and nuclear scan can help the surgeon identify the involved lobes. Final diagnosis is made by biopsy.

TREATMENT

Complete resection is the only curative therapy; only one third of tumors can be removed. Both hepatoblastoma and hepatocellular carcinoma are resistant to radiation; chemotherapy has a temporary effect on hepatoblastoma.

PROGNOSIS

Overall survival is 35% for hepatoblastoma and 13% for hepatocellular carcinoma. Less than complete resection always leads to local recurrence and death.

GONADAL AND GERM CELL NEOPLASMS
(*NELSON TEXTBOOK*, SEC. 17.24)

EPIDEMIOLOGY

These tumors generally are uncommon in children. Sacrococcygeal teratoma is the most common solid tumor in newborn infants (1:40,000 live births), and is found more often in girls than boys. Ovarian and testicular tumors peak in incidence at <2 yr of age, with a second peak after 6 yr for ovarian and 14 yr for testicular tumors. Children with cryptorchid testes have a 50-fold higher chance of malignancy; 20% of these tumors occur in the descended testicle.

Gonadal dysgenesis underlies the development of gonad-oblastoma.

PATHOLOGY

Tumors usually arise in the gonads but may occur in the retroperitoneum, mediastinum, sacrococcygeum, or CNS. Tumors express variable degrees of multipotential differentiation (see *Nelson Textbook*, Figure 17–9).

Choriocarcinoma

This is often present in both gonadal and extragonadal germ cell tumors but usually is not the major component of the tumor. It occurs after puberty in males and before and after puberty in females.

Yolk Sac Carcinoma (Endodermal Sinus Tumor)

This tumor resembles the endodermal sinuses of the placenta. It can differentiate to all three germ cell layers (teratoma or teratocarcinoma) or have malignant features (embryonal carcinoma).

Seminoma and Dysgerminoma

Seminoma is a testicular tumor of the 2nd decade and later. Clear cells aggregate in lobules separated by fibrous stroma. *Dysgerminoma* is the female version of the seminoma; cells appear as primordial germ cells.

Both seminoma and dysgerminoma metastasize to regional lymph nodes, lung, and bone. Dysgerminoma can metastasize locally to peritoneal surfaces.

CLINICAL MANIFESTATIONS

In the infant, *testicular tumor* presents as a nonpainful, scrotal mass, without inflammation. There may be an accompanying hydrocele, which often delays diagnosis. In older boys, gradual swelling of the teste occurs over weeks, often with pain and tenderness. Testicular tumor may present with metastatic symptoms (lung or retroperitoneal), weight loss, anorexia, or lethargy. It may cause gynecomastia as a result of chorionic gonadotropin secretion by the tumor.

Ovarian tumors present with pain, nausea, and vomiting; an abdominal mass or fullness; or signs of a sudden acute abdomen (ovarian torsion). Ovarian germ cell tumors rarely present with metastatic disease. Ninety-five percent are benign cystic teratomas; the younger the patient the more likely there is a malignant lesion.

Sacrococcygeal teratoma or *teratocarcinoma* usually presents with a buttocks or scrotal mass at birth or soon after. Ten percent of neonatal tumors are malignant, but this increases to 50–70% for older age at presentation. Tumor can interfere with normal genitourinary or gastrointestinal function. It is associated with congenital anomalies of the lower vertebrae, genitourinary system, or anorectum.

DIAGNOSIS

Careful examination is critical: testicular tumors are opaque to transillumination. Ultrasound helps detect scrotal or pelvic/abdominal masses.

A sacrococcygeal tumor suggests teratoma but could also be meningocele, chordoma, rectal duplication, neurogenic tumor, lipoma, rhabdomyosarcoma, or hemangioma; it also may suggest perirectal abscess. It may be mainly intrapelvic; these tend to present with anuria and constipation.

Work-up should include chest roentgenogram and CT, bone scan, abdominal CT (to check for retroperitoneal node metastasis), serum chorionic gonadotropin, and α-feto-protein.

TREATMENT

Surgical resection of the primary tumor is indicated. Radiation is used for dysgerminoma and seminoma, and all patients should receive chemotherapy.

PROGNOSIS

Prognosis worsens with widespread disease, so early treatment is critical. Extraembryonal elements in the tumor have a worse prognosis. Cure is possible, even after recurrence.

OTHER TUMORS OF THE GONADS

Sertoli tumors of the testicle are benign; they arise from sustentacular cells of the gonadal mesenchyme. They can be associated with sexual precocity or gynecomastia, and occur usually at 1–2 yr. *Treatment* is by surgical removal.

Benign ovarian cysts represent over half of ovarian tumors. They may cause acute abdomen, nausea, and vomiting if torsion of the ovary occurs. *Granulosa–theca cell tumor* is rare. It arises in ovarian stromal cells and is associated with precocious puberty and a lower abdominal mass. It is rarely malignant, and removal corrects the endocrine disorder. *Cystadenocarcinoma* is a rare malignant ovarian tumor. *Hemangiomas* may involve the ovary. *Lymphoma* can present initially in the ovary.

Gonadoblastoma occurs exclusively in children with gonadal dysgenesis. Eighty percent of patients are phenotypic females, some with virilization; others are phenotypic males, often with cryptorchidism, hypospadias, or female internal or secondary sex organs. Gonadoblastoma is cancer in situ; germinomas can develop. It presents as a growing abdominal mass that may be bilateral, and it may enhance virilization. *Treatment* is surgical removal of the tumor and the normal gonad and uterus. The patient should then receive hormone treatments, but increased risk of second cancer is associated with these.

MISCELLANEOUS CARCINOMAS
(*NELSON TEXTBOOK*, SEC. 17.25)

VAGINA AND CERVIX ADENOCARCINOMA

This is rare except in children exposed to diethylstilbestrol in utero. It is associated with genitourinary anomalies.

THYROID CARCINOMA

This is more frequent following radiation to the neck. Spontaneous carcinoma is more common in girls than boys, and the *papillary* type grows slower and is more common. *Medullary* carcinoma is either sporadic or familial; the latter is associated with Marfan-like features, pheochromocytoma, hyperparathyroidism, and mucosal neuromas.

ADRENAL GLAND CARCINOMA

This is more common in the first years of life. It may be associated with skin hemangiomas and genitourinary anomalies; it is more common in girls than boys. Patients present with endocrine adrenal hyperfunction, Cushing syndrome, and virilization and/or feminization.

SKIN CANCER

This is rare in children.

Malignant melanoma is a rapidly growing, fragile, ulcerated lesion, with dark pigment or altered color. It appears on any body part. There is an increased frequency with giant hairy cell nevus syndrome or dysplastic nevus syndrome. Initially, an excisional biopsy should be done; if positive, wide local resection is done. Regional lymph nodes also should be examined. For metastatic disease, treatment is with doxorubicin and cyclophosphamide.

Xeroderma pigmentosum is an autosomal recessive condition of defective DNA repair. Skin damage from ultraviolet light leads to malignant transformation at multiple sites. Surgical resection of tumors is indicated, and skin should be protected from the sun.

MISCELLANEOUS BENIGN TUMORS
(*NELSON TEXTBOOK*, SECS. 17.26–17.30)

BENIGN TUMORS AND TUMOR-LIKE PROCESSES IN BONE

Osteoid Osteoma

This usually occurs in adolescents, and is more common in boys than girls. It involves the femur or tibia, and less often the spine, humerus, and phalanges. The patient presents with dull pain, worse at night and after weight-bearing; pain is relieved by aspirin. There is local tenderness, but usually no inflammation.

Roentgenograms show a sharply edged radiolucent osteoid nidus with surrounding sclerotic bone.

Treatment is by surgical removal of the nidus.

Osteoblastoma is a similar tumor, although larger, with little sclerosis.

Fibrous (Benign) Cortical Defects

These eccentric lesions arise from the periosteum and erode the cortex. They occur in 53% of boys and 31% of girls, ages 4–8 yr. These asymptomatic lesions may persist into adulthood. They occur in the metaphyses of cylindrical bones, often the knees.

Diagnosis is made by roentgenogram, and they should not be treated.

Nonossifying Fibroma or Fibroxanthoma

This is most common in late childhood/early adolescence. Fifty percent are found incidentally; they may be associated with chronic bone pain. Pathologic fractures may occur. Usually these tumors are at the ends of long bones.

This tumor appears on roentgenograms as a rarefied scalloped lesion. It usually does not require treatment, but weakened bones may need curettage.

Osteochondroma (Cartilaginous Exostosis)

This is a single lesion similar to those of osteochondromatosis (hereditary multiple exostoses). It occurs in any cartilagine-derived bone, usually near the ends of the femur or tibia at the knee. It starts in childhood/early adolescence and ceases with growth plate closure. Patients may have a mass or pain with fracture. Roentgenograms show a pedunculated or sessile lesion.

Growth rarely may reactivate the lesion, sometimes after a fracture. These growths should be biopsied to check for malignancy, and lesions should be removed prophylactically.

Enchondroma

This is the solitary form of multiple enchondromatosis (Ollier disease). It is rare, usually involving the metacarpals, metatarsals, or phalanges. It presents as a deforming mass or the cause of pathologic fractures. Roentgenograms show rarefied bone with thinning and bulging of the cortex and stippled calcification.

Hand and feet lesions are benign, but those in large long bones, diaphyses, or membranous bones have malignant potential and can be difficult to discern histologically. Benign lesions should be curettaged, and others should be widely excised.

Solitary Unicameral Cyst

This begins close to the epiphyseal plate and grows toward the diaphysis. The cavity is uni- or multilocular, containing fluid or blood. Possibly these cysts follow traumatic hematomas. They usually occur without symptoms, but they may cause pathologic fractures. Roentgenograms show an area of rarefaction with pseudoloculation; it does not cross the epiphyseal plate.

These cysts may resolve spontaneously, but leg lesions should be curettaged or excised to prevent fracture.

HEMANGIOMA

This is one of the most common neoplasms in children; most occur in the skin. Rarely, they grow rapidly to a large size and can cause deformity or threaten life, especially if they occur in the head or neck. They can cause airway obstruction, pressure necrosis, difficulty in feeding, and ear canal obstruction. Tumors can develop bacterial superinfections. Large arteriovenous shunts can cause cardiac failure. Hemangiomas usually are obvious at less than 6 mo of age, grow during 1–2 yr of age, and slowly regress later, but their history is unpredictable. Surgical resection usually is very difficult; growth may respond to steroids, but they can recur with drug withdrawal.

Liver Hemangioma

This tumor appears before 6 mo of age. The patient may present with jaundice, vomiting, diarrhea, or simply increased abdominal girth in infants. Arteriovenous fistulas can cause cardiac insufficiency.

Abdominal roentgenograms show an enlarged liver and, occasionally, calcifications. Radionuclide and CT scans show a defect in the liver; an arteriogram shows an abnormal vascular pattern. *Treatment* initially is with prednisone; a unilobar lesion can be resected.

Cavernous hemangioma can cause hemolysis, intralesional clotting, thrombocytopenia, and hypofibrinogenemia with bleeding.

LYMPHANGIOMA (Cystic Hygroma)

This tumor usually occurs in the head and neck region. It appears early, usually by 3 yr, and is of unknown embryonic origin. It is a single or multicystic mass with thin, often transparent walls, containing straw-colored fluid. It presents as a compressible mass, not tender or painful. There may be some skin thinning but generally no erythema.

Lesions do not regress and should be resected as soon as possible. The lesion may involve intrathoracic extension in 10% of cases, and tumor may compress the trachea as it grows. Resection may require extensive surgery and reconstruction.

THYMOMA

This is rare in children, and occurs with equal frequency in boys and girls. It occurs in the anterior mediastinum, and sometimes is found inadvertently on chest roentgenogram. Growth of the tumor compresses neighboring tissues, causing cough, dyspnea, dysphagia, and superior vena cava syndrome.

Thymoma is associated with paraneoplastic syndromes such as myasthenia gravis, hypogammaglobulinemia, pure red blood cell aplasia; these may be due to disruption of the immune system. The tumor rarely metastasizes, but does extend locally.

Treatment is surgical resection. The tumor is sensitive to radiation, and recurrence can respond to doxorubicin, cyclophosphamide, and cisplatin.

SPLENIC CYSTS

These cause splenomegaly, and should be investigated by abdominal ultrasound or CT or both.

16

NEPHROLOGIC DISEASES AND UROGENITAL DISORDERS

ANATOMY
(NELSON TEXTBOOK, SEC. 18.1)

Placed retroperitoneally, each kidney has 1 million nephrons and consists of an outer cortex (glomeruli, proximal and distal convoluted tubules, collecting ducts) and an inner medulla (straight portions of tubules, loops of Henle, vasa recta, terminal collecting ducts). The blood supply includes the renal artery, arising from the abdominal aorta, and the renal vein, draining into the inferior vena cava.

PHYSIOLOGY
(NELSON TEXTBOOK, SEC. 18.2)

Renal function includes glomerular filtration and tubular secretion and absorption, which constitute the major mechanisms by which the urine is formed. Other renal functions include the metabolism of vitamin D and the production of renin and erythropoietin.

CONDITIONS ASSOCIATED WITH HEMATURIA
(NELSON TEXTBOOK, SECS. 18.3–18.23)

GLOMERULAR DISEASES
(NELSON TEXTBOOK, SECS. 18.3–18.13)

Etiologies (see Table 16–1)

Recurrent Gross Hematuria or Persistent Microscopic Hematuria

Recurrent episodes of painless gross hematuria may occur 1–2 days following the onset of an upper respiratory infection not associated with symptoms of renal disease, such as hypertension, edema, or elevated blood urea nitrogen (BUN) and creatinine. Some patients have microscopic hematuria or intermittent gross hematuria with microscopic hematuria. Evaluation of these children should proceed as described in Table 16–2.

   IMMUNOGLOBULIN A (IgA) NEPHROPATHY (Berger Nephropathy).   This is a common cause of gross hematuria. It usually occurs after the preschool years and is character-

TABLE 16–1. CAUSES OF HEMATURIA IN CHILDREN*

Glomerular Diseases
 Recurrent gross hematuria syndrome
  IgA nephropathy
  Idiopathic (benign familial) hematuria
  Alport syndrome
 Acute poststreptococcal glomerulonephritis
 Membranous glomerulopathy
 Systemic lupus erythematosus
 Membranoproliferative glomerulonephritis
 Nephritis of chronic infection
 Rapidly progressive glomerulonephritis
 Goodpasture disease
 Anaphylactoid purpura
 Hemolytic–uremic syndrome

Infection
 Bacterial
 Tuberculosis
 Viral

Hematologic
 Coagulopathies
 Thrombocytopenia
 Sickle cell disease
 Renal vein thrombosis

Stones and Hypercalciuria

Anatomic Abnormalities
 Congenital anomalies
 Trauma
 Polycystic kidneys
 Vascular abnormalities
 Tumors

Exercise

Drugs

---

* From Behrman RE (ed): Nelson Textbook of Pediatrics, 14th ed. Philadelphia, WB Saunders Company, 1992, p 1326.

ized by recurrent gross hematuria with persistent microscopic hematuria, generally without proteinuria, edema, hypertension, or renal insufficiency.

Laboratory examination reveals normal renal function, normal complement levels, and normal serum albumin. There is mesangial hypercellularity and deposition of IgA in the mesangium.

The outcome generally is favorable in most patients; however, about 20% progress to end-stage renal disease. Proteinuria, edema, hypertension, and azotemia are poor prognostic signs.

No *treatment* is established, although immunotherapy may benefit some patients. The disease may recur in a transplanted kidney.

IDIOPATHIC HEMATURIA. Recurrent episodes of gross hematuria occur without evidence of renal disease. Benign and familial disease occurs. Normal glomeruli are

TABLE 16–2. EVALUATION OF THE CHILD WITH HEMATURIA*

Step 1: Studies Performed in All Patients
Complete blood count
Urine culture
Serum creatinine level
24-hr urine collection for:
   creatinine
   protein
   calcium
Serum C3 level
Ultrasound or intravenous pyelography

Step 2: Studies Performed in Selected Patients
DNase B titer or streptozyme test if hematuria is of less than 6 mo
   duration
Skin or throat cultures when appropriate
Antinuclear antibody titer
Urine erythrocyte morphology
Coagulation studies/platelet count when suggested by history
Sickle cell screen in all black patients
Voiding cystourethrography with infection, or when a lower tract
   lesion is suspected

Step 3: Invasive Procedure
Renal biopsy indicated for:
   Persistent high-grade microscopic hematuria
   Microscopic hematuria plus any of the following:
   a. diminished renal function
   b. proteinuria exceeding 150 mg/24 hr (0.15 g/24 hr)
   c. hypertension
   Second episode of gross hematuria
Cystoscopy indicated for:
   pink to red hematuria, dysuria, and sterile urine culture

* From Behrman RE (ed): Nelson Textbook of Pediatrics, 14th ed. Philadelphia, WB Saunders Company, 1992, p 1328.

noted without evidence of immune complex disease; occasionally thinning of the glomerular basement membrane is seen.

No treatment is indicated, but close follow-up is required. The prognosis is excellent.

ALPORT SYNDROME. This occurs in children of all ages, although generally it is seen from the 2nd decade onward. It is associated with sensorineural deafness in 30–40% of patients and ocular manifestations in 15% of patients. Males are more severely affected than females. The mode of inheritance is variable; X-linked dominant is most common, although autosomal dominant with variable expression is seen.

Glomeruli may be normal or manifest minimal mesangial proliferation; capillary wall thickening may occur, leading to glomerular sclerosis. Glomerular basement membrane thickening with splitting and lamellation is a characteristic feature.

No ameliorative *treatment* is available. Genetic counseling and supportive care are indicated. Dialysis and transplantation in the 2nd or 3rd decade of life may be required.

Acute Poststreptococcal Glomerulonephritis

This is the second most common cause of gross hematuria in children. It is rare before age 3 yr and develops 1–2 wk following a streptococcal infection. The disease follows throat or skin infection by "nephritogenic" group A β-hemolytic streptococci. Staphylococcus, *Streptococcus pneumoniae*, gram-negative bacteria, viruses, fungus, and rickettsial diseases also may cause glomerulonephritis.

CLINICAL MANIFESTATIONS. These may range from mild asymptomatic microscopic or gross hematuria to acute renal failure, hypertension, edema, oliguria, and frank nephrotic syndrome. Resolution by 1 mo is the rule, although urinary abnormalities may persist for more than 1 yr.

PATHOLOGY. This is characterized by diffuse mesangial enlargement with crescents in the epithelial side of the glomerulus. Lumpy-bumpy deposits of immunoglobulin and complement are deposited on the epithelial side of the glomerulus.

DIAGNOSIS. *Laboratory studies of urine* show red blood cells, red blood cell casts, and often proteinuria. Evidence of recent streptococcal infection includes a positive antideoxyribonuclease B (anti-DNase) antibody or streptozyme test. Antistreptolysin O titers rise later and may be negative in skin infections. Serum complement C3 level is low transiently and returns to normal in about 6 wk.

Renal *biopsy* rarely is indicated, but should be considered when there is acute renal failure, nephrotic syndrome, or persistent hypocomplementemia.

TREATMENT. Early treatment of the streptococcal infection does not eliminate the risk of glomerulonephritis, in contrast to rheumatic fever. Supportive treatment consists of the management of complications of oliguria, acute renal failure, hypertension, edema, congestive heart failure, and electrolyte imbalances such as hyperkalemia, hypocalcemia, and acidosis. Complete recovery occurs in 95% of patients. Those with severe renal involvement may develop chronic renal failure. Recurrences are rare.

Membranous Glomerulopathy
(Glomerulonephritis)

This is a very rare cause of hematuria in children, although it is the most common cause of nephrotic syndrome in adults. In children, it presents in the teens as a nephrotic syndrome associated with microscopic, and sometimes gross, hematuria; there is no associated hypertension or depression of C3. It may be associated with systemic lupus erythematosus, syphilis, gold and penicillamine therapy, and hepatitis B. Treatment of the primary disease results in resolution of the glomerulonephritis.

Renal biopsy is indicated when a child who is more than 8 yr old presents with a nephrotic syndrome with hematuria or hematuria and proteinuria.

Pathologic diagnosis reveals diffuse thickening of the basement membrane resulting from immunocomplex deposition (IgG and C3) on the epithelial side. Spontaneous resolution usually occurs, although there may be persistent proteinuria.

Treatment is nonspecific. Nephrotic syndrome is treated in the usual manner; immunosuppressive therapy may retard its progression.

Systemic Lupus Erythematosus

Renal manifestations of systemic lupus erythematosus (SLE) are the most common presentation in childhood. Patients may present with asymptomatic microscopic hematuria or gross hematuria, with or without proteinuria, renal insufficiency, frank nephrotic syndrome, or acute renal failure.

The WHO classification is based on morphologic features of the renal biopsy:

Class I—no histologic abnormalities

Class II-A (mesangial)—light microscopy is normal but there are mesangial deposits of immunoglobulin and complement in some glomeruli

Class II-B (mesangial)—focal segmental glomerulosclerosis is seen along with mesangial deposits

Class III (focal proliferative)—mesangial deposits occur in all glomeruli, with focal and segmental mesangial changes and crescent formation

Class IV (diffuse proliferative)—this is the most common and severe form; there is thickening of the basement membrane creating "wire loop" lesions, necrosis, crescent formation, and scarring

Class V (membranous)—this is the least common form and resembles idiopathic membranous glomerulopathy

The *clinical manifestations* of renal disorders usually present in adolescent girls who have evidence of systemic disease and may include hematuria, proteinuria, reduced renal function, nephrotic syndrome, or acute renal failure.

Diagnosis is confirmed by demonstrating that circulating antinuclear antibodies react with double-stranded DNA. Complement levels (C3 and C4) are low. Biopsy is indicated because clinical manifestations do not correlate with the severity of renal involvement.

Immunosuppressive therapy is the mainstay of treatment, with the goal of clinical and serologic remission. Prednisone and azathioprine commonly are used.

Membranoproliferative (Mesangiocapillary) Glomerulonephritis

This is the most common cause of chronic glomerulonephritis. It usually presents in the 2nd decade of life with a mild nephrotic syndrome, microscopic or gross hematuria, and proteinuria. Renal function is normal. Hypertension is common. Persistent hypocomplementemia also is seen.

There are three types:

Type I—most common; involves mesangial proliferation with immune complex and mesangial matrix deposition between the endothelial cells

Type II—characterized by an irregular ribbon-like thinning of the basement membrane

Type III—findings similar to type I but with disruption of the basement membrane

The disease should be suspected when there is a late-onset nephrotic syndrome with hematuria and low serum complement levels, without preceding streptococcal disease. Renal biopsy is diagnostic.

No *treatment* is available. Long-term alternate-day prednisone and platelet inhibitors have been shown to stabilize the course of the disease. Types I and II recur in transplanted kidney. Outcome is generally poor. Type II has the worst prognosis, with eventual progression to end-stage renal disease.

Glomerulonephritis of Chronic Infection

Infection caused by *Streptococcus viridans*, *Staphylococcus epidermidis*, syphilis, hepatitis B, candidiasis, and malaria may cause immune complex disease–mediated glomerulonephritis. The *clinical manifestations* are those of acute glomerulonephritis or nephrotic syndrome.

Treatment consists of appropriate antibiotic therapy and elimination of the source of chronic microbial antigen. The condition rarely progresses to chronic renal failure.

Rapidly Progressive (Crescentic) Glomerulonephritis

This is a fulminant form of glomerulonephritis. The primary cause may be acute poststreptococcal disease, lupus, anaphylactoid purpura, or idiopathic glomerulonephritis.

Acute renal failure is the common presentation, following a nephritic or a nephrotic picture. There is a high incidence of progression to end-stage renal disease.

Crescents are seen inside of the Bowman capsule in addition to the pathologic changes of the primary disease. Laboratory evaluation includes streptozyme, antinuclear antibody, C3 and C4, and anti-DNase B titers. Kidney biopsy is confirmatory.

Outcome is poor except in poststreptococcal glomerulitis. Steroids and azathioprine have been useful in lupus and anaphylactic purpura. Immunosuppressive agents, anticoagulants, and plasmapheresis have helped a few patients.

Goodpasture Disease

This is a rare childhood disorder consisting of pulmonary hemorrhage and glomerulonephritis. It is due to antibodies against lung and glomerular basement membrane.

Clinically, it should be distinguished from Goodpasture syndrome, which may present similarly in association with several systemic disorders such as SLE and anaphylactoid purpura. Hemoptysis usually precedes hematuria, proteinuria, and progressive renal failure.

Goodpasture disease is similar to rapidly progressive glomerulonephritis, with IgG deposition in the basement membrane seen on biopsy. However, other diseases are excluded by the presence of serum anti–glomerular basement membrane antibody with normal complement levels.

Prognosis is poor, with progression to end-stage renal disease. Mortality is due to pulmonary hemorrhage. Immunosuppression and plasmapheresis may be helpful.

Anaphylactoid (Henoch–Schönlein) Purpura Glomerulonephritis

This is the most common form of vasculitis in children. The *etiology* is unknown, but most likely it is immune mediated.

Clinical manifestations include characteristic rash (urticarial or purpuric on buttocks and lower extremities), abdominal pain, and arthritis or arthralgias. Renal manifestations (usually gross or microscopic hematuria and/or proteinuria) occur in 50% of the cases. Nephrotic syndrome and acute renal failure also occur.

Pathologically, there is infiltration of leukocytes in the perivascular region with mesangial cell proliferation. Occasionally, crescents are seen.

Diagnosis is based solely on the clinical presentation, with normal platelet counts and C3 level and absence of serum antinuclear antibodies. Renal biopsy is indicated with severe renal involvement.

Prognosis is good, and usually there is spontaneous resolution. Presence of nephrotic syndrome, renal insufficiency, and a rapidly progressing glomerulonephritis on biopsy carries a poor outcome, with progression to end-stage renal disease.

Hemolytic–Uremic Syndrome

This is the most common cause of acute renal failure in young children. There usually is multiorgan system involvement. The *etiology* is unknown. *Escherichia coli* 0157:H7, *Shigella*, *Salmonella*, coxsackievirus, and some viral infections have been implicated. Endothelial cell injury leads to damage to the circulating cells, causing the characteristic microangiopathic changes and thrombocytopenia.

Clinical manifestations are most common under age 4 yr. The prodrome consists of gastroenteritis (often with bloody diarrhea) or upper respiratory tract infection, which is followed by sudden onset of severe pallor, irritability, weakness, lethargy, and oliguria. There may be dehydration, edema, petechiae and hepatosplenomegaly. Hypertension is common, and varying degrees of renal failure may occur.

Laboratory findings include microangiopathic hemolytic anemia, hematuria, thrombocytopenia, proteinuria, and findings of acute renal failure. *Differential diagnosis* includes hemolytic anemias, disseminated intravascular coagulation, SLE, malignant hypertension, and bilateral renal vein thrombosis.

Complete recovery is expected in milder cases. The mortality in the acute phase is about 10%. Complications include anemia, acidosis, hyperkalemia, congestive heart failure, hypertension, uremia, seizures, and coma. Recurrence are rare, but long term follow-up is indicated.

Treatment is supportive, including management of fluids and electrolytes; dialysis may be indicated. Use of plasmapheresis and fresh frozen plasma may be beneficial.

INFECTIONS CAUSING HEMATURIA
(*NELSON TEXTBOOK*, SEC. 18.14)

Lower urinary tract infections resulting from bacteria, microbacteria, or viruses can cause gross or microscopic hematuria. Patients usually have symptoms such as urgency, dysuria, or urethral discomfort. Trauma is also an important cause of hematuria that must be ruled out in such cases. Resolution of the hematuria generally is spontaneous. However, antibiotic treatment may be necessary.

HEMATOLOGIC DISEASES CAUSING HEMATURIA
(*NELSON TEXTBOOK*, SEC. 18.15)

Sickle Cell Nephropathy

Hematuria may occur in sickle cell anemia or trait. Spontaneous resolution of hematuria usually occurs. The cause of hematuria includes sickling of red cells in the medulla because of low oxygen tension, which also may cause papillary necrosis and interstitial fibrosis. Other symptoms include poor urine-concentrating ability, renal tubular acidosis, and, rarely, nephrotic syndrome.

Renal Vein Thrombosis

In the neonate, this occurs in association with dehydration, asphyxia, shock, and sepsis; it also occurs in infants of diabetic mothers. In older patients, it is seen in nephrotic syndrome, congestive heart failure, and following intravenous administration of hyperosmolar contrast agents.

Clinical manifestations include the sudden onset of gross hematuria, the appearance of unilateral flank pain, and identification of an enlarged kidney(s). Acute renal failure occurs when both renal veins are involved.

Renal ultrasound shows bilateral enlarged kidneys. There may be diminished blood flow detected on radionuclide scan. Doppler studies may confirm the presence of no or decreased blood flow. *Differential diagnosis* includes hemolytic uremic syndrome and other causes of hematuria with renal enlargement (i.e., hydronephrosis, cystic kidney disease, and Wilms tumor).

Supportive therapy is indicated. Spontaneous recovery of the kidney is seen. Bilateral disease is associated with chronic renal insufficiency, and thrombectomy or use of thrombolytic agents may be considered.

ANATOMIC ABNORMALITIES ASSOCIATED WITH HEMATURIA
(*NELSON TEXTBOOK*, SECS. 18.16–18.19)

Congenital Anomalies

Sudden onset of painless, gross hematuria or microscopic hematuria, especially following trauma to the flank, is associated with ureteropelvic junction obstruction of the urinary tract or cystic kidneys.

Trauma

Blunt or penetrating trauma to the abdomen can injure the kidney. Gross hematuria, abdominal rigidity, and flank pain may occur.

Infantile Polycystic Kidney Disease

This autosomal recessive disorder may be associated with significant liver disease. Bilateral flank masses typically are detected at birth. Gross hematuria and significant hypertension may be present. Oligohydramnios may be diagnosed in utero and may produce Potter syndrome (pulmonary hypoplasia, limb abnormalities, and characteristic facial features). Renal function may be impaired at birth. Nephrogenic diabetes insipidus with renal insufficiency also may be seen.

Pathologically, cysts are noted in the cortex and medulla, representing dilation of the collecting ducts. Renal failure is due to fibrosis of the interstitium and tubular atrophy. Associated liver abnormalities include cirrhosis, portal hypertension, and cholestasis. Infantile polycystic kidney disease and congenital hepatic fibrosis may be considered similar diseases with different manifestations.

The kidneys are enlarged bilaterally; increased echogenecity of both kidneys and the liver may be noted. Intravenous pyelography (IVP) demonstrates opacification of the collecting ducts and the presence of "radial streaks," which are diagnostic.

Treatment consists of supportive care, including management of hypertension and chronic renal insufficiency. Transplant is indicated for end-stage renal disease. Portal hypertension and cirrhosis are common complications.

Adult Polycystic Kidney Disease

This autosomal dominant disorder is rare in childhood. *Clinical manifestations* include microscopic or gross hematuria, hypertension, and flank pain or flank masses in the 4th or 5th decade of life. Children may present with unilateral or bilateral flank masses. End-stage renal disease occurs in the 6th or 7th decade.

Kidney Stones and Hypercalcinuria

These are uncommon cause of hematuria in pediatric patients. Usually they are associated with abdominal or flank pain as well as hematuria.

MISCELLANEOUS CAUSES OF HEMATURIA
(*NELSON TEXTBOOK*, SECS. 18.20–18.22)

Vascular malformations and *hemangiomas* are rare causes of hematuria. Frank blood clots may be noted. Angiography confirms the diagnosis.

Wilms tumor is the most common tumor causing hematuria, although a flank mass is usually the presenting sign. Other tumors, mostly extrarenal, such as leukemias, lymphomas, and neuroblastomas, also may cause hematuria.

Microscopic or gross hematuria may follow *vigorous exercise*. This rare condition usually is benign and resolves in 48 hr.

EVALUATION OF HEMATURIA
(*NELSON TEXTBOOK*, SEC. 18.23)

History and Physical Examination

Recent throat or skin infection or gastrointestinal symptoms should suggest acute poststreptococcal glomerulonephritis or hemolytic–uremic syndrome. An abdominal mass should suggest hydronephrosis, cystic disease, renal vein thrombosis, or tumor. Recent episodes of gross hematuria should suggest IgA nephropathy, idiopathic hematuria, Alport syndrome, or hypercalciuria. Rash and joint pains should suggest SLE or anaphylactoid purpura.

A family history of trauma, bleeding diathesis, drug usage, and hypertension should be queried.

Laboratory Evaluation (see Table 16–2)

PROTEINURIA
(*NELSON TEXTBOOK*, SECS. 18.25–18.27)

The presence of more than 150 mg of protein in the urine per day is considered abnormal. It can be detected by a urine dipstick test. However, high pH, highly concentrated urine, contamination with blood, and various drugs may give false-positive readings.

NONPATHOLOGIC PROTEINURIA

Postural (Orthostatic) Proteinuria

This is a benign condition. Generally, it is asymptomatic and is discovered on routine urinalysis. Proteinuria is less than 1 g/24 hr. The urine is free of protein or has a minimal amount on rising, but increases 10-fold or more in the upright position.

Diagnosis is established by detection of protein in the upright position and no protein in the supine position.

No *treatment* is necessary, but these children need close follow-up.

Febrile Proteinuria and Exercise Proteinuria

Fevers greater than 101°F and strenuous exercise are associated with low-grade proteinuria. They resolve spontaneously—in the case of exercise, after 48 hr, and for fever, after the temperature returns to normal.

PATHOLOGIC PROTEINURIA

Tubular Proteinuria

This is a rare cause of persistent low-grade proteinuria. It is associated with defects of the proximal tubules seen in a variety of acquired and inherited diseases (Table 16–3). Patients are asymptomatic, and usually signs of proximal tubular dysfunction, such as glycosurias, phosphaturia, aminoaciduria, and bicarbonate wasting, are associated.

Diagnosis of the underlying disease usually is made before proteinuria is detected. Electrophoresis of urine shows the absence of albumin and the presence of low-molecular-weight proteins.

TABLE 16–3. CLASSIFICATION OF PROTEINURIA*

Nonpathologic Proteinuria
  Postural (orthostatic)
  Febrile
  Exercise

Pathologic Proteinuria
  Tubular
    Hereditary
      Cystinosis
      Wilson disease
      Lowe syndrome
      Proximal renal tubular acidosis
      Galactosemia
    Acquired
      Analgesic abuse
      Vitamin D intoxication
      Hypokalemia
      Antibiotics
      Interstitial nephritis
      Acute tubular necrosis
      Sarcoidosis
      Cystic diseases
      Homograft rejection
      Penicillamine
      Heavy metal poisoning (mercury, gold, lead, bismuth, cadmium, chromium, copper)
  Glomerular
    Persistent asymptomatic
    Nephrotic syndrome
      Idiopathic nephrotic syndrome
        Minimal change
        Mesangial proliferation
        Focal sclerosis
    Glomerulonephritis
    Tumors
    Drugs
    Congenital

* From Behrman RE (ed): Nelson Textbook of Pediatrics, 14th ed. Philadelphia, WB Saunders Company, 1992, p 1340.

Glomerular Proteinuria

PERSISTENT ASYMPTOMATIC PROTEINURIA.
This is defined as the presence for more than 3 mo of asymptomatic proteinuria without hematuria. The incidence in
school-age children is about 6%. It is not associated with
edema and the proteinuria is less than 2 g/day.

Evaluation should include urine culture, 24-hr urine protein excretion, serum albumin, and renal ultrasound. Renal
biopsy is indicated when proteinuria is severe (more than 1
g/24 hr) or in the presence of hematuria, hypertension, or
abnormal renal function.

Differential diagnosis includes postural proteinuria, membranous glomerulonephritis, membranoproliferative glomerulonephritis, pyelonephritis, hereditary nephritis, developmental anomalies, and benign proteinuria.

No *treatment* indicated. Annual urinalysis and re-evaluation of blood pressure and renal function are recommended.

NEPHROTIC SYNDROME (Nephrosis)

This disorder is characterized by proteinuria, hypoproteinemia, edema, and hyperlipidemia. Idiopathic nephrotic syndrome occurs in about 90% of children who have nephrosis.
In the remainder, nephrosis is due to some form of glomerulonephritis, usually membranous glomerulonephritis and
membranoproliferative glomerulonephritis.

Increased permeability of the glomerular capillary as a result of loss of a negative charge on the basement membrane
is one of the mechanisms of protein loss in the nephrotic
syndrome. Proteinuria is composed mainly of albumin and
can exceed more than 2 g/24 hr. A decrease in plasma oncotic
pressure resulting from hypoalbuminemia may cause transudation of fluid into the interstitial space. Decreased intravascular volume stimulates the renin–angiotensin system
and the release of antidiuretic hormone, which increases absorption of sodium and fluids, worsening the edema. Capillary permeability also may be increased. Hyperlipidemia
(most serum lipids and lipoproteins) is due to excess production by the liver and decreased lipid catabolism from decreased levels of lipoprotein lipase.

Idiopathic Nephrotic Syndrome

The *etiology* is unknown. This disease is immune mediated
through several factors, including abnormal function of the
T lymphocyte. This nonhereditary disorder is more common
in boys than girls and occurs between 2 and 6 yr of age.
Usually, it follows viral infections.

CLINICAL MANIFESTATIONS. Usually the child presents with pitting edema. There may be ascites, pleural effusion, and weight gain. Anorexia, abdominal pain, and diarrhea are common; hypertension is uncommon. The typical
course is that of several relapses and remission per year in
patients responsive to steroid treatment.

LABORATORY FINDINGS. Urinalysis reveals a high
level of proteinuria and, rarely, hematuria. Serum albumin

is low. Hypercholesterolemia and triglyceridemia are seen. Complement levels are normal, serum calcium may be low, and there may be hypovolemia with decreased creatinine clearance.

PATHOLOGY. The most common lesion, *minimal change disease,* is found in 85% of patients. Glomeruli appear normal or may show a slight increase in mesangial cells and matrix. Immunofluorescent studies are normal. Retraction of the epithelial cell foot processes is seen on electron microscopy.

Increased mesangial cells and matrix are seen in the *mesangial proliferative* form (5% of patients). In the *focal sclerotic* group (10%) most of the glomeruli are normal or show proliferation. Others show areas of scarring in a segment of the glomerulus.

COMPLICATIONS. These include bacterial infections during a relapse, increased incidence of thrombosis, and peritonitis caused by *S. pneumoniae* (common). Reasons for this immunocompromise status include decreased immunoglobulin levels, edema fluid acting as a culture medium, protein deficiency, decreased bactericidal activity of leukocytes, and loss of complement factors that aid in opsonization.

TREATMENT. *Immunosuppressive* (steroids or alkylating agents) *therapy* is the mainstay of treatment. These agents prolong the duration of remission, but leukopenia is a common side effect. Prednisone dose is 60 mg/m^2/24 hr (max. 60 mg). Cyclophosphamide dose is 3 mg/kg/ 24 hr, given daily for 8 wk. Indications for cyclophosphamide treatment are:

steroid dependency or resistance
steroid toxicity—cushingoid facies, hypertension, growth failure

Treatment of relapses is the same as above. Supportive treatment is important.

Prognosis is excellent for the large majority of children with steroid-responsive nephrosis. Spontaneous resolution usually occurs in the 2nd decade of life, without residual renal dysfunction.

Congenital Nephrotic Syndrome

This is a rare cause of nephrotic syndrome in the first 6 mo of life. Congenital infections (syphilis, toxoplasmosis, and cytomegalovirus) and Wilms tumor may cause nephrotic syndrome.

An autosomal recessive form is common in populations of Scandinavian descent: enlarged placenta, prematurity, respiratory distress, proteinuria, and massive edema may be present at birth. There is dilation of the proximal convoluted tubules, mesangial proliferation, and sclerosis. Antenatal diagnosis is made by measuring α-fetoprotein levels.

Kidney transplantation is the only definitive *treatment.* Steroid and alkylating agents are of no benefit. Renal failure usually occurs by 5 yr of age.

Other Causes

Other causes of nephrotic syndrome include lymphomas, carcinomas, and drugs.

TUBULAR DISORDERS
(*NELSON TEXTBOOK*, SECS. 18.28–18.31)

Tubular function includes modification of ultrafiltrate, maintenance of the electrolyte balance, acidification, and concentration or dilution of the urine.

RENAL TUBULAR ACIDOSIS

In renal tubular acidosis (RTA) there is impaired capacity of the tubules to acidify the urine. This results in hyperchloremic normal anion gap metabolic acidosis (see Table 16–4 for basic types).

Proximal RTA

The primary defect is the reduced ability of the proximal tubule to reabsorb bicarbonate, presumably as a result of deficient carbonic anhydrase production. It is a more severe form of acidosis than distal RTA. Electrolyte abnormalities include hyperchloremia and hypokalemic acidosis. The urine can be acidified to as low as pH 5.5. Proximal RTA can be primary or due to other diseases (Table 16–4). Treatment includes large doses of sodium bicarbonate.

Distal Tubular RTA

A deficiency of hydrogen ion secretion in the distal tubule and collecting duct is the primary mechanism causing the disorder. Usually the acid–base and electrolyte consequences are similar but less severe than in proximal RTA. There is a high incidence of nephrocalcinosis. Urine pH cannot be reduced below 5.8. This disorder may be primary or secondary (Table 16–4).

Mineralocorticoid Deficiency

Inadequate production or decreased responsiveness of the distal tubule to mineralocorticoid hormone is the mechanism causing the disorder. Electrolyte abnormalities include hyperkalemia and hyperchloremic acidosis. The urine may be acidic to less than pH 5.5.

Clinical Features

Growth failure occurs in the 1st yr of life. Distal RTA is associated with hypercalciuria, nephrolithiasis, nephrocalcinosis, and renal paranchymal destruction. Some patients present with gastrointestinal symptoms.

Diagnosis

A normal anion gap is noted, and other causes of systemic acidosis (diarrhea, diabetes, renal failure, etc.) should be excluded. Hyperchloremia, hypokalemia, and low serum bicarbonate level are the features of proximal and distal RTA, whereas in mineralocorticoid deficiency there is acidosis with hyperkalemia. In proximal RTA the urine pH may be as low as 5.5 in the presence of systemic bicarbonate of 16 mEq/L or less. In distal RTA the urine pH is greater than 5.8 at a similar bicarbonate level.

TABLE 16–4. CLASSIFICATION OF RENAL TUBULAR ACIDOSIS*

Proximal	Distal	Mineralocorticoid Deficiency†
Isolated	Isolated	Adrenal disorders ($\downarrow$A, $\uparrow$R)
Sporadic	Sporadic	Addison disease
Hereditary	Hereditary	Congenital hyperplasia
Fanconi syndrome	Secondary	Primary hypoaldosteronism
Primary	Interstitial nephritis	Hyporeninemic
Secondary	Obstructive	hypoaldosteronism ($\downarrow$A, $\downarrow$R)
Inherited	Pyelonephritis	Obstruction
Cystinosis	Transplant rejection	Pyelonephritis
Lowe syndrome	Sickle cell nephropathy	Interstitial nephritis
Galactosemia	Lupus nephritis	Diabetes mellitus
Hereditary fructose	Ehlers–Danlos syndrome	Nephrosclerosis
intolerance	Nephrocalcinosis	Pseudohypoaldosteronism
Tyrosinemia	Hepatic cirrhosis	($\uparrow$A, $\uparrow$R)
Wilson disease	Elliptocytosis	
Medullary cystic disease	Medullary sponge kidney	
Acquired	Toxins	
Heavy metals	Amphotericin B	
Outdated tetracycline	Lithium	
Proteinuria	Toluene	
Interstitial nephritis		
Hyperparathyroidism		
Vitamin D–deficiency		
rickets		

* From Behrman RE (ed): Nelson Textbook of Pediatrics, 14th ed. Philadelphia, WB Saunders Company, 1992, p 1345.
† A = aldosterone; R = renin.

Other tests include fractional excretion bicarbonate and the ammonium chloride loading test to differentiate between distal and proximal RTA.

Treatment

Bicarbonate replacement is the mainstay of therapy. Acidosis and electrolyte abnormalities should be corrected.

Prognosis

Generally, the prognosis is excellent. Proximal RTA is transient and less severe than distal RTA, which is life long. Obstructive uropathy can cause a variety of RTA that is transient and resolves after the obstruction is corrected. Renal failure is a rare complication of distal RTA.

NEPHROGENIC DIABETES INSIPIDUS

This disorder is caused by failure of the kidney to respond to antidiuretic hormone despite elevated levels of this hormone.

Etiology

Primary nephrogenic disease is a rare, usually X-linked recessive inherited disorder. There is complete tubular unresponsiveness to antidiuretic hormone. *Secondary* diabetes insipidus is due to decreased response of the tubules to antidiuretic hormone (hypokalemia, hypercalcemia, lithium) or loss of medullary concentration gradient (postobstructive uropathy, vesicoureteral reflux, interstitial nephritis, nephrocalcinosis, and osmotic diuresis).

Clinical Manifestations

Males are more severely affected than females; they present with polyuria and polydipsia and may develop hypernatremic dehydration. Females may become symptomatic later in life.

Diagnosis

This is suspected by history (esp. a positive family history in males), hypernatremia, dilute urine, and a serum osmolality exceeding 295 mOsm/kg H_2O, with a lower urine osmolality. A water deprivation test may be needed to confirm the diagnosis in some patients.

Complications

Mental retardation occurs as a result of repeated episodes of hypernatremia. There is also growth failure. Dilation of the collecting system, including hydronephrosis, may occur.

Treatment

Adequate fluid and calories and a decrease in the solute load is the goal of therapy. A low-sodium diet with caloric intake optimal for growth, frequent liquid intake, and use of diuretics are indicated.

Prognosis

Generally this is good, although it is a life-long disease.

BARTTER SYNDROME

This rare autosomal recessive disorder manifests as hypokalemia and normal blood pressure in the presence of high renin and aldosterone levels. Electrolyte abnormalities include hypokalemia, hypochloremia, metabolic alkalosis, hypercalciuria, and hypomagnesemia. Urine abnormalities include high potassium chloride and sodium. Hyperplasia of the juxtaglomerular apparatus is seen.

Clinical Manifestations

Growth failure, muscle weakness, polyuria, polydipsia, and dehydration resulting from water and salt wasting may be seen. Older patients may develop signs of hypokalemia. Diuretic, licorice, and laxative abuse can mimic this syndrome.

Treatment

Potassium supplements are indicated in the form of potassium chloride to maintain serum potassium above 3.5 mEq/L. Use of triamterene may be indicated in difficult cases. The prostaglandin inhibitor indomethacin also has been used.

INTERSTITIAL NEPHRITIS
(NELSON TEXTBOOK, SEC. 18.32)

The space between the glomeruli in the areas surrounding the tubules is inflamed in this disorder.

ACUTE INTERSTITIAL NEPHRITIS

Drug reactions are the most common cause of acute interstitial nephritis. There is infiltration of lymphocytes, plasma cells, and neutrophils in the interstitium; tubular edema; degeneration; and necrosis. Immunologic mechanisms and other factors may play a role.

Fever, maculopapular rash, eosinophilia, and eosinophiluria develop about 1 wk following the drug administration. Urine output, renal function, and tubular function usually are normal. Renal failure may develop.

Renal biopsy is the most definitive way to confirm the *diagnosis*.

Treatment is supportive. Spontaneous resolution usually occurs after withdrawal of the offending drug. High-dose corticosteroids are reserved for patients with acute renal failure and severe injury.

CHRONIC INTERSTITIAL NEPHRITIS

Chronic interstitial nephritis usually is seen in patients with underlying structural abnormalities of the kidney or lower urinary tract, such as cystic disease, reflux, or obstruction.

Inflammatory infiltrates consist of lymphocytes and plasma cells as well as fibrosis and areas of glomerular sclerosis.

The *clinical manifestations* are those of chronic renal failure or the underlying disorder.

Treatment is mainly supportive. There is a high likelihood of progression to end-stage renal disease.

TOXIC NEPHROPATHIES (see *NELSON TEXTBOOK*, Table 18.7)

KIDNEY PROBLEMS IN THE NEWBORN INFANT
(*NELSON TEXTBOOK*, SEC. 18.34)

RENAL DYSGENESIS

Renal Aplasia or Agenesis

Bilateral agenesis is incompatible with life. Unilateral agenesis may be associated with other congenital abnormalities or may be asymptomatic; the eventual risk of development of hypertension or proteinuria requires close follow-up.

Hypoplasia

Unilateral or bilateral hypoplasia is not an inherited disorder. Unilateral hypoplastic kidney is the most common cause of hypertension in the 1st decade of life. Bilateral hypoplasia usually manifests as chronic renal failure and progresses to end-stage renal disease in the 1st decade of life.

Dysplasia

Cysts, abnormal ducts, undifferentiated mesenchyme, and nonrenal elements such as cartilage are seen in these kidneys. The lesion can be unilateral or bilateral and present as a flank mass, infection, or uncontrollable hypertension. It may result from intrauterine obstruction of the urinary tract; this usually is bilateral and leads to end-stage renal disease.

Bilateral *multicystic dysplasia* is associated with Potter facies at birth and may progress to chronic renal failure.

CORTICAL NECROSIS

This lesion has a multifactorial *etiology*, involves the cortex and medulla, and is bilateral. It may be secondary to dehydration, asphyxia, shock, disseminated intravascular coagulation, renal vein thrombosis, and hemolytic–uremic syndrome in older patients.

There is acute renal failure with hematuria and oliguria. Endothelial cell injury resulting from toxins and other factors initiates thrombosis and cortical necrosis. Decreased blood flow to the cortex leads to cortical infarction.

Diagnosis is made by demonstrating enlarged, nonobstructed kidneys on renal ultrasound and diminished or no renal blood flow on renal isotope scan.

Treatment is supportive. Prompt correction of dehydration, shock, and asphyxia and treatment of sepsis are essential.

RENAL FAILURE
(*NELSON TEXTBOOK*, SECS. 18.35–18.37)

ACUTE RENAL FAILURE

The inability of the kidneys to maintain normal homeostasis with or without diminished urine output is defined as renal failure. Acute renal failure is divided into three categories based on the etiology:

Prerenal: decreased renal perfusion resulting from several factors, such as diminished intravascular volume, poor cardiac function causing decreased renal perfusion, and hypoxia

Renal: renal parenchymal involvement may be due to a variety of disorders, including acute glomerulonephritis, hemolytic–uremic syndrome, hereditary nephritis, developmental abnormalities, and tubular disorders such as acute tubular necrosis

Postrenal: obstruction to the outflow of urine also may lead to the development of acute renal failure; the obstruction must be bilateral

Clinical Manifestations

In addition to the signs and symptoms of the precipitating causes of the acute renal failure, there may be oliguria, pallor (anemia), edema, hypertension, vomiting, and lethargy. Complications include congestive heart failure (volume overload), pulmonary edema, arrhythmias, gastrointestinal bleeding, seizures, and coma.

Differential Diagnosis

Anemia may suggest renal vein thrombosis, hemolytic–uremic syndrome, or SLE. Electrolyte abnormalities include hyponatremia, hypocalcemia, hyperkalemia, acidosis, and elevated levels of BUN, serum creatinine, phosphate, and uric acid. Serum complement C3 level may be depressed in acute poststreptococcal nephritis, SLE, membranoproliferative glomerulonephritis, and chronic antigenemia. Antibasement antibodies may be detected in Goodpasture disease. Chest roentgenography may reveal cardiomegaly and pulmonary congestion resulting from fluid overload. Roentgenographic studies, including renal ultrasound and radioisotope scan, should be done to detect the presence of obstruction of the urinary tract.

Treatment

This includes fluid restriction for oliguria, the use of dopamine to improve renal perfusion, and careful monitoring of serum electrolytes to avoid hyperkalemia and other abnormalities.

Complications and Their Management

HYPERKALEMIA. This is potentially a life-threatening situation. Avoidance of fluids, medications, and foods containing potassium is important in the presence of acute renal failure. Electrocardiography should be used to detect early signs of hyperkalemia. Procedures to deplete potassium stores include the use of Kayexalate, either orally or per rectum, at the dose of 1 g/kg mixed with sorbitol (for potassium levels of 5.5 mEq/L or more). Agents employed to decrease the serum potassium when serum potassium rises above 7 mEq/L (but that do not affect the total body potassium) are:

calcium gluconate (10%) at 0.5 mL/kg given IV
sodium bicarbonate (7.5%) at 3 mEq/kg given IV
glucose solution (50%) 1 mL/kg given with regular insulin,
   1 U/5 g of glucose given IV over 1 hr (glucose and insulin
   facilitate movement of potassium from the extracellular
   compartment to the intracellular compartment)

Dialysis is the only definitive mode of therapy for removal of potassium.

ACIDOSIS. Moderate acidosis is common in acute renal failure and rarely requires treatment. Severe acidosis requires treatment with sodium bicarbonate. It is important to avoid tetany produced by hypocalcemia resulting from rapid correction of acidosis. Only partial correction of acidosis is recommended, using the following formula:

mEq/L $NaHCO_3$ required =

$\quad$ 0.3 × weight (kg) × (12 − serum bicarbonate, mEq/L)

HYPOCALCEMIA. Avoidance of high phosphorus and calcium is important in preventing precipitation of calcium phosphorus when their product is above 70 mg/dL. Use of phosphate binders, like calcium carbonate, mixed with food will help decrease the absorption of phosphorus and increase its excretion.

HYPONATREMIA. This usually follows hypotonic fluid administration and, therefore, fluid restriction is indicated. Hyponatremia below 120 mEq/L may require correction with hypertonic (3%) sodium chloride:

mEq/L of sodium required =

$\quad$ 0.6 × weight (kg) × (125 − serum sodium, mEq/L)

Dialysis to correct hyponatremia may be required when there is congestive heart failure and hypertension from extreme volume overload, which may be a contraindication to hypertonic saline administration.

HYPERTENSION. High blood pressure is seen in acute renal failure as a result of volume overload, primary renal disorder, or both. Prompt treatment of hypertension is important. Diazoxide or nifedipine is used for acute episodes of hypertension; continuous intravenous drip of sodium nitroprusside or labetalol is reserved for severe hypertension. For chronic hypertension, propranolol or apresoline are effective.

SEIZURES. This is an uncommon complication that may be secondary to primary renal disease, uremia, hyponatremia, hypocalcemia, and hypertension. Diazepam is the drug of choice for controlling the seizures. Other common agents such as phenobarbital, paraldehyde, or phenytoin have a limited value.

ANEMIA. This is mild and does not require treatment.

Dialysis

Indications for dialysis in acute renal failure may include acidosis, electrolyte imbalance (especially hyperkalemia), central nervous system disturbances, hypertension, fluid overload, congestive heart failure, and a uremic state causing complications such as hemorrhage, central nervous system abnormalities, or pericarditis.

Prognosis

This depends on the primary renal problem. It usually is good in hemolytic–uremic syndrome, acute tubular necrosis, acute interstitial nephritis, or uric acid nephropathy. Rapidly progressive glomerulonephritis, bilateral renal vein thrombosis, or bilateral cortical necrosis usually is not associated with complete recovery.

CHRONIC RENAL FAILURE

The etiology of chronic renal failure correlates closely with the age of the patient. In patients with chronic renal failure before 5 yr of age the cause usually is an anatomic defect. After 5 yr the cause usually is acquired glomerular disease.

Clinical Manifestations

Once a critical level of renal functional deterioration occurs, whatever the cause, progression to end-stage renal failure is inevitable. When the glomerular filtration rate falls below 20%, the signs and symptoms of a uremic state develop.

Anatomic abnormalities may result in the insidious onset of renal failure characterized by fatigue, headache, lethargy, anorexia, vomiting, polydipsia, polyuria, and growth failure. Patients may present with hypertension and anemia. Glomerular or hereditary diseases usually result in clinical manifestations before the onset of renal insufficiency.

Treatment

This requires meticulous attention to various aspects of the disease.

DIET. Inadequate caloric intake once renal function falls below 50% is a major cause of growth failure in children. Protein restriction is important in severe uremia. Water-soluble vitamins are recommended to avoid deficiency states.

WATER AND ELECTROLYTE BALANCE. This usually is not a problem in chronic renal failure. Hyperkalemia can be a potentially life-threatening situation and can be a treated with an oral potassium exchange resin.

ACIDOSIS. Development of acidosis is a late phenomenon and is easily treated with either Bicitra or sodium bicarbonate at approximately 2 mEq/kg/24 hr.

RENAL OSTEODYSTROPHY. Excretion of phosphorus occurs exclusively in the kidney. Secondary hyperparathyroidism occurs in response to hyperphosphatemia as a result of diminishing renal function. Parathyroid hormone causes an increase in the serum calcium level at the expense of the bones. Inadequate production of 1,25dihydroxy vitamin D worsens the renal osteodystrophy.

ANEMIA. This occurs mainly as a result of inadequate erythropoietin production. In addition, iron deficiency is seen. Recombinant human erythropoietin is given subcutaneously or intravenously if the child is on dialysis.

HYPERTENSION. Nifedipine or diazoxide is given for acute hypertension, and β-blockers, diuretics, salt restriction, and hydralazine may be indicated.

DRUG DOSAGES. Renal excretion is a major route of excretion for many drugs; their dosages must be modified in chronic renal failure.

END-STAGE RENAL DISEASE

When the renal function is unable to sustain a stable milieu or serum creatinine is at 10 mg/dL, dialysis or renal transplantation is considered. Continuous ambulatory peritoneal dialysis is the most common renal replacement therapy. Hemodialysis is another important method of replacing renal function. Renal transplantation has been very successful in children, even in those less than 1 yr of age. Living related donor kidney transplantation has the best outcome. The reason for better survival is the advent of antirejection drug therapy.

UROLOGIC DISORDERS OF INFANTS AND CHILDREN
(*NELSON TEXTBOOK*, SECS. 18.38–18.48)

CONGENITAL ANOMALIES OF THE KIDNEYS

Renal Agenesis

Bilateral renal agenesis is incompatible with life. The infant is stillborn, with the classic features of Potter syndrome (associated with oligohydramnios), which include pulmonary hypoplasia, limb abnormalities, low-set ears, flattened nose, epicanthic folds, receding chin, and widely separated eyes. Unilateral renal dysplasia may be asymptomatic and often is discovered during a work-up for other congenital abnormalities. There is compensatory hypertrophy of the normal kidney. These children are at risk for developing hypertension or proteinuria and need follow-up.

Anomalies of Shape or Position

Horseshoe kidney is a common anomaly of shape and position. It is associated with Turner syndrome, and there is an increased risk of development of Wilms tumor.

URINARY TRACT INFECTIONS

The incidence of urinary tract infections varies with the age and sex of patients. In the newborn period, there is a male preponderance and the patients usually are asymptomatic. In the school-age group, females predominate. *E. coli* is the most common organism, followed by *Klebsiella* and *Proteus*. Viruses also can cause urinary tract infections.

In the neonate, the urinary tract infection generally is blood borne, unlike an older patient, in whom ascending infection is the most common mode of infection. In addition, other risk factors include urinary stasis, vesicoureteral reflux, and bladder overdistention.

Clinical Manifestations

In the neonate these commonly include failure to thrive, jaundice, weight loss, fever, diarrhea, and vomiting. In older children, fever of unknown origin, incontinence with urgency, bed-wetting, dysuria, frequency, foul-smelling urine, and abnormal pain may occur. Hematuria, hypertension, and sepsis also are noted. There may be asymptomatic bacteriuria.

Diagnosis

A midstream urine sample, collected after cleaning the external genitalia, that grows 10^5/mL colonies is significant for the diagnosis of a urinary tract infection. Other methods of collection include catheterization and suprapubic puncture in younger patients. Urinalysis indicating leukocytes only suggests an infection.

Anatomic or functional underlying abnormalities must be identified. Renal ultrasound is indicated if there is failure to eradicate the infection. Renal scanning (DMSA) is used when pyelonephritis is suspected. A voiding cystourethrogram should be done about 3 wk after the infection is treated. Cystoscopies rarely are indicated.

Treatment

Acute cystitis should be treated promptly with a 7–10-day course of sulfisoxazole, 100–125 mg/kg/24 hr qid or nitrofurantoin at 5–7 mg/kg/24 hr tid or qid. Amoxicillin also may be used. If pyelonephritis is suspected, parenteral antibiotics, cefotaxime, or ampicillin with an aminoglycoside are used.

Prophylactic antibiotics (low-dose sulfamethoxazole–trimethoprim or nitrofurantoin) are indicated in the presence of vesicoureteral reflux or repeated urinary tract infections.

VESICOURETERAL REFLUX

Incompetence of the valvular mechanism at the vesicoureteral junction leads to antegrade movement of urine into the ureter and pelvis. Reflux nephropathy is an important cause of end-stage renal disease in children and young adults. Renal scarring resulting from reflux and/or infection is a common complication of reflux and leads to hypertension.

Primary reflux is due to congenital malformations such as abnormal insertion of the ureter into the bladder, duplicated collecting system, ureteral ectopia, or paraurethral diverticula. *Secondary* reflux is due to increases in intravesicular pressure (e.g., neurogenic bladder, bladder dysfunction or outlet obstruction); inflammatory processes (e.g., severe bacterial cystitis, foreign body calculi, chemical cystitis); or surgical procedures at the ureterovesical junction.

Clinical Manifestations

The degree of renal dysfunction is directly related to the degree of reflux, and the chance of spontaneous recovery with severe degrees of reflux is minimal. Reflux often is silent and is detected during a work-up of urinary tract infection, hypertension, renal insufficiency, failure to thrive, or voiding dysfunction.

Diagnosis

Baseline blood pressure measurements, creatinine clearance, and urodynamics (voiding cystourethrogram) are indicated to distinguish between primary and secondary causes of reflux. Renal ultrasound is indicated to evaluate renal size, and renal scanning is indicated to detect the presence of scars (IVP and tomography yield similar results). Cystoscopy is not recommended.

Treatment

Medical management is indicated for lesser grades of reflux, especially grades I and II, and secondary reflux resulting from duplications. Medication for urinary tract prophylaxis usually includes trimethoprim–sulfamethoxazole or nitrofurantoin.

Surgical treatment is indicated for severe grades of reflux, particularly grades IV and V; reflux associated with recurrent urinary tract infections despite prophylactic treatment; reflux in infants and young children; and reflux in the presence of diverticulum of the bladder.

OBSTRUCTION OF THE URINARY TRACT

Obstructions may occur at any level of the urinary tract, and in children may be congenital or caused by trauma, neoplasm, calculi, inflammatory processes, or surgical procedures. Congenital obstruction is the most frequent obstructive lesion in childhood. Chronic obstruction can lead to dilation of the ureters, hydronephrosis, renal hypoplasia, tubular dysfunction, and renal scarring. A patent urachus results from urethral obstruction in utero. Bilateral ureteral or urethral obstruction can lead to oligohydramnios and pulmonary hypoplasia.

Clinical Manifestations

Obstructive lesions may be asymptomatic (esp. if unilateral). They often present as an abdominal mass in the newborn. Ascites, patent urachus, or oligohydramnios should suggest the presence of urinary tract obstruction. Infection and sepsis resulting from contamination of the obstructed urinary system can occur in the neonatal period. In addition, failure to thrive, vomiting, diarrhea, polyuria or polydipsia, and voiding dysfunction in older children are nonspecific symptoms of an obstructed and infected urinary tract.

Diagnosis

Renal ultrasound usually detects hydronephrosis and hydroureter, can indicate renal size, and may suggest parenchyma and bladder abnormalities. Renal isotope DTPA scan, with or without furosemide, estimates renal function. IVP also provides the same information in older children. In addition, it is useful in detecting renal calculi, spinal abnormalities, and an abnormal intestinal gas pattern. A voiding cystourethrogram is helpful in detecting the presence of reflux.

Specific Types of Obstruction

URETEROPELVIC JUNCTION OBSTRUCTION. This is the most common cause of urinary obstruction in childhood. It presents as fetal hydronephrosis, an abdominal mass in the neonatal period, abdominal or flank pain, or febrile illness. Renal ultrasound, voiding cystourethrogram, renal isotope scan, and IVP in older children are indicated for the work-up.

When there are mild to moderate degrees of hydronephrosis by imaging, no surgical correction is indicated. However, if there is severe obstruction, diminished renal function, cortical thinning, or a palpable mass, prompt surgical correction is indicated.

MIDURETERAL OBSTRUCTION. This lesion may be congenital or acquired (tumor, postsurgical, fibrosis, inflammation, radiation). Surgical correction is indicated only if functional obstruction is demonstrated.

URETERAL ECTOPIA (Ectopic Ureteral Orifice). This usually is associated with a duplicated collecting system (particularly in females), with the ureter of the upper system always inserted caudal to the ureteral insertion of the lower collecting system. In males, ectopic ureters usually are single and associated with high-grade obstruction and urinary tract infections or epididymitis.

URETEROCELE. Congenital cystic dilation of the ureter occurs at the level of its insertion into the bladder. It protrudes into the bladder wall and has a small orifice. Simple ureteroceles are associated with nonduplicated collecting systems. More commonly, ureteroceles are associated with ureteral duplication. In this situation the ureter that has formed the ureterocele drains the upper pole of the kidney and is prone to obstruction, and the ureter that is inserted cephalad drains the lower pole and has a tendency to reflux.

Treatment of an ectopic ureterocele consists of excision of the upper collecting system, partial nephrectomy, and ureterectomy.

MEGAURETER. This may be secondary to obstruction or nonobstructed. The former requires surgical treatment.

PRUNE BELLY SYNDROME. This rare disease is characterized by deficient abdominal muscles, urinary tract anomalies, and undescended testes. Massive hydroureter, enlarged bladder, patent urachus, and vesicoureteral reflux are the common urinary tract abnormalities. Posterior urethral valves, urethral obstruction, and urethral stenosis or atresia are associated. Renal dysplasia may occur, and there may be varying degrees of renal dysfunction, including frank renal failure.

Surgical correction of obstruction is indicated. If no obstruction is noted, urinary prophylaxis to prevent urinary tract infections is indicated. Renal transplantation has shown good results.

BLADDER NECK OBSTRUCTION. This is due to extrinsic causes, including bladder neck calculi, tumors, and ureteroceles. Urinary retention, urinary tract infections, voiding difficulty, and bladder neck obstruction with overflow incontinence occur.

POSTERIOR URETHRAL VALVES. This is the most common type of urethral valvular obstruction. It occurs in males and causes urinary obstruction and/or vesicoureteral reflux. Depending on the degree of obstruction and the time of fetal onset, the renal changes can range from mild hydronephrosis to renal dysplasia. If the obstruction is severe and goes unrecognized during the neonatal period, infants present later in life with failure to thrive and sepsis.

On prenatal ultrasonography, if there is bilateral hydronephrosis, hydroureter, and a distended bladder, posterior urethral valves with obstruction can be diagnosed. Voiding cystourethrogram is the definitive diagnostic test.

Treatment is surgical, with supportive measures for drainage and to prevent sepsis.

URETHRAL STRICTURES. This is an acquired disease following urethral trauma or procedures in males. The stricture typically develops gradually, and manifestations include dysuria, hematuria, and bladder instability. IVP and voiding film suggest the diagnosis, and retrograde urethrography confirms it. Short strictures may respond to dilation or internal urethrotomy.

ANTERIOR URETHRAL STRICTURE. These are associated with congenital urethral diverticulum. They are rare and cause symptoms similar to those of posterior valves.

MALE URETHRAL MEATAL STENOSIS. This rare lesion usually results from inflammation associated with ammoniacal dermatitis of the glans following neonatal circumcision. Alternatively, a thin ventral membrane may partially cover the meatus. *Treatment* is meatoplasty.

BLADDER ANOMALIES

Bladder Exstrophy

Bladder exstrophy is an uncommon congenital condition occurring in the neonatal period. It is more common in males than females and occurs with varying degrees of severity. The bladder mucosa is exposed by protrusion of the bladder through a defect that ranges from a small cutaneous fistula in the abdominal wall to complete exstrophy of the cloaca, exposing the entire hindgut and bladder. There are associated bony abnormalities of the pelvis and deformities of the external genitalia.

Repair is started as early as possible after birth, with coverage of the defect to prevent desiccation of the mucosa and allow urinary drainage. Closure of the defect and reconstruction often is possible within 48 hr of life. The repair of other anomalies may be achieved at a later date. Chronic urinary tract infections, vesicoureteral reflux, and urinary incontinence are complications.

Neurogenic Bladder

This dysfunction of the bladder and its sphincters is due to aberrant or abnormal innervation. Congenital forms of neurogenic bladder may result from myelomeningocele, lipomeningocele, sacral agenesis, and other spinal abnormalities. Acquired diseases and traumatic lesions of the spinal cord are less frequent etiologies. Cerebral palsy, central nervous system tumors and their treatment, and pelvic operations also can produce a neurogenic bladder.

Two important consequences of neurogenic bladder are functional loss and urinary incontinence. Recurrent urinary tract infections and reflux are common.

Urodynamic studies and roentgenographic evaluation are helpful in predicting the outcome. In patients with an atonic bladder or denervated sphincters there is lower risk of developing vesicoureteral reflux. In patients with high intravesicular pressure or reflux, treatment may include antibiotics, intermittent catheterization, anticholinergics, and surgical correction (such as bladder augmentation), depending on the severity of the manifestations.

Voiding Dysfunction

NOCTURNAL ENURESIS. Involuntary voiding at an age when volitional control of micturition is expected is defined as enuresis. It is more common in males and tends to run in families. Involuntary voiding at nighttime with daytime continence is defined as nocturnal enuresis. It is believed to be due to delayed maturation of cortical areas in the brain that control micturition. It may be primary when the patient has never attained continence or secondary when incontinence has occurred after a period of continence.

Evaluation of nocturnal enuresis includes a detailed family history, including a history pertaining to the presence of polyuria and polydipsia. Physical examination includes examination of the spine and a search for anomalies that might account for the incontinence. Urinalysis is indicated to rule out the presence of urinary tract infections, defects in concentrating urine, and glucosuria.

Treatment in the absence of any structural abnormalities generally is supportive, with reassurance and avoidance of punitive measures.

UNSTABLE BLADDER. This common entity is not related to neurologic abnormalities or dysfunctions and is characterized by frequency, urgency, and episodes of diurnal urinary incontinence with or without bladder pain. An evaluation for significant urinary tract pathology is indicated.

ABNORMALITIES OF THE PENIS AND URETHRA

Hypospadias

This is the abnormal location of the urethral opening. It occurs with varying degrees of severity, including the mildest form, wherein the meatal opening is noted at the ventral aspect of the glans. With greater severity of hypospadias there is ventral curving of the penis, described as *chordee*. In a severe form the urinary meatus may open at the penoscrotal junction. Undescended testes and inguinal hernias are associated with hypospadias. In extreme cases there may be ambiguous genitalia.

Evaluation of the upper urinary tract is not indicated in all cases of hypospadias but is appropriate in the most severe forms.

Mild forms of hypospadias are repaired mainly for cosmetic reasons. The severe forms require extensive surgery in order to preserve sexual function, and this should be done as early as 1 yr of age.

Agenesis and Micropenis

Agenesis of the penis is rare and is associated with other anomalies. If the patient survives the neonatal period, rearing the patient as a female is recommended.

Micropenis develops as a result of testicular failure during fetal life. It can be associated with other syndromes such as Prader–Willi, Noonan, Kallman, and anencephaly.

Treatment is not satisfactory and includes rearing the patient as a female and a trial of hormonal stimulation. Normal sexual function is achieved in some patients.

Phimosis and Paraphimosis

Phimosis is the inability to retract the prepuce at an age when it normally should be retractable. There is a physiologic phimosis in infants until the age of 3 yr.

Treatment is circumcision. Excessive removal of the foreskin, sepsis, amputation of the glans, and development of ureterocutaneous fistula are some of the potential complications of this procedure.

DISORDERS OF THE SCROTUM AND ITS CONTENTS

Undescended Testes

Undescended testes are testes that fail to descend into the scrotum and remain anywhere in the path of descent. The most common site of ectopic testes is lateral to the external inguinal ring. Spontaneous descent does not occur after the 1st yr of life. Malignant changes (especially seminoma), infertility, hernias, torsion, and untoward psychological effects are complications noted if the condition is not treated.

Human chorionic gonadotrophins and luteinizing hormone–releasing hormone have been used, but orchiopexy is the treatment of choice and should be done before 2½ yr of age.

TABLE 16–5. LABORATORY TESTS SUGGESTED TO EVALUATE UROLITHIASIS*

Serum
  Calcium
  Phosphorus
  Uric acid
  Electrolytes and acid–base balance
  Creatinine
  Alkaline phosphatase
Urine
  Urinalysis
  Urine culture
  Urinary pH
  Calcium/creatinine ratio
  Spot test for cystinuria
  24-hr collection for:
    creatinine clearance
    calcium
    phosphorus
    oxalate
    uric acid
    dibasic amino acids (if cystine spot test is positive)

* From Behrman RE (ed): Nelson Textbook of Pediatrics, 14th ed. Philadelphia, WB Saunders Company, 1992, p 1381.

Other Disorders

Other scrotal conditions include *varicoceles*, which are rare before 10 yr of age; *hydroceles*, which are common in the 1st yr of life; and *epididymitis*, which is rare in the prepubertal age and is treated with oral antibiotics. *Torsion of the testes* requires prompt diagnosis and treatment if the gonad is to survive. It presents with acute pain and swelling. Surgery is indicated.

UROLITHIASIS

Urinary Tract Calculi

These may present with hematuria (gross or microscopic), abdominal pain, dysuria, or voiding abnormalities.

The laboratory evaluation of urolithiasis is detailed in Table 16–5. Plain abdominal roentgenograms, renal ultrasound, and voiding cystourethrogram also are indicated.

Treatment includes avoidance of dehydration. Alkalization of the urine can prevent some types of stones. Thiazides, allopurinol, sodium bicarbonate for the treatment of renal tubular acidosis, and *N*-acetylcysteine are indicated for specific disorders. The extracorporeal lithotripter has made surgery for renal lithiasis unnecessary in most children.

GYNECOLOGIC PROBLEMS OF CHILDHOOD
(*NELSON TEXTBOOK*, SECS. 18.49–18.54)

VULVOVAGINITIS

This is the most common gynecologic problem in childhood or adolescence.

Clinical Manifestations

There is a normal physiologic increase in the vaginal discharge 6–12 mo prior to the onset of menarche. A pathologic discharge is a common presenting complaint of vulvitis, vaginitis, or vulvovaginitis. Pruritus, urinary frequency, dysuria, or enuresis may be associated findings.

Nonspecific vulvovaginitis is associated with poor perineal hygiene and primarily coliform bacteria. It is characterized by a brown or green discharge with a fetid odor. Basic *treatment* is improved hygiene.

Specific vulvovaginitis commonly is due to *Gardnerella vaginalis, Candida,* or *Trichomonas.* Antimicrobial *treatment* depends on the organism.

Molluscum contagiosum is a common perineal skin infection by the pox virus group that causes an umbilical dome-shaped papule. *Treatment* usually involves curettage and silver nitrate.

Lichen sclerosus is a chronic atrophic skin disease of unknown etiology resulting in anogenital papules, vesicles, and bullae. *Treatment* is symptomatic.

Other lesions include lichen planus, seborrheic dermatitis, atopic dermatitis, vulvar psoriasis, enterobiasis, shigellosis, and vitiligo.

Labial adhesions, which commonly occur in children under 6 yr of age, often are associated with local inflammation. *Treatment* with topical estrogen cream usually is effective.

Clitoritis may be caused by the same local conditions as vulvovaginitis and by organisms that cause vulvovaginitis. It should be treated similarly.

Foreign bodies may cause inflammation and vaginal bleeding.

BREAST DISORDERS

Instruction in self-examination should be given at the first gynecologic evaluation in adolescence.

Congenital Anomalies include amastia (rare), supernumerary breasts and nipples (relatively common), and hypoplasia.

Neonatal breast abnormalities include hypertrophy, which may be associated with discharge; enlargement secondary to endogenous steroids in late gestation; and mastitis secondary to staphylococcal infection.

Mastodynia (pain) may be associated with ovulatory cycles.

Breast masses in childhood and adolescence may be due to virginal hypertrophy (macromastia), fibroadenomas, fibrocystic disease, rhabdomyosarcoma, neuroblastoma, non-Hodgkin lymphoma, mastitis, henangioma, fat neurosis, lymph nodes, cancer (rare), cystosarcoma phylloides, and other rare tumors.

Nipple discharge may consist of galactorrhea or blood and requires careful evaluation.

HIRSUTISM

Excessive androgen production before puberty may cause excessive hair growth (hirsutism) and should be distinguished from virilization, which involves additional physical changes (e.g., body habitus, voice change, acne, clitoromegally). Most often hirsutism in an adolescent is idiopathic and associated with normal circulating androgen levels. However, it may respond to hormonal efforts to decrease androgens. Other causes of hirsutism include androgen-producing tumors of adrenal or gonadal origin, HAIR-AN syndrome, hyperprolactinemia, polycystic ovarian syndrome (chronic anovulation, Stein–Leventhal syndrome), and congenital adrenal hyperplasia. *Treatments* must be appropriate to the disorder.

GYNECOLOGIC NEOPLASMS

Ovarian neoplasm is the most common form of gynecologic tumor in children, and the most common presentation is abdominal pain, a mass, or both. Excision followed by chemotherapy and radiotherapy often are required.

Ovarian follicular cysts also may occur from birth to puberty and usually disappear spontaneously. Torsion may require surgical intervention.

Cervical intraepithelial neoplasm occurs in sexually active teenagers.

Adenocarcinoma of the uterus is rare in children and adolescents.

Gartner duct cyst of the vagina is a relatively common disorder usually not requiring therapy. Excision may be indicated for dyspareunia.

PREMATURE OVARIAN FAILURE
(*NELSON TEXTBOOK*, SEC. 18.55)

This may occur in adolescent females as a result of gonadal dysgenesis, gonadotropin-resistant ovarian syndrome, ovarian tumors, and extirpation of the ovaries secondary to surgery, radiation, or chemotherapy. *Treatment* is hormone replacement.

DEVELOPMENTAL ANOMALIES
(*NELSON TEXTBOOK*, SEC. 18.56)

A large variety of uncommon uterine and vaginal anomalies of the müllerian duct, as well as hereditary disorders associated with such anomalies, may occur in childhood. Prominent among these anomalies are congenital absence of the vagina, incomplete fusion of the vagina, transverse vaginal septa, and unobstructed and obstructed lateral fusion of the vagina (e.g., hemivagina, hydrocolpos, hydrosalpinx, atresia of the uterine cervix, and didelphic, bicornuate and unicornuate uteri).

THE ENDOCRINE SYSTEM

DISORDERS OF THE HYPOTHALAMUS AND PITUITARY GLAND
(*NELSON TEXTBOOK*, SECS. 19.1–19.9)

ANTERIOR PITUITARY

The anterior pituitary gland originates from the Rathke pouch (oral endoderm). Persistent fetal rests of the Rathke pouch can develop into craniopharyngiomas. The anterior pituitary is under the control of hypothalamic secretions, each of which regulates specific pituitary cells.

Anterior Pituitary Hormones

Growth hormone (GH) is controlled by two hypothalamic hormones: growth hormone–releasing hormone (GHRH), which stimulates release of (GH); and somatostatin, which inhibits release of GH as well as insulin, glucagon, secretin, gastrin, and vasoactive intestinal peptide. GH circulates bound to protein and is mediated through synthesis of insulin-like growth factor-1 (IGF-1). Secretion of GH is rhythmic, with highest levels during sleep.

Prolactin has an unidentified releasing factor. Dopamine is the major prolactin-inhibiting factor. The major role of prolactin is initiation and maintenance of lactation.

Thyrotropin (*TSH*) has a structure similar to those of luteinizing hormone, follicle-stimulating hormone, and human chorionic gonadotropin. TSH increases iodine uptake, iodide clearance, iodotyrosine and iodothyronine formation, thyroglobulin proteolysis, and release of thyroxine (T_4) and triiodothyronine (T_3).

Corticotropin (*ACTH*) release has a diurnal rhythm with a peak at 8 A.M. Its secretion is regulated by corticotropin-releasing hormone (CRH). During pregnancy, levels rise dramatically, probably from placental sources.

Gonadotropic hormones include luteinizing hormone (LH) and follicle-stimulating hormone (FSH). FSH receptors are on ovarian granulosa cells (stimulates follicular development) and testicular Sertoli cells (gametogenesis). LH receptors are on theca cells (luteinization of ovary) and Leydig cells (function of the testis). LH and FSH are controlled by luteinizing hormone–releasing hormone (LHRH).

Posterior Lobe (Neurohypophysis)

This lobe is the source of arginine vasopressin, which has pressor and antidiuretic activities, and Oxytocin.

371

HYPOPITUITARISM

GH deficiency is the most common manifestation of hypopituitarism. In infancy it presents with hypoglycemia, microphallus, and a neonatal hepatitis syndrome.

Etiology

Etiologies include:

congenital defects—aplasia/hypoplasia are rare and associated with other central nervous system (CNS) defects (anencephaly, septo-optic dysplasia)

empty-sella syndrome—idiopathic, occurs after surgery or radiation therapy

hypogammaglobulinemia/GH deficiency association—an X-linked trait

destructive lesions—craniopharyngioma, CNS germinoma, tuberculosis, sarcoidosis, toxoplasmosis, aneurysms, histiocytosis, trauma including traction at delivery, cranial irradiation

idiopathic hypopituitarism—involves one or more hormone deficiencies

Clinical Manifestations

These include normal birth size but slow growth later, apnea, cyanosis, hypoglycemia, microphallus, characteristic facial features, fine hair, and normal intelligence.

Diagnosis

Laboratory evaluation includes provocative growth hormone testing, IGF-1, TSH, T$_4$, ACTH, cortisol, dehydroepiandrosterone sulfate (DHEAS), gonadotropins, and gonadal steroids. Roentgenograms show small sella, delayed bone age, and delayed closure of fontanels.

Differential diagnosis for abnormal growth includes inflammatory bowel disease, renal disease, Turner syndrome, IGF-1 deficiency, and:

constitutional growth delay—normal at birth then deceleration in growth, but with subsequent normal adult height; bone age is consistent with height but not with chronologic age; there is a family history of delay of puberty and growth

primary hypothyroidism—causes decreased levels of GH

emotional deprivation—psychosocial dwarfism; when removed from home situation, growth improves

Silver–Russell syndrome—short stature, frontal bossing, triangular facies, incurved 5th finger, and hemihypertrophy

Treatment

Classic GH deficiency: growth hormone therapy until closure of epiphyses

TSH deficiency: thyroid hormone

ACTH deficiency: hydrocortisone

Gonadotropin deficiency: gonadal steroids

DIABETES INSIPIDUS

This results from a lack of antidiuretic hormone. *Etiology* includes tumors of the suprasellar and chiasmatic regions (esp. craniopharyngiomas, germinomas, and optic gliomas), histiocytosis X, autosomal dominant heredity, and a possible autoimmune etiology.

Clinical manifestations include polyuria, polydipsia, hyperthermia, weight loss, vomiting, constipation, growth failure, and dehydration.

Laboratory findings include a urine specific gravity of 1.001–1.005, with osmolality of 50–200 mOsm/kg water. There is normal serum osmolality with adequate hydration. Skull roentgenograms may reveal calcifications, enlarged sella, and widened suture lines. *Differential diagnosis* is that of neurogenic versus nephrogenic diabetes insipidus; other renal disorders (i.e., familial nephronophthisis), which usually have elevated blood urea nitrogen (BUN)/creatinine, anemia, and isotonic urine; and psychogenic polydipsia, in which patients have concentrated urine when fluid deprived.

Treatment is desmopressin (dDAVP). The usual dose is 5–15 µg/24 hr in one or two doses intranasally. For children <2 yr old, the dose is 0.15–0.5 µg/kg/24 hr.

INAPPROPRIATE SECRETION OF ANTIDIURETIC HORMONE

Etiology includes CNS infections, head trauma, Guillain–Barré syndrome, pneumonia, tuberculosis, cystic fibrosis, infantile botulism, asphyxia, medications, and oat cell carcinoma of the lung.

Clinical manifestations include loss of appetite, nausea, irritability, and personality changes. Stupor and seizures occur with worsening hyponatremia.

Laboratory findings include hyponatremia, hypochloremia, normal serum bicarbonate, serum hypo-osmolarity, elevated urine osmolality compared to serum tonicity, and hypouricemia.

Treatment involves restriction of fluids and sodium replacement; in rare cases hypertonic saline and Lasix are indicated.

HYPERPITUITARISM

The most common pituitary tumors secrete corticotropin, prolactin, or GH.

Pituitary Gigantism and Acromegaly

Pituitary adenoma is the most common cause. GH-secreting adenomas are associated with McCune–Albright syndrome.

Clinical manifestations include height of 8 feet or taller in gigantism; acromegaly consists of a broad nose, large tongue, large distal body parts, coarse facial features, and thick fingers and toes.

Laboratory findings include elevated GH and IGF-1 levels, hyperprolactinemia, and possible impairment of secretion of other hormones. Roentgenograms show enlargement of the sella turcica and paranasal sinuses; there is normal bone age. *Differential diagnosis* includes hereditary tall stature, precocious puberty, Marfan syndrome, and cerebral gigantism (Sotos syndrome).

Treatment includes surgery, irradiation, and medications such as bromocriptine and octreotide (a long-acting somatostatin analogue).

Prolactinoma

This is the most common pituitary tumor in adults. Children present with headache, decreased growth rate and delayed puberty, primary or secondary amenorrhea, gynecomastia, galactorrhea, and advanced puberty. In children, most are macroadenomas with an enlarged sella and sometimes visual field defects.

Treatment is surgical resection and bromocriptine.

PUBERTY

Prepubertal children have suppression of the hypothalamus and pituitary by low levels of gonadal steroids. One to 2 yr prior to puberty, low levels of LH during sleep occur in a pulsatile manner. This increases in frequency and amplitude as clinical puberty approaches.

FSH and LH are secreted in a pulsatile fashion and together stimulate gonadal maturation. Females in midadolescence exhibit a positive feedback mechanism in which estrogen causes a rise in LH. Adrenarche occurs in response to elevation of adrenal cortical androgens (dehydroepiandrosterone [DHEA]).

In girls, onset of puberty occurs with breast bud development at 10–11 yr. Menarche is 2–2.5 yr after onset of puberty and is preceded by a growth spurt. Athletes may exhibit marked delay in puberty. *In boys,* onset of puberty occurs with growth of the testes, followed by pigmentation and thinning of the scrotum and growth of the penis. The peak height velocity is attained after puberty is advanced, at 14–16 yr of age.

DISORDERS OF PUBERTAL DEVELOPMENT

Puberty is consider precocious in girls <8 yr and in boys <9 yr of age.

Precocious Puberty without Other Pathologic Findings (Constitutional)

In girls the first sign is breast development, then pubic hair. In boys, enlargement of the penis and testes, pubic hair, acne, and erections occur. Height, weight, and bone maturation are advanced, leading to a final height that is less than full potential.

Laboratory findings include FSH/LH that is elevated for age, increased response to LHRH, elevated levels of testosterone (males) and estradiol (females), advanced bone age, and enlarged ovaries on ultrasound.

LHRH analogue suppresses pulsatile secretion of gonado-tropins. With treatment, breast development regresses or does not advance, growth returns to normal rates, and bone maturation decreases. Discontinuation of treatment results in puberty.

Precocious Puberty Resulting from Organic Brain Lesions

Forty percent of boys and 10% girls with true precocious puberty have a brain tumor. Meningitis, hydrocephalus, tuberous sclerosis, head trauma, tumors, neurofibromas, and hypothalamic hamartoma are other associated lesions. Other endocrinopathies and neurologic symptoms may accompany precocious puberty.

Syndrome of Precocious Puberty and Hypothyroidism

Prolonged and severe hypothyroidism may cause precocious puberty with growth retardation and delayed bone age. TSH and gonadotropins have similar structure, causing "overlap" syndrome and subsequent stimulation of ovaries and testes. Treatment of hypothyroidism causes regression of precocious puberty.

Gonadotropin-Secreting Tumors

Hepatic tumors produce human chorionic gonadotropin (hCG), causing precocious maturation of the testes. FSH is low but LH levels are high as a result of cross-reactivity with hCG on radioimmunoassay. Choriocarcinomas, teratocarcinomas, or teratomas located in the CNS, mediastinum, or gonads also may cause precocious puberty.

Precocious Pseudopuberty

McCune–Albright syndrome consists of precocious puberty, polyostotic fibrous dysplasia, and abnormal pigmentation. It is seen primarily in girls, with average age at onset of 3 yr. LH/FSH is suppressed, with normal to high estradiol levels. The syndrome is caused by functioning luteinized follicle cysts of the ovary (gonadotropin independent). Other endocrinopathies may be associated.

Familial Male Gonadotropin-Independent Precocious Puberty

This is autosomal dominant, occurring in males only. The testes are slightly enlarged, with Leydig cell maturation. Testosterone is markedly elevated, there are prepubertal levels of LH, and the condition does not respond to LHRH. Treatment consists of ketoconazole (inhibits C-17,20 lyase and testosterone synthesis), spironolactone (blocks androgen action), and testolactone (competitive inhibitor of aromatase).

INCOMPLETE (PARTIAL) PRECOCIOUS DEVELOPMENT

Premature thelarche is isolated breast development. Usually it occurs in the first 2 yr of life with no other evidence of estrogenization. The breasts may regress or persist—subsequent puberty and menarche are normal.

Premature adrenarche is isolated growth of sexual hair before 8 yr in girls or 9 yr in boys. No other evidence of maturation occurs but there may be slightly advanced bone and height age. It is much more frequent in girls, especially black girls. The cause is an early maturation event of adrenal androgen production not related to ACTH stimulation.

MEDICATIONAL PRECOCITY

Estrogens (over-the-counter cosmetics, hair creams, breast augmentation creams, and estrogens used in animal husbandry) and anabolic steroids may cause precocious puberty. This regresses with cessation of the exposure.

DISORDERS OF THE THYROID GLAND
(*NELSON TEXTBOOK*, SECS. 19.10–19.16)

Production of thyroid hormone occurs by iodination of tyrosine to form mono- or diiodotyrosine. Molecules of T_4 or T_3 are formed, then stored as thyroglobulin in the lumen of the follicle. These are then released by activation of proteases and peptidases. T_3 has metabolic potency 3–4 times that of T_4 and is responsible for most of the physiologic actions, although the T_4 level is 50 times greater than that of T_3.

Effects of thyroid hormone include increased oxygen consumption, stimulation of protein synthesis and growth, and effects on carbohydrate, lipid, and vitamin metabolism. Seventy percent of thyroid hormones are bound to thyroxine-binding globulin (TBG); however, TBG levels can be altered with certain disease states, which one must consider when interpreting T_4 and T_3 values. Thyrotropin-releasing hormone (TRH) from the hypothalamus stimulates release of TSH, which then stimulates the thyroid gland to synthesize and release thyroid hormone.

THYROID HORMONE STUDIES

Methods are available to measure T_4, free T_4, T_3, free T_3, reverse T_3, and thyroglobulin. The physician must take age into consideration when interpreting results.

At birth TSH increases up to 70 µU/mL, with subsequent rapid decline over 24 hr followed by a more gradual decline over 2 days to below 10 µU/mL. T_3 increases to approximately 300 ng/dL as a result of the TSH surge, with gradual decline during the 1st wk of life. TBG transports thyroid hormones in plasma and bind 75% of T_4 and 70% of T_3. TBG levels increase with pregnancy, during the neonatal period, and with estrogens, and also may be altered by several drugs.

TBG deficiency occurs as an X-linked dominant disorder. Affected patients have low T_4, normal free T_4 and TSH, and low TBG levels. *Elevated TBG* is an X-linked dominant disorder. T_4 is elevated, T_3 is variably elevated, TSH and free

T_4 are normal, and resin triioclothyronine uptake (RT3U) is decreased. Affected patients are euthyroid.

HYPOTHYROIDISM

Congenital Hypothyroidism

One in 4,000 infants are affected worldwide. *Etiology* includes:

- Thyroid dysgenesis

    causes 90% of congenital hypothyroidism

    one third of infants have aplasia, two thirds have thyroid remnants

    ectopic thyroid tissue may provide enough thyroid hormone for many years or may fail in early childhood (such children have a midline mass at the neck or base of the tongue)

- TSH-binding inhibitory antibody (TBIAb)

    maternal antibodies inhibit binding of TSH to its receptor.

- Thyrotropin deficiency

    associated with developmental defects of pituitary/hypothalamus

    usually due to TRH deficiency but there may be other pituitary deficiencies

- Thyrotropin hormone unresponsiveness

    caused by impairment of cyclic adenosine monophosphate activation

    seen in type Ia pseudohypoparathyroidism

- Defective synthesis of thyroxine

    may involve defects of iodide transport, organification, thyroglobulin synthesis, or deiodination

- Thyroid hormone unresponsiveness

    characterized by resistance to endogenous and exogenous T_3 and T_4

    goiter is present; T_4, free T_4, T_3, and free T_3 are elevated; and TSH is normal or moderately elevated

    most patients are clinically euthyroid

Other causes of hypothyroidism include fetal exposure to iodides or antithyroid drugs and neonatal exposure to iodine-containing antiseptics.

CLINICAL MANIFESTATIONS. In the *neonate*, there is heavier birth weight, prolonged jaundice (delayed maturation of glucuronide conjugation), feeding problems, lethargy, choking, respiratory difficulties (due to large tongue), hypothermia, cold and mottled skin, edema of genitals and extremities, bradycardia, heart murmurs and cardiomegaly, anemia, and wide fontanels. In the *child*, there is stunted growth, normal or large head size, wide fontanels, widespread eyes, depressed nasal bridge, thick tongue, delayed dentition, dry and scaly skin, myxedema, coarse brittle hair, retarded development, and hypotonia.

LABORATORY FINDINGS. Most newborn screens measure T_4; TSH should be tested if there is an abnormal T_4. Roentgenograms reveal delayed bone development (i.e., absent distal femoral epiphysis). Electrocardiographic (ECG) abnormalities include depressed P and T waves and QRS complexes. The electroencephalogram (EEG) shows low voltage.

PROGNOSIS. When diagnosed and treated within the first few weeks of life, there is normal growth and intelligence.

TREATMENT. L-Thyroxine is the drug of choice. Doses are: neonates, 10–15 μg/kg/24 hr; children, 4 μg/kg/24 hr; and adults, 2 μg/kg/24 hr. Side effects in older children may include pseudotumor cerebri during the first 4 mo of treatment.

Juvenile Hypothyroidism (Acquired Hypothyroidism)

The most common cause is lymphocytic thyroiditis. Other causes include defects in thyroid hormone synthesis, thyroid dysgenesis, thyroidectomy for cancer, thyrotoxicosis or removal of ectopic tissue, irradiation and ingestion of iodide-containing medications.

Clinical manifestations include growth deceleration, skin changes, constipation, cold intolerance, less energy, increased sleep, and delayed bone age. Some children present with headaches, visual problems, precocious puberty, or galactorrhea. These manifestations return to normal with treatment; with long-standing hypothyroidism adult height may be impaired.

THYROIDITIS

Lymphocytic Thyroiditis (Hashimoto Thyroiditis/Autoimmune Thyroiditis)

This is the most common cause of thyroid disease and hypothyroidism in children. The *etiology* in 90% of children is lymphocytic infiltration of the thyroid gland with thyroid antimicrosomal antibodies. Antithyroglobulin antibodies and blocking TSH antibodies also are seen.

CLINICAL MANIFESTATIONS. It is more frequent in girls and peaks during adolescence. The thyroid is diffusely enlarged, firm, and nontender and there is insidious onset of goiter. Most patients are clinically euthyroid. The goiter may disappear spontaneously.

Familial clusters are common, as is association with chromosomal aberrations, including Down and Turner syndromes and congenital rubella. It also is associated with other autoimmune diseases (i.e., diabetes mellitus, Addison disease).

LABORATORY FINDINGS. Thyroid function often is normal but there may be slightly elevated TSH. Positive antimicrosomal antibodies occur in the majority of cases; antithyroglobulin antibodies are positive in <50%.

TREATMENT. This includes replacement of thyroxine, if indicated. Prominent nodules should be biopsied to rule out thyroid cancer.

Other Causes of Thyroiditis

These include tuberculosis, sarcoidosis, mumps, cat-scratch disease, acute suppurative thyroiditis (may be related to thyroglossal duct remnant or pyriform sinus fistula), and subacute nonsuppurative thyroidits (probable viral etiology).

GOITER

This may result from increased TSH or an infiltrative, inflammatory, or neoplastic process.

Congenital goiter may be the result of maternal Graves disease, antithyroid drugs, or ingestion of iodides during pregnancy (asthma medications, amiodarone, propylthiouracil [PTU]), which readily cross the placenta and interfere with thyroid hormone synthesis. It usually is transient but can cause respiratory distress at birth. Other causes include a defect in the synthesis of thyroid hormone or iodine deficiency.

Endemic goiter occurs in areas of relative deficiency of iodine (i.e., developing countries). Clinical hypothyroidism is rare but T_4 levels may be low.

Endemic cretinism occurs in a neurologic type and a myxedematous type, and is related to iodine deficiency and endemic goiter.

Sporadic goiter is caused by lymphocytic thyroiditis, iodide goiter (prolonged use of an iodide-containing drug), lithium, and amiodarone.

Simple goiter occurs in an idiopathic, euthyroid state, usually in girls, and may progress to multinodular goiter.

Multinodular goiter is associated with McCune–Albright syndrome, but malignancy must be ruled out.

HYPERTHYROIDISM

Graves Disease

This presents as infiltration of the thyroid gland and retroorbital tissues with lymphocytes and plasma cells, as well as enlargement of the thymus, spleen, and lymph nodes. Thyroid-stimulating antibodies are produced that stimulate the thyroid gland. It is associated with Addison disease, insulin-dependent diabetes mellitus (IDDM), myasthenia gravis, and celiac disease.

CLINICAL MANIFESTATIONS. Peak incidence is in female adolescents. Emotional lability, tremor, increased appetite, weight loss, exophthalmos, eyelid lag, sweating, and tachycardia are common features. Thyroid "crisis" is an acute onset of hyperthermia, tachycardia, and restlessness.

LABORATORY FINDINGS. Elevated T_4, T_3, free T_4, and free T_3, suppressed TSH, and positive TSH receptor–stimulating antibodies are found.

TREATMENT. PTU and methimazole are used to inhibit iodine incorporation. PTU also inhibits conversion of T_4 to

T_3 and is the preferred drug during pregnancy. Response to medication occurs in 2–3 wk, with control at 1–3 mo. Surgery and radioactive iodine are used infrequently in children. β-Adrenergic blockers also are used for symptomatic patients.

Congenital Hyperthyroidism

This occurs a few days after birth to infants of mothers with Graves disease. Symptoms include prematurity, goiter, hyperactivity, exophthalmia, tachycardia, and hyperthermia. Treatment is with Lugol solution and PTU. Digitalis and propranolol sometimes are required.

CARCINOMA OF THE THYROID

This is rare in children, and usually is related to irradiation of the neck area. Hashimoto thyroiditis is associated with thyroid cancer. A painless nodule in the thyroid or neck is the usual first symptom. The survival rate is high in localized disease.

Solitary Thyroid Nodules

These are uncommon in children but 15% are malignant. Benign adenomas, lymphocytic thyroiditis, thyroglossal duct cyst, and ectopic thyroid tissue may present as a solitary nodule. *Diagnosis* is made with ultrasound and technetium scan.

Medullary Carcinoma

This arises from the parafollicular cells (C cells) and is responsible for 10% of thyroid cancer. The patient presents with goiter or thyroid nodule. When medullary carcinoma is diagnosed, the physician also should look for other tumors (esp. pheochromocytoma).

MULTIPLE ENDOCRINE NEOPLASIA (MEN) TYPE IIa. This is a carcinoma/hyperplasia of thyroid C cells with adrenal medullary hyperplasia or pheochromocytoma and parathyroid hyperplasia. A defect in the neural crest causes the syndrome.

MEN TYPE IIb (Mucosal Neuroma Syndrome). Multiple neuromas, medullary carcinoma, and pheochromocytoma occur along with a characteristic phenotype.

DISORDERS OF THE PARATHYROID GLANDS
(*NELSON TEXTBOOK*, SECS. 19.17–19.20)

Calcium homeostasis is regulated by parathyroid hormone (PTH), vitamin D, and calcitonin. Low serum calcium stimulates PTH secretion, which increases 1α-hydroxylase in the kidney, with subsequent increased production of 1,25-dihydroxycholecalciferol (1,25-[OH]$_2$D$_3$). Calbindin-D, a calcium-binding protein in the intestinal mucosa, is synthesized and causes absorption of calcium. PTH in conjunction with 1,25-dihydroxy vitamin D also increases calcium by increasing bone resorption. Calcitonin is secreted by parafollicular cells

(C cells) of the thyroid gland and acts by inhibiting bone resorption. It is independent of PTH and vitamin D.

HYPOPARATHYROIDISM

The *etiology* includes:

maternal hyperparathyroidism

functional immaturity of parathyroid gland (in neonates)

aplasia of the parathyroid glands, associated with defects of the 3rd and 4th pharyngeal pouches (DiGeorge syndrome)

familial congenital hypoparathyroidism, which presents as seizures at 2 wk to 6 mo, low calcium and PTH, and high PO_4

surgical condition associated with thyroidectomy

deposition of copper or iron

autoimmune disorder, frequently associated with Addison disease and chronic mucocutaneous candidiasis (polyglandular autoimmune disease, type I)

Clinical manifestations include muscle pain, cramps, numbness, tingling, and convulsions. The teeth are soft and erupt late, there is dry and scaly skin, and cataracts may occur.

Laboratory findings include low calcium (5–7 mg/dL), elevated phosphorus (7–12 mg/dL), normal or low alkaline phosphatase, low 1,25-dihydroxy vitamin D, normal magnesium, and low PTH. Roentgenograms show increased metaphyseal thickening. There is a prolonged Q-T interval on the ECG and EEG slowing. *Differential diagnosis* includes hypomagnesemia (possibly by impaired release of PTH and PTH resistance), inorganic phosphate poisoning, and acute lymphoblastic leukemia.

Treatment may include calcium gluconate and calcitriol (1,25-dihydroxy vitamin D) in addition to an adequate calcium dietary intake and low-phosphorus diet.

PSEUDOHYPOPARATHYROIDISM

This results from a defect in the hormone receptor–adenylate cyclase system, causing PTH resistance.

Type Ia, resulting from a defect of the guanine nucleotide–binding protein (G protein), is an autosomal dominant trait, and is associated with resistance to TSH, gonadotropins, and glucagon. *Clinical manifestations* include sexual immaturity, infertility, amenorrhea, skeletal abnormalities, cataracts, and mental retardation. *Laboratory findings* include high PTH, PO_4, and alkaline phosphatase and low calcium. In **Type Ib,** there are normal levels of G protein, a normal phenotype, and resistance to PTH but not to other hormones.

HYPERPARATHYROIDISM

This usually is secondary to other conditions (i.e., Vitamin D–deficient rickets, malabsorption states, chronic renal disease). Primary hyperparathyroidism is due to adenoma or idiopathic hyperplasia. MEN type I, with hyperplasia/adenoma of the pancreatic islets, anterior pituitary, and parathyroids, is a rare cause. Transient neonatal hyperparathyroidism associated with maternal hypoparathyroidism also occurs. *Other causes of hypercalcemia* include familial hypocalciuric hypercalcemia, granulomatous disease, malignancy, vitamin D intoxication, subcutaneous fat necrosis, hypophosphatasia, and parenteral nutrition.

Clinical manifestations include muscle weakness, constipation, polydipsia, polyuria, weight loss, fever, renal stone, skeletal abnormalities, and pancreatitis.

Laboratory findings include a high calcium level, low phosphorus and magnesium, high PTH, and normal calcitonin after prolonged hypercalcemia. Roentgenograms show resorption of subperiosteal bone.

Treatment includes surgical exploration and treatment of the underlying disease.

DISORDERS OF THE ADRENAL GLANDS
(*NELSON TEXTBOOK*, SECS. 19.21–19.28)

The adrenal gland is composed of the medullary and cortical systems. The mesoderm forms the adrenal cortex, gonads, and the liver, all of which are active in steroid metabolism. During fetal life the adrenals are comparatively large, with a "fetal cortex" that produces DHEA and DHEAS and then involutes after birth.

The *adrenal cortex* is composed of the zona fasciculata, which secretes cortisol and androgens under the control of ACTH, and the zona glomerulosa, which synthesizes aldosterone independently of ACTH. ACTH is regulated by CRH, with cortisol exerting negative feedback on ACTH. Aldosterone secretion is regulated by the renin–angiotensin system; in rare cases ACTH affects aldosterone. Changes in sodium and blood volume stimulate the juxtaglomerular apparatus to alter renin and aldosterone, which controls sodium and water reabsorption.

Androgens promote growth, secondary male sex characteristics, and female axillary and pubic hair. Glucocorticoids affect the metabolism of tissues, increase protein and glycogen content in the liver, and have effects on the immune and nervous systems.

The *adrenal medulla* secretes catecholamines: dopamine, norepinephrine, and epinephrine.

ADRENOCORTICAL INSUFFICIENCY

The *etiology* includes:

> *corticotropin deficiency*—caused by congenital hypoplasia/aplasia of pituitary, craniopharyngioma, other pituitary lesions, autoimmune hypophysitis, and CRH deficiency
> *congenital pituitary hypoplasia*—associated with secondary adrenal hypoplasia as well as other hormonal deficiencies

primary adrenal aplasia/hypoplasia—a defect in organogenesis; corticotropin is present and both cortisol and aldosterone are affected

X-linked inheritance—sometimes associated with glycerol kinase deficiency and/or Duchenne muscular dystrophy

familial glucocorticoid deficiency—consists of a deficiency of glucocorticoids, elevated ACTH, and normal aldosterone; presents with hypoglycemia, seizures, and pigmentation in first decade of life; autosomal recessive defect is in the responsiveness of the adrenals to ACTH

inborn defects of steroidogenesis—21-hydroxylase, 3β-hydroxysteroid dehydrogenase, and lipoid adrenal hyperplasia all have a deficiency in the synthesis of cortisol and aldosterone

isolated deficiency of aldosterone

pseudohypoaldosteronism—elevated aldosterone with target-organ unresponsiveness

Addison disease—may be due to destruction of the adrenal cortex by an autoimmune process, tuberculosis, and autoimmune polyendocrinopathy type I (chronic mucocutaneous candidiasis, hypoparathyroidism, Addison disease) and type II (Addison disease with autoimmune thyroid disease or IDDM); most patients have antiadrenal cytoplasmic antibodies

adrenoleukodystrophy—a disorder of very-long-chain fatty acid metabolism associated with neurologic deterioration

Hemorrhage in adrenal glands—may be due to difficult delivery, asphyxia, and Waterhouse–Friderichsen syndrome

Abrupt cessation of corticotropin or corticosteroids—may cause insufficiency

Drugs—rifampin, ketoconazole, phenytoin, phenobarbital

Clinical Manifestations

In neonates/young children, failure to thrive, vomiting, lethargy, anorexia, dehydration, and shock may occur. In older children there is a gradual onset of muscular weakness, anorexia, weight loss, low blood pressure, increased skin pigmentation (esp. in the genitals, umbilicus, axillae, nipples, and joints), and bluish brown buccal mucosa.

Laboratory Findings

Low sodium and chloride, elevated potassium and renin levels, hypoglycemia, and ECG changes consistent with potassium level may be noted. On the ACTH stimulation test (measurement of cortisol before and after administration of ACTH), if no increase in cortisol occurs after ACTH, there is most likely a primary adrenal disorder.

Treatment

For acute adrenal insufficiency, high-dose IV hydrocortisone (infants, 25 mg q6hr; older children, 75 mg q6hr) and desoxycorticosterone acetate (DOCA), a salt-retaining hormone (in a dose of 1–5 mg/24 hr IM) are given. After stabilization, treatment changes to oral cortisol and fluorohydrocortisone.

Stress steroid doses must be given for infection and operations. For non–salt losers, hydrocortisone alone is adequate.

ADRENOCORTICAL HYPERFUNCTION

Adrenogenital Syndrome

CONGENITAL ADRENAL HYPERPLASIA (CAH) (AUTOSOMAL RECESSIVE)

21-Hydroxylase Deficiency. Occurs in 95% of cases; the majority have a salt-losing, virilizing form. Female salt losers present with virilized genitalia, weight loss, dehydration, vomiting, and anorexia; male salt losers have normal genitalia but other manifestations are the same. Female non–salt losers have virilized genitalia with progressive masculinization (premature pubic and axillary hair, acne, lack of breast development and menarche). Male non–salt losers develop premature isosexual development with enlarged penis and scrotum, pubic hair, and acne but with relatively small testicles.

Laboratory findings include low sodium, high potassium, elevated 17-hydroxyprogesterone (17-OHP) and renin, and low aldosterone. In the late-onset variant of CAH, elevated 17-OHP is seen only after ACTH stimulation.

Treatment is with hydrocortisone and 9α-fluorocortisol; response can be monitored with serum 17-OHP, renin, androstenedione, and testosterone levels as well as growth, bone age, and pubertal development.

11β-Hydroxylase Deficiency. Hypertension is common, and there is virilization and non–salt losing.

3β-Hydroxysteroid Dehydrogenase Deficiency. In the classic form, there is salt wasting, boys are incompletely virilized and have hypospadius, and there is mild virilization in girls. In the incomplete form, the patient presents with hirsutism, menstrual disorder, and polycystic ovaries.

17α-Hydroxylase Deficiency. This results in hypertension, hypokalemia, and suppressed renin and aldosterone. Males are unvirilized and females present with failure of sexual development at puberty.

VIRILIZING ADRENOCORTICAL TUMORS. These cause masculinization in girls and precocious puberty in boys; they are associated with hypertension. They also may be associated with hemihypertrophy and Beckwith–Wiedemann syndrome. Carcinoma is 3 times more common than adenoma.

Cushing Syndrome

In infants, a functioning adrenocortical tumor is the most common (malignant) cause of Cushing syndrome in children over 7 yr, ACTH-dependent bilateral adrenal hyperplasia is most commonly found; it may be due to pituitary adenoma or ectopic production of ACTH.

Clinical manifestations in young children include moon facies, double chin, buffalo hump, obesity, masculinization, hypertrichosis on face and trunk, pubic hair, acne, clitoral enlargement, impaired growth, and hypertension. In older children, purplish striae, delayed puberty, weakness, headache, and emotional lability occur.

Laboratory findings include polycythemia, lymphopenia, eosinopenia, abnormal glucose tolerance, lack of diurnal rhythm, elevated urinary and serum cortisol, osteoporosis, variable bone maturation, and suppressed growth hormone. Magnetic resonance imaging screening for pituitary adenoma is indicated.

Treatment includes removal of adenoma/carcinoma. Total adrenalectomy can cause postoperative pituitary tumor expansion with elevated ACTH and an enlarged sella turcica (Nelson syndrome). Transphenoidal pituitary microsurgery/ pituitary external radiation and cyproheptadine (blocks ACTH release) are additional therapies.

Excess Mineralocorticoid Secretion

PRIMARY ALDOSTERONISM. This is characterized by hypertension, hypokalemia, and a suppressed renin–angiotensin system (i.e., adenoma). The *etiology* includes:

overproduction of desoxycorticosterone (11- and 17-hydroxylase deficiencies)
aldosterone-secreting adenoma
bilateral micronodular adrenocortical hyperplasia
glucocorticoid-suppressible hyperaldosteronism—aldosterone controlled by ACTH

Clinical manifestations include headache, dizziness, visual changes, hypokalemia, muscle weakness, fatigue, growth failure, polyuria, polydipsia, and hypertension. *Laboratory findings* include elevated pH, CO_2, and sodium; decreased chloride and magnesium; and elevated plasma/urine levels of aldosterone with low renin level.

SECONDARY HYPERALDOSTERONISM. High aldosterone and renin levels may be due to a low-salt diet, nephrotic syndrome, congestive heart failure, and cirrhosis of the liver. The etiology includes pseudohypoaldosteronism, which is caused by abnormal aldosterone receptors; and Bartter syndrome (defect in the ascending limb of the loop of Henle), which is characterized by hypokalemic alkalosis, hypochloremia, hyperaldosteronism, and elevated renin.

TREATMENT. This includes glucocorticoids if indicated, bilateral adrenalectomy, and treatment of the underlying disorder in cases of secondary hyperaldosteronism.

Feminizing Adrenal Tumors

These are associated with excess estrogen production, causing precocious puberty (in males it causes gynecomastia). Gonadotropin levels are suppressed even with GNRH stimulation.

EXCESSIVE SECRETION OF CATECHOLAMINES

Pheochromocytoma arises from chromaffin cells of the adrenal medulla and abdominal sympathetic chain and is associated with neurofibromatosis and MEN types IIa and IIb. *Clinical manifestations* include hypertension, attacks of headache, palpitations, pallor, vomiting, and sweating. *Laboratory findings* include elevated plasma/urinary catecholamines and metabolites (i.e., vanillylmandelic acid and metanephrine). Tumors usually are seen on CT scan. *Treatment* is surgical removal using preoperative α- and β-adrenergic blockade.

DISORDERS OF THE GONADS
(*NELSON TEXTBOOK*, SECS. 19.29–19.43)

FUNCTION OF THE TESTES

During the 1st trimester of pregnancy, placental hCG stimulates fetal Leydig cells to secrete testosterone. This is critical for normal virilization of the XY fetus. The fetal testosterone levels decrease to low continuous levels after masculinization occurs. Müllerian-inhibiting factor is secreted by Sertoli cells of the fetal testes and causes the embryologic precursors of the cervix, uterus, and fallopian tubes to involute during sexual differentiation.

In 95% of boys puberty occurs between 9½ and 13½ yr, with the growth spurt occurring later than in girls. Sperm productions begins in midpuberty at approximately 14 yr.

FUNCTION OF THE OVARIES

Estradiol-17β (E_2) and estrone (E_1) are produced by the ovary. Estrogens also arise from androgen conversion. The ovary, adrenal cortex, and testis synthesize progesterone. Estrogens inhibit LH/FSH secretion but also provoke the LH surge in midmenstrual cycle. E_2 level increases with rising FSH, pubertal development, and skeletal age. The average age at menarche is 12½ to 13 yr.

HYPOFUNCTION OF THE TESTES
(*NELSON TEXTBOOK*, SECS. 19.30–19.33)

Hypergonadotropic Hypogonadism in the Male
(Primary Hypogonadism)

The *etiology* includes:

congenital anorchia—normal external genitalia are present, and therefore some noxious event damaged the fetal testes after sexual differentiation (14th wk of fetal life); there is low testosterone with elevated LH and FSH; hCG does not evoke increase in testosterone

atrophy of the testes—surgical manipulation or torsion

acute orchitis—mumps occurring in pubertal or adult males

chemotherapy/radiation—dependent on dosage, duration, and agent used

germinal cell aplasia—normal sexual maturation and testosterone, but with azoospermia and infertility

chromosomal aberrations—Klinefelter or XX males

The condition often is not noted until adolescence, when secondary sex characteristics fail to develop. Facial, pubic, and axillary hair is scant, there is no acne, and the voice remains high pitched. There is fat accumulation and long extremities as a result of delayed epiphyseal closure (eunuchism). At birth males may have abnormally small testes and penis. *Diagnosis* is made by elevated LH and FSH levels and a low testosterone level with no rise following hCG.

NOONAN SYNDROME. There are normal karyotypes in boys and girls. The phenotype similar to that of Turner syndrome: short stature, neck webbing, pectus excavatum, cubitum valgum, congenital heart disease, and characteristic facies. There is moderate mental retardation in 25% of cases. Males frequently have cryptorchidism, small testes, and delayed puberty; in females premature ovarian failure can occur.

KLINEFELTER SYNDROME. The chromosome complement is 47,XXY but mosaic patterns also are common; it occurs in 1:1,000 newborn males. Maternal age predisposes to the syndrome.

The syndrome usually is not diagnosed in childhood. Patients exhibit behavioral/psychiatric disorders, mental retardation, and learning and school adjustment disorders, and they may engage in antisocial acts, and be very shy or aggressive. Patients are tall and slim, with long legs, and the testes and phallus are small for age. Delayed puberty, gynecomastia, azoospermia, and infertility are common. Patients have a higher incidence of pulmonary disease, varicose veins, breast cancer, and extragonadal germ cell neoplasms.

Laboratory findings include abnormal chromosomes and, prior to 10 yr, normal response to GnRH and hCG. There is normal testicular growth in early puberty but growth stops, gonadotropins elevate, and testosterone levels decrease in midpuberty. Azoospermia and infertility occur in adults.

Treatment is by testosterone replacement.

XX MALES. These individuals have a male phenotype, small testes, small phallus, and no ovarian or müllerian duct tissue. Hypergonadotropic hypogonadism occurs secondary to testicular failure. In this disorder the testicular-determining factor (TDF) is exchanged from the Y to the X chromosome during paternal meiosis, and XX males inherit one maternal X and one paternal X with the translocated male-determining gene.

XYY MALES. Hypogonadism is not present in these individuals. Adults are impulsive and antisocial but not aggressive, are tall, and have severe nodulocystic acne.

Hypogonadotropic Hypogonadism in the Male
(Secondary Hypogonadism)

There is a deficiency of FSH or LH with normal testes present. The *etiology* includes:

- Hypopituitarism
    may be due to organic lesions in or near the pituitary or may be hypothalamic, with deficiency of LHRH microphallus and growth hormone deficiency in the newborn male suggests hypopituitarism

- Isolated deficiency of gonadotropin

    there is LHRH deficiency, sometimes in association with anosmia (Kallman syndrome)

    cleft palate, hypotelorism, median facial clefts also are found in Kallman syndrome

- Congenital adrenal hypoplasia

Diagnosis includes gonadotropins and gonadal steroids in the prepubertal range, no nocturnal pulsatile secretion of LH, and a blunted LHRH stimulation test. A gonadotropin deficiency is likely if evidence of other hormone deficiencies are present. Constitutional delayed puberty must be differentiated from hypopituitarism.

Treatment is with testosterone and hCG.

Pseudoprecocity Resulting from Tumors of the Testes

Leydig cell tumors are rare, and usually are unilateral and benign. There is elevated testosterone, suppressed FSH/LH levels, and no response to LHRH. Puberty occurs at from 5 to 9 yr of age. *Treatment* is surgical removal of the affected testis.

Testicular adrenal rests occur in patients with congenital adrenal hyperplasia during adolescence with poor steroid suppression. *Treatment* is with adequate doses of corticosteroids.

Fragile X syndrome includes testicular enlargement, mental retardation, and normal hormonal and testicular studies.

GYNECOMASTIA. This is a common condition that is a sign of estrogen–androgen imbalance. It occurs in most male newborns; two thirds of boys develop it during midpuberty. FSH, LH, prolactin, testosterone, E_1, and E_2 are all within normal limits for the stage of puberty. Spontaneous regression usually occurs within a few mo. In young children, an exogenous source of estrogens must be ruled out, and when associated with galactorrhea, prolactinoma must be ruled out. Gynecomastia also occurs with liver cirrhosis, digitalis, bronchogenic carcinoma, nonsteroidal agents, heavy marijuana use, and ketoconazole.

HYPOFUNCTION OF THE OVARIES
(*NELSON TEXTBOOK*, SECS. 19.34–19.36)

Hypergonadotropic Hypogonadism in the Female

TURNER SYNDROME. Patients are females with a single X chromosome (45,X); 30% of Turner females have mosaics or partial deletion of one X chromosome. It occurs in 1:3,000 live-born females. The Turner karyotype is responsible for 5–10% of all spontaneous abortions. An *etiology* of ovarian hypofunction is related to acceleration of oocyte degeneration, with nearly all oocytes gone by 2 yr of age. The ovaries then appear as "streaks" consisting of connective tissue, with few germ cells.

Clinical manifestations include edema of the hands and feet, loose skinfolds at the nape of the neck, low birth weight, decreased length, neck webbing, low posterior hairline, small mandible, prominent ears, epicanthic folds, high-arched palate, broad chest, cubitum valgum, hyperconvex fingernails, short stature, shortened 4th metacarpal, Madelung deformity, and scoliosis. The growth rate in the first 3 yr is normal, then decelerates. There is failure of sexual maturation. Average height is 143 cm.

Cardiac defects, especially nonstenotic bicuspid aortic valves, and renal defects are common. Recurrent bilateral otitis media, sensorineural hearing deficits, and delayed development are common. Some girls may have breast development and menstruation, but this is uncommon. Intelligence is normal. The risk of lymphocytic thyroiditis, inflammatory bowel disease, and gastrointestinal telangiectasia is increased.

Laboratory findings include chromosomal deficit; abnormalities on ultrasound of the heart, kidneys, and ovaries; elevated FSH/LH and low estrogen; and antimicrosomal thyroid antibodies.

Treatment includes GH, with or without anabolic steroid, which may increase height up to 150 cm or more. Estrogen replacement with progesterone cycling is indicated. Pregnancy is possible with in vitro fertilization.

XX GONADAL DYSGENESIS (Pure Ovarian Dysgenesis).   These girls have a normal phenotype and genotype, normal external genitalia, and normal growth but fail to mature sexually. Gonadotropins are elevated, and pelvic ultrasound shows streak ovaries. *Treatment* is with estrogen replacement.

45X/46,XY GONADAL DYSGENESIS (Mixed Gonadal Dysgenesis).   The phenotype is very variable, ranging from Turner-like to a male phenotype with penile urethra. Many patients present with ambiguous genitalia. Short stature is a major finding. The fallopian tubes and uterus are present, but the gonads are intra-abdominal undifferentiated streaks or there may be an intra-abdominal testis and contralateral streak. Gonadal tumors occur in 25% of cases; therefore, the gonads should be removed.

XXX FEMALES.   This is the most frequent X chromosomal abnormality in females, occurring in 1:1,000. The phenotype, sexual development, and menarche are normal. Patients have speech delay, poor school performance, and immature behavior.

XXXX AND XXXXX FEMALES.   These individuals have mental retardation, congenital heart disease, and a typical phenotype. Sexual maturation often is incomplete.

NOONAN SYNDROME.   Girls with Noonan syndrome are similar to girls with Turners syndrome except that they have mental retardation, pulmonary valve defect or atrial septal defect, and normal sexual maturation.

OVARIAN DEFECTS.   These may be due to cytotoxic drugs, radiation, autoimmune ovarian failure (i.e., type 1 autoimmune polyendocrinopathy), galactosemia, and ataxia–telangiectasia.

Hypogonadotropic Hypogonadism in the Female
(Secondary Hypogonadism)

The *etiology* includes:

- Hypopituitarism

  due to a destructive lesion in or near the pituitary
  idiopathic hypopituitarism probably is due to a defect
  in the hypothalamus

- Isolated deficiency of gonadotropins

  some cases are associated with anosmia (i.e., Kallman
  syndrome)
  severe thalassemia may cause pituitary damage as a
  result of chronic iron overload

This condition is difficult to differentiate from physiologic
delay of puberty. In the presence of other hormone deficiencies it is easy to make the diagnosis. Measurements of FSH
and LH may be helpful.

Polycystic Ovaries (Stein–Leventhal Syndrome)

This is the most common cause of anovulatory infertility.
The *etiology* includes idiopathic, late-onset 21-hydroxylase
deficiency; partial 3β-hydroxysteroid dehydrogenase deficiency; Cushing syndrome; and 17-ketoreductase deficiency.
Patients have an increased ratio of LH to FSH and exaggerated response to LHRH. Abnormal LH secretion causes hyperplasia of theca cells, arrested follicular development, and
impaired E_2 production, which leads to hyperandrogenemia
and irregular cycles. Insulin-resistant hyperinsulinemia and
acanthosis nigricans are associated. *Clinical manifestations* include obesity, hirsutism, and secondary amenorrhea with
bilaterally enlarged ovaries. *Treatment* is with oral contraceptives, which suppress the ovaries. Testolactone also is used.

PSEUDOPRECOCITY OWING TO LESIONS OF THE OVARY
(*NELSON TEXTBOOK*, SECS. 19.37–19.39)

Estrogenic Lesions of the Ovary

These cause isosexual precocious sexual development.
JUVENILE GRANULOSA-CELL TUMOR. This is the
most common lesion; most occur before 10 yr and are unilateral. The breasts enlarge, external genitalia are estrogenized,
the uterus is enlarged, and there is a white vaginal discharge
and irregular or cyclic menstruation. Pubic hair usually is
absent. An abdominal mass usually is palpable by the time
sexual precocity is noted. E_2 is elevated; gonadotropins are
suppressed and do not respond to LHRH. Fewer than 5% of
tumors are malignant; therefore, the prognosis is excellent.

Sex-cord tumor with annular tubules is seen in
Peutz–Jeghers syndrome.

Chorionepithelioma arises from a pre-existing teratoma.
It is very malignant and produces a large amount of hCG.

FOLLICULAR CYST. Autonomously functioning cysts
occur in the absence of LH/FSH and can cause precocious

puberty. Ultrasound of the ovaries is used to diagnose follicular cysts. In some cases spontaneous resolution of the cyst occurs, with regression of pubertal signs.

Androgenic Lesions of the Ovary

These are a rare cause of virilization. Gonadoblastoma occurs in dysgenetic gonads, especially with Y chromosome, leading to accelerated growth, acne, clitoral enlargement, sexual hair, and elevated testosterone and androstenediones; LH/FSH are suppressed. Tumors should be surgically removed. Prophylactic removal of the gonads with Y chromosome may be indicated.

HERMAPHRODITISM
(*NELSON TEXTBOOK*, SECS. 19.40–19.43)

In hermaphroditism a discrepancy between the morphology of gonads and the external genitalia occurs. The short arm of the Y chromosome is critical for development of the male phenotype because TDF is located there. TDF induces the genital ridge to develop into a testis. The testis then produces müllerian-inhibiting factor (MIF), causing the müllerian ducts to regress. Testosterone then initiates virilization of the wolffian duct into the epididymis, vas deferens, and seminal vesicle.

During male meiosis the X and Y chromosomes segregate; there is a small region of sequences that X and Y share, and pairing occurs at that site. Therefore it is possible to have exchange at that site (the sex-determining region of the Y chromosome).

In the XX fetus the ovary develops at the 12th week only in the absence of testosterone and MIF.

Female Pseudohermaphroditism

This is an XX genotype with ovaries, uterus, and fallopian tubes, but the external genitalia are virilized. Most cases are due to excessive exposure to androgens:

> *congenital adrenal hyperplasia*—the most common cause
> *placental aromatase deficiency*—androgens are converted to estrogens by aromatase; in its absence virilization occurs
> *masculinizing maternal tumors*—benign adrenal adenoma or ovarian tumors; maternal virilization also is present
> *administration of androgenic drugs* to women during pregnancy (progestational drugs, testosterone)

Male Pseudohermaphroditism

This is an XY genotype but the external genitalia are incompletely virilized or completely female.

DEFECTS IN TESTICULAR DIFFERENTIATION.

XY Pure Gonadal Dysgenesis. These patients present with normal stature and female phenotype, including vagina, uterus, and fallopian tubes, but with hypergonadotropic primary amenorrhea resulting from deletion of the short arm of the Y chromosome, TDF gene mutation, inactive TDF, or TDF receptor defects. The gonads are undifferentiated streaks and do not suppress müllerian ducts.

XY Gonadal Agenesis Syndrome (Embryonic Testicular Regression Syndrome). In these patients the external genitals are slightly ambiguous; there is no uterus, gonadal tissue, or vagina. No sexual development occurs at pubertal age, and LH/FSH are elevated. Testicular tissue was active long enough for MIF to inhibit müllerian structures but not long enough for testosterone production to cause virilization.

DEFECTS IN TESTICULAR HORMONES.

- Leydig cell aplasia

    usually a female phenotype with testes, epidiymis, and vas present but with no uterus or fallopian tubes

    no pubertal changes occur but there is normal pubic hair

    testosterone is low and does not respond to hCG

    LH/FSH are elevated as a result of absent/deficient Leydig cells—may involve hCG or LH receptor defects

- 20,22-Desmolase deficiency

    high defect in steroid synthesis that leads to lipoid adrenal hyperplasia

    males have female phenotype but male genital ducts

- 3β-Hydroxysteroid dehydrogenase deficiency

    varying degrees of virilization

- Deficiency of 17-hydroxylase/17,20-lyase

- Deficiency of 17-ketosteroid reductase

    males have female phenotype or severe genital ambiguity

    müllerian ducts are absent but shallow vagina is present

    at puberty very high levels of DHEA and androstenedione occur and virilization occurs

    some patients initially raised as females adopt a male gender role after puberty and virilization occurs

- Uterine hernia syndrome

    persistence of müllerian duct derivatives in otherwise completely virilized males

    cryptorchidism is common

    defect usually is found at surgery for hernia or cryptorchidism

    testicular function is normal, but there may be an isolated deficiency of MIF or an MIF receptor defect

    treatment consists of removal of müllerian structures.

DEFECTS IN ANDROGEN ACTION.

5α-Reductase Deficiency. Decreased production of dihydrotestosterone from testosterone causes severe ambiguity of external genitalia of males: small phallus, bifid scrotum, urogenital sinus with perineal hypospadias, and blind vaginal pouch. No müllerian structures are present but the vas deferens, epididymis, and seminal vesicles are present. At puberty, masculinization occurs normally with phallic enlargement, descent of testes, and spermatogenesis.

Testicular Feminization Syndrome. Genetic males appear female, with female external genitalia, blind vaginal pouch, absent uterus, and intra-abdominal testes. At puberty, breast development occurs without menses or pubic hair. Testes in adults produce normal levels of testosterone and dihydrotestosterone but a receptor or postreceptor defect is present. The testes should be removed to prevent malignant transformation.

True Hermaphroditism

In this condition, both ovarian and testicular tissues are present and the external genitalia are ambiguous. Testicular tissue is defective in androgen and MIF secretion. Usually these patients are reared as females, with removal of testicular tissue.

Diagnosis and Management of Genital Ambiguity

It is important to decide the sex of rearing as soon as possible. Analysis of chromosomes, pelvic ultrasound, and measurement of adrenal hormones should be undertaken. When receptor disorders in XY male are suspected, testosterone injection may aid in diagnosis.

18

THE NERVOUS SYSTEM

NEUROLOGIC EVALUATION
(*NELSON TEXTBOOK*, SEC. 20.1)

HISTORY

The history is the most important component of the evaluation of a child with a neurologic problem. It should carefully document in chronologic order the onset of symptoms and a thorough description of their frequency, duration, and associated characteristics. A comprehensive review of systems also is essential.

It is important to start with a concise description of the chief complaint within its developmental context. A comprehensive understanding of developmental milestones is essential in order to ascertain the relative importance of the parents' observations.

Following the chief complaint and history of present illness, a review of pregnancy, labor, and delivery is indicated, particularly if a congenital disorder is suspected. Maternal exposure to infections, drugs, cigarettes, and alcohol during the pregnancy is important. Decreased or absent fetal activity may be associated with the congenital myopathies and other neuromuscular disorders.

The history of birth weight, length, and head circumference are particularly important. Apgars scores, need for ventilatory assistance, and history of feeding difficulties should be noted.

The most important component of a neurologic history is the child's developmental assessment. An abnormality in development from birth suggests an intrauterine or perinatal cause. A slowing of the rate of acquisition of skills later in infancy or childhood suggests an acquired abnormality of the nervous system. A loss of skills over time strongly suggests an underlying degenerative disease of the central nervous system (CNS).

The family history is extremely helpful in the neurologic evaluation of the child. The history should document the presence of neurologic disease, including epilepsy, migraine, strokes, and heredofamilial disorders. It also should be determined whether the parents are related.

NEUROLOGIC EXAMINATION

Observation of the child's behavior and play provides useful information. The neurologic examination must be modified for infants and children of various ages. The examination should be conducted in a setting that is nonthreatening and enjoyable for the child. The more it seems like a game the greater will be the degree of cooperation. Evaluation of the motor function, gait, and coordination should precede the more threatening head and cranial nerve examination.

Head

The size and shape of the head should be documented carefully. Head circumference should be documented on every patient, at every visit, and should be recorded on a suitable head growth chart. The fontanels and cranial sutures should be examined. Auscultation of the skull for cranial bruits is performed to look for vascular malformations.

Cranial Nerves

OLFACTORY NERVE (1).   The sense of smell is not routinely tested in infants and young children.

OPTIC NERVE (2).   Examination of the optic disk and retina is an important component of the neurologic examination.

Papilledema rarely occurs in infancy because the skull sutures are capable of separating to accommodate the expanding brain. Papilledema in the older child is characterized by hyperemic optic nerve, dilation of the larger veins, indistinct border of the optic nerve, and subhyaloid, flame-shaped hemorrhages surrounding the optic nerve. Visual acuity remains intact but the blind spot is increased.

Visual acuity and *visual fields* are other important components in the examination of the optic nerve. Peripheral vision may be tested in an infant by bringing a colorful toy from behind the patient into the peripheral field of vision.

OCULOMOTOR (3), TROCHLEAR (4), AND ABDUCENS (6) NERVES.   The *oculomotor nerve* innervates the superior, inferior, and medial rectus as well as the inferior oblique and the levator palpebri muscles. Complete paralysis of the oculomotor nerve causes ptosis, dilation of the pupil, and displacement of the eye outward and downward.

The *trochlear nerve* supplies the superior oblique muscle, and isolated paralysis causes the eye to deviate upward and outward, often with an associated head tilt.

The *abducens nerve* innervates the lateral rectus muscle so that its paralysis causes medial deviation of the eye and the inability to abduct beyond the midline.

Complete ocular movement may be demonstrated in newborns utilizing the **doll's eye maneuver.** The *pupils* are assessed for their size and reaction to light and accommodation.

TRIGEMINAL NERVE (5).   The sensory distribution of the face is divided into the ophthalmic area, the maxillary area, and the mandibular area. Each region may be tested by light touch and by pinprick. The corneal response is elicited by touching the cornea with cotton and observing eye closure response. Motor function may be tested by examination of the masseter and temporalis muscles during mastication.

FACIAL NERVE (7).   Decreased voluntary movement of the lower face with flattening of the nasolabial angle indicates an upper motor neuron or supranuclear corticospinal lesion. A lower motor neuron lesion tends to involve equally upper and lower facial muscles.

AUDITORY NERVE (8). Screening for hearing loss is an important component of the neurologic examination. A normal newborn will pause briefly during sucking when a bell is presented. By 3 mo a normal infant will turn its head toward a bell or rattle.

GLOSSOPHARYNGEAL (9) AND VAGUS (10) NERVES. These nerves are tested by observing the gag response to tactile stimulation of the posterior pharyngeal wall. A unilateral injury of the vagus nerve produces weakness and asymmetry of the ipsilateral soft palate and a hoarse voice resulting from paralysis of a vocal cord.

ACCESSORY NERVE (11). The strength of the sterno-mastoid and trapezius muscles is tested.

HYPOGLOSSAL NERVE (12). This nerve innervates the tongue. Abnormalities of the hypoglossal nucleus or nerve produce wasting, weakness, and fasciculation of the tongue.

Motor Examination

The components of the motor examination include testing of power, muscle bulk, tone, posture, locomotion and motility, deep tendon reflexes, and the presence of primitive reflexes, when applicable.

POWER. The muscle appearance should be examined for bulk, atrophy, and fasciculations. The testing of muscle power is straightforward in the cooperative child.

Shoulder girdle strength may be evaluated in the newborn or infant by supporting the child by the axillae. The patient with weakness will be unable to support body weight and will "slip through" the examiner's hands.

Examination of the pelvic girdle or proximal lower extremity strength is performed by observing the child climb steps or stand up from a prone position. Weakness in these muscle causes the child to use the hands to "climb up" the legs to assume an upright position, a maneuver called **Gower sign.**

TONE. Muscle tone is tested by assessing the degree of resistance when an individual joint is moved passively.

Spasticity results from upper motor neuron lesions and is characterized by initial resistance to passive movement, followed by a sudden release called the **clasp-knife phenomenon.** Spasticity is most apparent in the upper extremity flexors and lower extremity extensor muscles. It is associated with brisk tendon reflexes and an extensor plantar reflex and clonus.

Rigidity, the result of a basal ganglia lesion, is characterized by constant resistance to passive movement of both extensor and flexor muscles.

Hypotonia refers to abnormally diminished tone and is the most common abnormality of tone in the neurologically compromised premature neonate.

MOTILITY AND LOCOMOTION. Observation of crawling, cruising, walking, or running may uncover movement disorders.

Ataxia refers to incoordination of movement or a disturbance of balance. Truncal ataxia is characterized by unsteadiness during sitting or standing and results primarily from involvement of the cerebellar vermis. Ataxia may be demonstrated by the finger-to-nose and heel-to-shin test, and tandem walking. Abnormalities of the cerebellar hemispheres characteristically cause *intention tremor*.

DEEP TENDON REFLEXES. The deep tendon reflexes are absent or decreased in myopathies, neuropathies, and abnormalities of the cerebellum. They are characteristically increased in upper motor neuron lesions. Asymmetry of deep tendon reflexes suggests a lateralizing lesion.

The **plantar response** is obtained by stimulation of the external portion of the sole of the foot, beginning at the heel and extending to the base of the toes.

The **Babinski reflex** is characterized by extension of the great toe and by fanning of the remaining toes. Stimulation may produce withdrawal, which may be misinterpreted as a Babinski response.

PRIMITIVE REFLEXES. Primitive reflexes appear and disappear in sequence during specific periods of development.

The **Moro reflex** is obtained by placing the infant in a semi-upright position. The head is momentarily allowed to fall backward, with immediate resupport by the examiner's hand. The child will symmetrically abduct and extend the arms, followed by flexion and adduction of the upper extremities. An asymmetric response may signify a brachial plexus injury or hemiparesis.

The **grasp response** is elicited by placing a finger or object in the open palm of each hand. The normal infant will grasp the object.

The **tonic neck reflex** is produced by manually turning the head to one side while supine. Extension of the arm occurs on that side of the body corresponding to the direction of the face, and flexion develops in the contralateral extremities. An obligatory tonic neck response, by which the infant remains "locked" in the fencer's position, always is abnormal and implies a disorder of the CNS.

Sensory Examination

The sensory examination is difficult to interpret in the infant or uncooperative child. In the older cooperative child, light touch, pinprick, vibration, and joint position sensation can be tested.

Gait and Stance

Observation of a child's gait is an important aspect of the neurologic examination. The *spastic gait* is characterized by stiffness and a "tin soldier"–like steppage appearance. *Hemiparesis* is associated with a decreased arm swing on the affected side and a lateral circular motion of the leg (circumduction). Cerebellar ataxia produces a broad-based, unsteady gait. A *waddling gait* results from weakness of the proximal hip girdle.

SPECIAL DIAGNOSTIC PROCEDURES

Lumbar Puncture and Cerebrospinal Fluid Examination

An examination of the cerebrospinal fluid (CSF) is essential in confirming the diagnosis of meningitis, encephalitis, and subarachnoid hemorrhage. The primary contraindication for performing a lumbar puncture (LP) is any condition that may lead to herniation of intracranial contents following the procedure. Inspection of the eyegrounds for the presence of papilledema is mandatory before proceeding with a LP. Routine CSF studies include white and red blood cell counts, glucose, protein, Gram stain, and bacterial cultures.

Neuroradiologic Procedures

The *skull roentgenogram* is useful to detect fractures, craniosynostosis, or bony defects.

Computerized tomographic (CT) *scanning* is useful in demonstrating congenital malformations of the brain, subdural collections, cerebral atrophy, intracranial calcifications, intracerebral hematoma, brain tumors, infarction, and edema.

Magnetic resonance imaging (MRI) is a noninvasive procedure that does not utilize ionizing radiation. It is especially well suited for the study of neoplasm, cerebral edema, degenerative diseases, and congenital anomalies, particularly of the posterior fossa and spinal cord. Spine MRI is indicated for demonstration of congenital anomalies, tumors, and vascular malformation of the spinal cord.

Cerebral angiography is reserved for study of vascular disorders, such as arteriovenous malformations, aneurysms, arterial occlusions, and venous thrombosis.

Cranial ultrasound is used in neonates for the detection of intraventricular hemorrhage and hydrocephalus.

Electroencephalography

Electroencephalography (EEG) provides a continuous recording of electrocortical activity. EEG is useful for identification of epileptiform discharges (spikes and sharp waves), which are associated with epilepsy. Focal slow waves may be due to a circumscribed lesion such as a tumor; generalized slow waves suggest a metabolic, inflammatory, or more widespread process.

Evoked Potentials

An evoked potential is an electrical response that follows stimulation of the CNS by a specific stimulus of the visual, auditory, or sensory system. Abnormal evoked responses often are seen in neurodegenerative diseases. Brain stem auditory evoked potentials may be used to measure, objectively, hearing acuity, particularly in the neonate or uncooperative child.

CONGENITAL ANOMALIES OF THE CENTRAL NERVOUS SYSTEM
(*NELSON TEXTBOOK*, SECS. 20.2–20.16)

NEURAL TUBE DEFECTS (Dysraphism)
(*NELSON TEXTBOOK*, SECS. 20.2–20.7)

Neural tube defects account for most congenital anomalies of the CNS and result from failure of the neural tube to close spontaneously between the 3rd and 4th wk of gestation. The failure of closure of the neural tube allows the excretion of fetal substances (e.g., α-fetoprotein) into the amniotic fluid, serving as a biochemical marker for a neural tube defect.

Myelomeningocele

This is the most severe form of dysraphism involving vertebral columns and occurs in 1:1,000 live births. The etiology is unknown, but a genetic predisposition exists. Risk of recurrence after one affected child rises to 3–4%. Nutritional and environmental factors are thought to play a role.

CLINICAL MANIFESTATIONS. A lumbosacral location is most common. The myelomeningocele usually is covered by a sac-like cystic structure with neural tissue visible underneath. The membrane may rupture and leak CSF. The extent and degree of neurologic deficit depends on location. *Hydrocephalus* in association with type II Chiari defect develops in 80% of patients with myelomeningocele. Infants with hydrocephalus and Chiari II malformation may develop brain stem dysfunction, including difficulty feeding, choking, stridor, apnea, and vocal cord paralysis.

TREATMENT. Surgical repair of the myelomeningocele is performed during the neonatal period. Ventriculoperitoneal shunting may be needed for hydrocephalus.

PROGNOSIS. Many children will achieve functional ambulation. The mortality rate is 10–15%, and normal intelligence occurs in 70% of cases.

Encephalocele

Encephaloceles are protrusion of tissue through a bony midline defect, forming a sac with a pedunculated stalk. Encephaloceles contain neural tissue that often is abnormal. They most commonly occur in the occipital regions at or below the inion, but also occur in a frontal or nasofrontal location. Hydrocephalus may develop as a result of aqueductal stenosis or Dandy–Walker malformation. The sac may be covered completely with skin or denuded skin, but may rupture. CT or MRI may define the contents of the lesion. Children with cranial encephalocele are at risk for visual problems, microcephaly, mental retardation, and seizures.

Anencephaly

Anencephaly is due to failure of closure of the rostral neuropore, resulting in a large defect of the calvarium, meninges, and scalp. There is a rudimentary brain with absent cerebral hemispheres and cerebellum, and only a residue of the brain stem. Most anencephalic infants die within several days of birth. The incidence is.1:1,000 live births, and it is highest in Ireland and Wales. The recurrence risk is 4%. The etiology is unknown.

DISORDERS OF CELL MIGRATION
(*NELSON TEXTBOOK*, SECS. 20.8–20.11)

Lissencephaly

Lissencephaly is a disorder in which there is an absence of cerebral convolutions and a poorly formed Sylvian fissure. It may be due to faulty neuroblast migration during early embryonic life. Infants have failure to thrive, microcephaly, marked developmental delay, and a severe seizure disorder. Hypoplasia of the optic nerves and microphthalmia are common.

Schizencephaly

Unilateral or bilateral cleft within the cerebral hemispheres occurs in schizencephaly as a result of abnormal morphogenesis. The borders of the cleft are surrounded by abnormal gray matter, particularly microgyria. Many patients are severely retarded, with seizures that are difficult to control.

Porencephaly

Cysts or cavities within the brain may result from a developmental defect or acquired lesions, including infarction of tissue. Children with these lesions may have hemiparesis, focal seizures, or mental retardation.

AGENESIS OF THE CORPUS CALLOSUM

An insult to the commissural plate during early embryogenesis causes agenesis of the corpus callosum. When it is an isolated phenomenon, the patient may be normal. When associated with other brain anomalies, such as heterotopias, microgyria, and pachygyria (broad, wide gyri), mental retardation, seizures, and hemiparesis or diplegia may occur. MRI is the best test for diagnosis of this and other associated brain anomalies. Agenesis of the corpus callosum may be associated with specific chromosomal abnormalities, such as 8-trisomy and 18-trisomy.

Aicardi syndrome is a complex disorder that affects only girls and is associated with agenesis of the corpus callosum, infantile spasms, and abnormalities of the retina or optic nerve.

MICROCEPHALY

Microcephaly is defined as a head circumference that measures more than three standard deviations below the mean for age and sex. *Primary microcephaly* refers to a group of conditions that usually have no other malformation and follow a mendelian pattern of inheritance or are associated with a specific genetic syndrome. *Secondary microcephaly* results from a large number of noxious agents that may affect the fetus in utero or the infant during periods of rapid brain growth (first 2 yr of life). Both types may be associated with mental retardation. Serial measurement of head circumference and measurement of head circumferences of family member are important.

HYDROCEPHALUS

Hydrocephalus is a diverse group of conditions that result from impaired circulation and absorption of CSF. CSF is formed by the choroid plexus, primarily in the lateral ventricles. CSF is reabsorbed primarily by the arachnoid villi into the venous sinuses.

Pathophysiology and Etiology

Obstructive or noncommunicating hydrocephalus results from obstruction within the ventricular system. Causes include congenital aqueductal stenosis or acquired aqueductal gliosis (after a neonatal or congenital infection or intraventricular hemorrhage). Posterior fossa brain tumors, the Chiari malformation, and the Dandy–Walker malformation cause obstruction of the fourth ventricle.

Nonobstructive or communicating hydrocephalus results from obliteration of the subarachnoid cisterns or malfunction of the arachnoid villi. Communicating hydrocephalus may follow subarachnoid (intraventricular) hemorrhage, tuberculous and pneumococcal meningitis, or leukemic infiltration of the subarachnoid spaces.

Clinical Manifestations

In infants, an accelerated rate of head growth is the most prominent sign. A bulging anterior fontanel, separated cranial sutures, dilated scalp veins, broad forehead, and downward deviation of the eyes ("setting sun" sign) are present. In the older child, headache, personality change, and deterioration in school performance are common. Papilledema, abducens nerve palsy, and pyramidal tract signs are evident in most cases. Irritability, lethargy, poor appetite, and vomiting occur in both groups.

CHIARI MALFORMATION. The Chiari type II malformation consists of elongation of the fourth ventricle and kinking of the brain stem, with displacement of the inferior vermis and medulla into the cervical canal. It is associated with myelomeningocele. MRI is diagnostic. Surgical decompression is performed if there are signs of brain stem dysfunction.

DANDY–WALKER MALFORMATION. This malformation consists of a cystic expansion of the fourth ventricle in the posterior fossa, which results from developmental failure of the roof of the 4th ventricle during embryogenesis. About 90% of patients have hydrocephalus and a significant number have other brain anomalies. Long tract signs, cerebellar ataxia, and developmental delay are common.

Diagnosis and Differential Diagnosis

Papilledema is observed in older children but is rarely present in infants. CT or MRI scan is important in establishing the diagnosis and identifying the specific cause.

Treatment

Most cases require treatment with ventriculoperitoneal shunts.

MEGALENCEPHALY

Various metabolic and degenerative disorders of the CNS produce megalencephaly as a result of abnormal storage of substances within the brain parenchyma. These include lysosomal diseases (e.g., Tay–Sachs, gangliosidoses, mucopolysaccharidoses); aminoaciduria (maple syrup urine disease); and the leukodystrophies (e.g., metachromatic, Alexander disease, and Canavan disease). Familial megalencephaly is inherited as an autosomal dominant trait with normal or near-normal intelligence.

CRANIOSYNOSTOSIS

Premature closure of the cranial sutures is a developmental anomaly that causes skull deformities that are evident at birth. Fusion of the suture may be confirmed by plain skull roentgenograms. *Scaphocephaly* is the most common form of craniosynostosis and is due to premature closure of the sagittal suture, which produces a long and narrow skull. Premature fusion of a single suture rarely causes neurologic deficit. Craniosynostosis may be associated with genetic disorders such as Crouzon, Apert, Chotzen, and Pfeiffer syndromes.

SEIZURES IN CHILDHOOD
(*NELSON TEXTBOOK*, SECS. 20.17–20.34)

A *seizure (convulsion)* is defined as a paroxysmal involuntary disturbance of brain function that may be manifested as an impairment or loss of consciousness, abnormal motor activity, behavioral abnormalities, sensory disturbances, or autonomic dysfunction. *Epilepsy* is defined as recurrent seizures unrelated to fever or to an acute cerebral insult.

EVALUATION

The history should attempt to define factors that may have precipitated the seizures. It also should determine if the seizure had a focal onset. Presence of auras or postictal (Todd) paralysis on one side implies a focal onset.

The physical examination should focus on a search for organic causes. Head circumference and facial features are important. Birth marks such as café-au-lait spots or hypopigmented macules may point to a neurocutaneous syndrome. Funduscopy is important for identification of papilledema, chorioretinitis, retinal hamartomas, and other congenital anomalies.

CLASSIFICATION OF SEIZURES
(*NELSON TEXTBOOK*, SECS. 20.18–20.20)

Partial Seizures

Partial seizures account for up to 40% of childhood seizures.

SIMPLE PARTIAL SEIZURES (SPS). Consciousness is maintained during SPS. Motor activity is the most common sign of SPS. Asynchronous clonic or tonic movements are seen in the face, neck, and extremities. Automatisms do not occur in SPS, but an aura may be present. An average seizure lasts for 10–20 sec. The EEG may show spikes or sharp waves unilaterally or bilaterally in patients with SPS.

COMPLEX PARTIAL SEIZURES (CPS). A CPS may begin with a simple partial seizure with or without an aura, followed by impaired consciousness. An *aura* consisting of vague, unpleasant feelings is present in approximately one third of children with SPS and CPS. *Automatisms,* usually alimentary in nature, are a common feature of CPS in infants and children. CPS can evolve into a generalized tonic–clonic convulsion. Interictal EEG may show sharp waves or spikes in the anterior temporal lobes; spikes in the frontal, parietal, and occipital lobes are less common. MRI may show lesions in CPS, particularly in the temporal lobe.

BENIGN PARTIAL EPILEPSY WITH CENTROTEMPORAL SPIKES (BPEC). BPEC is a common type of partial epilepsy of childhood with an excellent prognosis. The onset peaks at 9–10 yr and remission occurs by 14–16 yr. Seizures usually are partial, with facial or tongue twitching, speech arrest, and drooling. Partial seizures may progress to hemiclonic or generalized seizures. Seizures often occur at night during sleep. The EEG shows a characteristic pattern of centrotemporal spikes with normal background activity.

Generalized Seizures

ABSENCE SEIZURES. Simple absence (petit mal) seizures are characterized by sudden cessation of motor activity or speech with a blank facial expression and flickering of the eyelids, rarely exceeding 30 sec. Absences are not associated with a postictal state, and the child resumes preseizure activity. Autonomic behavior may accompany absence seizures. Hyperventilation may induce an absence seizure. Absences are more common in girls and uncommon prior to 5 yr of age. The EEG shows characteristic, generalized 3/sec spike–wave discharges.

GENERALIZED TONIC–CLONIC SEIZURES. In primary generalized tonic–clonic seizures, there is a sudden loss of consciousness. The eyes roll back, the entire body undergoes tonic contractions, and the child becomes cyanotic in association with apnea. In the clonic phase, there are rhythmic clonic contractions alternating with relaxation of all muscle groups. Clonic activity slows after a few minutes. Postictally the child will initially be semicomatose, and typically remains in deep sleep from 30 min to 2 hr.

INFANTILE SPASMS. Infantile spasms usually begin between 4 and 8 mo and are characterized by brief symmetric contractions of the neck, trunk, and extremities. Spasms may be flexor, extensor, or mixed in type. Clusters or volleys of seizures tend to occur during drowsiness or on awakening. They persist for minutes with brief intervals between each spasm. The EEG shows characteristic hypsarrhythmia, a chaotic pattern of high-amplitude slow waves and spikes.

Symptomatic infantile spasms are related to several prenatal, perinatal, and postnatal factors, such as hypoxic–ischemic encephalopathy, congenital infections, metabolic disorders, and developmental brain anomalies. Only 10–20% of infantile spasms are classified as *cryptogenic*, in which the children have normal development and physical examination and no associated risk factors. Infants with cryptogenic infantile spasms have a good prognosis, whereas those with the symptomatic type have an 80–90% risk of mental retardation.

Febrile Seizures

CLINICAL MANIFESTATIONS. Febrile seizures typically consist of a generalized, tonic–clonic convulsion of a few seconds to 10 min in duration and occur with rapidly rising temperature (usually 39°C or greater). They occur from 9 mo to 5 yr of age, with peak onset at 14–28 mo of age. The incidence is 3–4% of young children. Febrile seizure may signify a serious underlying acute infectious disease such as bacterial meningitis. Complex febrile seizures include a seizure lasting for more than 15 min, repeated convulsions within a febrile illness, and focal seizures.

Approximately 50% of children with febrile seizure have a recurrent febrile seizures. The risk factors for development of epilepsy include a positive family history of epilepsy, initial febrile seizure prior to 9 mo of age, and complex febrile seizures. The incidence of epilepsy is 1% in those with no risk factors and up to 9% when several risk factors are present.

TREATMENT. Short-term anticonvulsant prophylaxis is not indicated. Prolonged anticonvulsant prophylaxis for prevention of recurrent febrile convulsion is controversial and no longer recommended routinely. Rectal diazepam or lorazepam is the drug of choice for the acute management of prolonged febrile seizures.

DIAGNOSIS OF SEIZURES

Investigation depends on the age of the patient, the type and frequency of seizure, and the presence or absence of neurologic findings. The minimum work-up for the first unprovoked seizure in an otherwise healthy child includes a fasting glucose, calcium, magnesium, serum electrolytes, and a routine EEG. Paroxysmal discharges on EEG support a diagnosis of epilepsy. However, a normal EEG does not exclude the diagnosis of epilepsy. MRI or CT scans in the investigation of seizures should be reserved for patients in whom an intracranial lesion is suspected on the basis of the history or an abnormal neurologic examination and those with prolonged partial seizures or medically intractable seizures.

TREATMENT OF EPILEPSY

Antiepileptics usually are withheld after a single unprovoked seizure in an otherwise healthy child. If there is a recurrent seizure disorder, the drug of choice depends on the classification of the seizure, as determined by history and EEG findings. The goal is monotherapy with the fewest possible side effects for the control of seizures.

Carbamazepine and *phenytoin* are used for partial seizures and some generalized tonic–clonic seizures. *Phenobarbital* and *primidone* are useful for generalized tonic–clonic seizures. *Valproic acid* is effective for many seizure types, including generalized tonic–clonic, absence, atypical absence, and myoclonic seizures. A rare side effect of valproic acid, idiosyncratic hepatotoxicity, is fatal.

NEONATAL SEIZURES

Clinical Manifestations and Classification

Generalized tonic–clonic seizures tend not to occur during the 1st mo of life. Clinical seizures are classified as focal clonic, multifocal clonic, tonic, myoclonic, and subtle seizures (consisting of chewing motions, excessive salivation, blinking, pedaling movements, and change of color). Nonepileptic movements are suppressed with gentle restraint, but true seizures are not.

Etiologies

Hypoxic–ischemic encephalopathy is the most common cause of neonatal seizures. Intracranial hemorrhage in preterm and term infants also is a common etiology. Metabolic disorders such as hypoglycemia, hypocalcemia, or hypomagnesemia can be diagnosed and treated easily. Inborn errors of metabolism cause generalized convulsions in the newborn period. Congenital TORCH infections and acute infections such as bacterial meningitis or viral encephalitis also may cause seizures. Cytoarchitectural abnormalities of the brain, including lissencephaly, schizencephaly, neonatal adrenoleukodystrophy, and Aicardi syndrome, also present with seizures.

Treatment

Benzodiazepines, phenobarbital, and phenytoin are the agents most commonly used for neonatal seizures when not associated with transient metabolic disturbances.

Prognosis

The prognosis depends on the underlying cause for seizure. Infants with seizures caused by hypoxic–ischemic encephalopathy or cytoarchitectural abnormalities of the brain have a poor prognosis.

STATUS EPILEPTICUS

Status epilepticus is defined as convulsions lasting greater than 30 min or the occurrence of serial convulsions between which there is no return of consciousness. Most status epilepticus cases consist of generalized tonic–clonic seizures.

Etiology

Prolonged febrile seizures are the most common cause of status epilepticus in children. Status epilepticus may be the initial presentation of epilepsy or may follow sudden withdrawal of anticonvulsants in epileptic patients. Mortality and morbidity in these two groups are low. Seizures occurring in association with long-standing neurologic disorders (*symptomatic status epilepticus*) are associated with much higher mortality and morbidity.

Pathophysiology

Status epilepticus is a medical emergency. A critical period exists during status epilepticus when irreversible neuronal changes may develop. Management of the child should be directed to supporting vital functions and to controlling the convulsions as expeditiously as possible.

Treatment

The initial management is to assess and manage the cardiorespiratory system. Blood is obtained for Dextrostix, complete blood count, electrolytes, glucose, creatinine, and anticonvulsant levels, if indicated. Blood and urine for toxicology are obtained when indicated. Physical and neurologic examination should be carried out concurrently to assess evidence of trauma, papilledema, a bulging fontanel, or lateralizing neurologic signs.

Medications always should be delivered intravenously. Either *diazepam* (0.3 mg/kg to a maximum of 10 mg) or *lorazepam* (0.05–0.1 mg/kg) is used initially. *Phenytoin* (15–20 mg/kg IV at a rate of 1 mg/kg/min) is given immediately after diazepam or lorazepam. *Phenobarbital* (10–15 mg/kg or, in the neonate, 20 mg/kg IV over 10–30 min) is given next if the seizures are not controlled. If seizures still are not controlled, the choices for further drug management include paraldehyde, a diazepam drip, lidocaine, pentobarbital coma, or general anesthesia.

Prognosis

The mortality rate of status epilepticus is approximately 5% in most series. Most deaths and morbidity occur in the symptomatic group.

CONDITIONS THAT MIMIC EPILEPSY
(*NELSON TEXTBOOK*, SECS. 20.24–20.34)

Night Terrors

Night terrors are common, particularly in boys between 5 and 7 yr of age. They occur in 1–3% of children. The attacks occur between midnight and 2 A.M., during stage 3 or 4 sleep. The child screams and appears frightened, with dilated pupils, tachycardia, and hyperventilation. The child may thrash violently and cannot be consoled. Sleep follows in a few minutes, and there is total amnesia the following morning. Patients also may experience somnambulism.

Breath-Holding Spells

CYANOTIC BREATH-HOLDING SPELLS. Cyanotic breath-holding spells are provoked by upsetting or scolding an infant. They begin with a brief, shrill cry, followed by forced expiration and apnea. There is rapid onset of cyanosis and loss of consciousness that may be associated with repeated generalized clonic jerks, opisthotonus, and bradycardia. Spells present after 6 mo of age, with a peak at 2 yr of age, and abate by 5 yr of age.

PALLID SPELLS. These spells are much less common than cyanotic breath-holding spells but share several of their characteristics. Pallid spells are initiated by a painful experience, such as falling and striking the head or a sudden startle. The child stops breathing, rapidly loses consciousness, becomes pale and hypotonic, and may have a tonic seizure. Spells are associated with asystole or severe bradycardia. Most children do well without treatment, but in refractory cases atropine can be used.

Syncope

Syncope results from vagal stimulation and is precipitated by pain, fear, excitement, and extended periods of standing. Decreased blood flow to the brain resulting from systemic hypotension causes a brief tonic contraction of the muscles of the face, trunk, and extremities. The EEG shows transient slowing during the attack but no seizure discharges. Syncope is most common among adolescent females.

HEADACHES
(*NELSON TEXTBOOK*, SECS. 20.35–20.38)

MIGRAINE

Migraine is a recurrent headache with symptom-free intervals and at least three of the following symptoms or findings: abdominal pain, nausea or vomiting, throbbing headache, unilateral location, associated aura (visual, sensory, motor), relief following sleep, and a positive family history. Girls are more likely to develop migraines as adolescents.

Clinical Manifestations and Classifications

COMMON MIGRAINE. This is the most prevalent type of migraine in children. The headache is throbbing or pounding, located in the bifrontal or temporal regions. Headaches usually last 1–3 hr. Intense nausea and vomiting occur during the headache. Photophobia, light-headedness, and paresthesias of the hands and feet may occur. A family history is present in approximately 90% of children with common migraine.

CLASSIC MIGRAINE. An aura precedes the onset of headache. A visual aura, rarely present in children, may take the form of blurred vision, scotomas, flashes of light, fortification spectra (brilliant white zig-zag lines), or irregular distortion of objects.

MIGRAINE VARIANTS. *Cyclic vomiting* is characterized by recurrent, sometimes monthly bouts of severe vomiting that may persist for several days. After a period of deep sleep, the child awakens and resumes normal play and eating habits. Headaches may be reported in older children.

Acute confusional states may be a manifestation of migraine characterized by confusion, disorientation, unresponsiveness, memory disturbances, vomiting, and lethargy. Confusion lasts for several hours and clears after sleep. Severe headache or visual symptoms may precede the acute attack of confusion.

COMPLICATED MIGRAINE. Migraines are classified as complicated when there are neurologic signs during a headache that persist following termination of the headache. *Hemiplegic migraine* refers to the onset of unilateral motor or sensory signs during an episode of migraine. Neurologic signs may be transient or may persist for days but rarely lead to a completed stroke. *Basilar migraine* attacks present with vertigo, tinnitus, diplopia, blurred vision, scotomas, ataxia, and an occipital headache.

Diagnosis and Differential Diagnosis

A thorough history and physical examination suffice to establish the diagnosis in most cases. MRI or CT scan is indicated if the headache is associated with an unusual constellation of symptoms (early morning headaches, focal seizures) or focal neurologic signs or when increased intracranial pressure is suspected.

Treatment

Children should avoid certain initiating stimuli such as stress, anxiety, and certain foods and drugs. Acute attacks are treated with analgesics (acetaminophen, ibuprofen) and antiemetics. Continuous daily medication (β-adrenergic blocker or tricyclic antidepressants) is used for severe and frequent headaches that affect the child's daily activities. Behavioral management is effective for treatment of migraine in some children.

ORGANIC HEADACHES

Headache may be the earliest symptom of increased intracranial pressure resulting from tension or traction of the cerebral blood vessels and dura. These headaches occur primarily in the early hours of the morning and may be enhanced by coughing, sneezing, or straining during a bowel movement. Causes of organic headaches include brain tumors, hydrocephalus, meningitis and encephalitis, cerebral abscess, subdural hematoma, and pseudotumor cerebri.

PSYCHOGENIC OR STRESS HEADACHES

Psychogenic, stress, or tension headaches usually occur in adolescents and often are difficult to differentiate from migraine headaches. Headaches usually are bifrontal and aching in quality. They usually are not associated with nausea and vomiting. Stress and anxiety often may provoke headaches.

NEUROCUTANEOUS SYNDROMES
(*NELSON TEXTBOOK*, SECS. 20.39–20.44)

This is a heterogeneous group of disorders characterized by abnormalities of both the integument and the CNS.

NEUROFIBROMATOSIS

Neurofibromatosis (NF) is a common autosomal dominant disorder, affecting approximately 1:4,000 of the population. NF may result from a new mutation in one half of all cases.

Clinical Manifestations and Diagnosis

NEUROFIBROMATOSIS 1. NF-1 is the most prevalent type; the gene is located on chromosome 17. *Clinical manifestations* include multiple café-au-lait spots, axillary or inguinal freckling, iris Lisch nodules, and neurofibromas or plexiform neurofibroma. Neurofibromas typically involve the skin, but they may be situated along peripheral nerves or blood vessels or within viscera. A distinctive osseous lesion, such as dysplasia of the sphenoid wing or bowing of the tibula, may occur. Optic gliomas are present in approximately 15% of patients with NF-1. Seizures and psychological disturbances may occur. Malignant neoplasms (neurofibrosarcoma, malignant schwannoma, pheochromocytoma, and rhabdomyosarcoma) also are a problem.

NEUROFIBROMATOSIS 2. NF-2 accounts for 10% of all cases of neurofibromatosis. Bilateral eighth nerve masses are the most distinctive feature of NF-2. The gene for NF-2 is located near the center of the long arm of chromosome 22.

TUBEROUS SCLEROSIS

Tuberous sclerosis (TS) is an autosomal dominant disorder with an estimated frequency of 1:30,000. The TS gene is located on chromosome 9, but at least one half of the cases are sporadic, due to new mutations. TS is a heterogeneous disease with a wide clinical spectrum. Disease affects many organs other than the skin and brain, including the heart, kidneys, eyes, lungs, and bone. Characteristically, tubers (hamartomas) are located in convolutions of the cerebral hemispheres and the subependymal region, where they undergo calcification.

Clinical Manifestations

TS may present in infancy with infantile spasms and a hysparrhythmic EEG pattern. Hypopigmented skin lesions ("ash leaf" spots) occur in more than 90% of cases. Seizures may be difficult to control. There is a high incidence of mental retardation in young patients with TS and infantile spasms.

During childhood, TS presents most often with a generalized seizure disorder and pathognomonic skin lesions (sebaceous adenomas of nose and cheeks and *shagreen patch*, a roughened, orange peel–like lesion located primarily in the lumbosacral region). Retinal hamartomas (mulberry tumors) may be present. Cardiac rhabdomyomas occur in 50% of TS patients. The kidneys are affected by hamartomas or polycystic disease.

STURGE–WEBER DISEASE

In this disease, there is a constellation of findings, including a facial nevus (port-wine stain), seizures, hemiparesis, intracranial calcifications, and in many cases mental retardation. It has a sporadic occurrence with an incidence of approximately 1:50,000. A facial nevus is present at birth, tends to be unilateral, and always involves the upper face and eyelid. Abnormally rich leptomeningeal vasculature leads to cortical atrophy and calcification in the underlying cortex. Glaucoma of the ipsilateral eye is a common complication. Focal tonic–clonic seizures develop in most patients during the 1st yr of life. A slowly progressive hemiparesis ensues. Seizures become refractory to anticonvulsants and may require hemispherectomy for control.

MOVEMENT DISORDERS
(*NELSON TEXTBOOK*, SECS. 20.45–20.48)

ATAXIAS

Congenital Anomalies of the Posterior Fossa

Dandy–Walker syndrome, the Chiari malformation, and encephalocele are prominently associated with ataxia because of their destruction or replacement of the cerebellum.

Acute Cerebellar Ataxia

Acute cerebellar ataxia occurs primarily in children 1–3 yr of age, often following a viral illness such as varicella, coxsackievirus, or echovirus infection by 2–3 wk. Truncal ataxia is severe, so that the child is unable to stand or sit. CSF reveals slight pleocytosis of lymphocytes (10–30/mm^3). Ataxia begins to improve in a few weeks, but may persist for a couple of months. The prognosis generally is good.

Toxic Causes

Alcohol, thallium, and anticonvulsants may cause ataxia.

Brain Tumors

Tumors of the cerebellum and frontal lobe may present with ataxia. Neuroblastoma may be associated with an encephalopathy characterized by progressive ataxia, myoclonic jerks, and opsoclonus.

Metabolic Disorders

Abetalipoproteinemia and aminoacidopathies such as arginosuccinic aciduria, Hartnup disease, and maple syrup urine disease also cause ataxia.

Degenerative Diseases

ATAXIA–TELANGECTASIA. This is an autosomal recessive condition characterized by ataxia that begins about 2 yr of age and progresses to loss of ambulation by adolescence. Telangectasias of the bulbar conjunctiva, over the bridge of the nose, and on the ears and exposed surfaces of the extremities are evident by mid-childhood. Abnormalities of immunologic function lead to frequent respiratory infections. Decreased serum and secretory immunoglobulin (Ig) A and diminished IgG_2, IgG_4, and IgE levels are present in more than 50% of patients. The serum α-fetoprotein is elevated. Patients also have a high risk of developing lymphoreticular tumors.

FRIEDREICH ATAXIA. Friedreich ataxia is inherited as an autosomal recessive or dominant trait. Ataxia, which develops prior to 10 yr of age, is slowly progressive and involves the lower extremities more than the upper extremities. Nystagmus, areflexia, a positive Romberg test, and extensor plantar responses are present. Intelligence is preserved. There is loss of vibration and position sense as a result of degeneration of the posterior columns. Pes cavus, hammer toes, and progressive kyphoscoliosis develop. Hypertrophic cardiomyopathy with progression to heart failure is the cause of death.

CHOREA

Sydenham Chorea

This is the most common acquired chorea of childhood and is a neurologic manifestation of rheumatic fever. The major features are rapid and jerky movements prominent in the face, trunk, and distal extremities that dart from one muscle group to another, are increased by stress, and disappear during sleep. The chorea may last for several months and usually remits spontaneously. The chorea usually does not require treatment with phenothiazines or haloperidol, but rheumatic fever requires appropriate management.

DYSTONIAS

Dystonia is a slow, intermittent twisting motion that produces exaggerated turning and posture of the extremities and trunk.

Dystonia Musculorum Deformans

This is a slowly progressive disorder that typically begins during childhood. There are autosomal dominant and autosomal recessive forms (the latter are more common among Ashkenazi Jews). Symptoms begin with unilateral dystonic posturing of the lower extremity, progressing to all four extremities and the axial musculature.

Drug-Induced Dystonia

Phenothiazines and other neuroleptics may produce idiosyncratic reactions characterized by acute dystonic posturing. Phenytoin and carbamazepine rarely may cause dystonia.

Wilson Disease

Wilson disease is a treatable autosomal recessive disorder that is due to an inborn error of copper metabolism characterized by cirrhosis of the liver and degenerative changes in the basal ganglia. The gene has been localized to chromosome 13. Neurologic manifestations occur after 10 yr of age, initially with progressive dystonia. Coarse tremors of the extremities develop (the so-called wing-beating tremor). Fixed smile and drooling occur as well. A Kayser–Fleischer ring resulting from copper deposition in the Descemet membrane is pathognomonic. An MRI or CT scan shows lesions of the basal ganglia and thalamus.

TICS

Tics are spasmodic, repetitive, stereotyped movements that are nonrhythmic and often exacerbated by stress. *Transient tic disorder* is a common, often familial, movement abnormality consisting of eye blinking or facial movements and occasional throat-clearing noises that lasts a few weeks to less than 1 yr.

Gilles de la Tourette syndrome is a lifelong condition that has its onset between 2 and 15 yr of age. Fluctuating tics of the face, eyes, neck, and shoulders are characteristic. Tics are accompanied by vocalizations, including throat clearing, sniffling, coughing, barking, coprolalia (obscene words), echolalia, palilalia, and echokinesis. Compulsive behavior and learning problems are common. Severe tics may be treated with haloperidol, pimozide, and in some cases clonidine.

ENCEPHALOPATHIES
(*NELSON TEXTBOOK*, SECS. 20.49–20.54)

Encephalopathy is defined as a generalized disorder of cerebral function that may be acute or chronic, progressive or static.

CEREBRAL PALSY

Cerebral palsy (CP) is a static encephalopathy that may be defined as a nonprogressive disorder of posture and movement (i.e., significant motor dysfunction), which may be associated with abnormalities of speech, vision, and intellect resulting from a defect or lesion of the developing brain. The prevalence is 2:1,000.

Epidemiology and Etiology

Most cases of CP are due to congenital, developmental, or genetic disorders. Birth asphyxia is an uncommon cause of CP.

Clinical Manifestations

CP commonly is associated with a spectrum of developmental disabilities, including mental retardation, epilepsy, and visual, hearing, speech, cognitive, and behavioral abnormalities.

Infants with *spastic hemiplegia* have decreased spontaneous movement on the affected side and show hand preference at a very early age. The arms are more involved than the legs. Walking is delayed until 18–24 mo, and a circumductive gait is apparent. Seizures occur in one third of children. A CT scan characteristically shows an atrophic cerebral hemisphere with a dilated lateral ventricle contralateral to the side of the affected extremity.

Spastic diplegia refers to bilateral spasticity of the legs with brisk reflexes, excessive adduction in the hips, and equinovarus position of the feet. The prognosis for normal intellectual development is good. Seizures are minimal. The most common neuropathologic finding is periventricular leukomalacia.

Spastic quadriplegia is the most severe form of CP because of the marked motor impairment of all extremities and the high association with mental retardation and seizures. It is characterized by increased tone and spasticity in all extremities, brisk reflexes, and plantar extensor responses.

ACQUIRED IMMUNODEFICIENCY SYNDROME ENCEPHALOPATHY

Neurologic signs in congenitally infected patients may appear during early infancy or may be delayed to as late as 5 yr of age. The encephalopathy may have an acute onset with a relentless progressive course, but in some cases the process is either static or characterized by insidious deterioration. Children display arrest in brain growth, evidence of developmental delay, and evolution of neurologic signs.

MITOCHONDRIAL ENCEPHALOMYOPATHIES

Mitochondrial encephalomyopathies are associated with defects in the mitochondrial DNA resulting in abnormalities in the mitochondrial electron chain transport system.

Mitochondrial Myopathy, Encephalopathy, Lactic Acidosis, and Stroke (MELAS)

MELAS is a progressive disorder with episodes of hemiparesis, hemianopia, cortical blindness, and dementia. CT scans show calcifications of the basal ganglia and lucencies in other regions (not corresponding to vascular distributions) that are compatible with the acute neurologic deficit. Seizures and delayed motor and cognitive development occur. Muscle bi-

opsy shows ragged-red fibers, suggesting an abnormality of
the electron chain transport system. Serum lactate levels are
elevated during an acute episode.

Myoclonic Epilepsy and Ragged-Red Fibers (MERRF)

MERRF begins in childhood with myoclonic epilepsy and
progressive ataxia associated with dysarthria and nystagmus. Intellectual deterioration is slowly progressive. Pathologic findings include elevated serum lactate levels, ragged-
red fibers in muscle biopsies, marked loss and degeneration
of neurons in the dentate nuclei, and degeneration of the
subcortical cerebellar white matter.

Kearns-Sayre Syndrome

Kearns-Sayre syndrome is characterized by ophthalmoplegia, retinal degeneration, ataxia, and sensorineural
hearing loss. Many children also have heart block. Ragged-
red fibers also are found in muscle biopsies.

Leigh Disease (Subacute Necrotizing Encephalomyelopathy)

Leigh disease is an autosomal recessive disorder characterized by feeding and swallowing difficulties, vomiting, developmental delay, seizures, hypotonia, ataxia, and nystagmus. Intermittent respirations and external ophthalmoplegia
occur. Pathologic findings consist of scattered foci of necrosis
and capillary proliferation of the basal ganglia, tegmental
gray matter, and periventricular and periaqueductal regions.
At least three known defects cause Leigh disease: pyruvate
dehydrogenase complex and deficiency of complex I, and of
complex IV of the respiratory chain. Elevated serum lactate
levels are the hallmark of Leigh disease.

COMA IN THE PEDIATRIC PATIENT
(*NELSON TEXTBOOK*, SECS. 20.55–20.56)

Coma is defined as a state of unconsciousness from which
the child cannot be aroused by ordinary verbal, sensory, or
physical stimuli. Coma is a medical emergency. The history
is important in determining possible drug ingestions or toxic
causes.

The child's level of consciousness and the response to
stimuli should be carefully documented. A modification of
the *Glasgow Coma Scale* (see Table 4–8), is useful for the grad-
ing of the degree of coma and the severity of the insult in
infants and children. A coma score of less than 5 is associated
with a grave prognosis, whereas a score of 5–8 may indicate
a better prognosis in the child than the adult.

The *physical examination* is helpful in distinguishing between a metabolic and a structural cause for the coma. A
slow irregular pulse combined with systemic hypertension
indicates increased intracranial pressure or hypertensive encephalopathy. CSF rhinorrhea, hematotypmanum, and **Battle sign** (bruising over the mastoid) are suggestive of a basilar

skull fracture. Nuchal rigidity may indicate meningitis, encephalitis, subarachnoid bleeding, or herniation of the cerebellar tonsils. *Pinpoint pupils* are associated with narcotics and barbiturate toxicity. Small and irregular pupils suggest a lesion in the pons, and dilated and unresponsive pupils are seen with certain drugs, including amphetamine, atropine, cocaine, ethanol, and mydriatics. A unilaterally dilated and unresponsive pupil in the comatose child indicates herniation of the uncus of the ipsilateral temporal lobe. The integrity of the extraocular muscles may be tested by the doll's eye maneuver. The fundi must be examined for the presence of papilledema and retinal hemorrhage. Brain stem function may be evaluated by *ice water calorics*. In a comatose child with an intact brain stem the eyes deviate toward the side of the stimulus. Focal neurologic signs may be difficult to elicit in the comatose patient. The *hemiparetic* extremity has altered reflexes and tone, and an extensor plantar reflex.

During the initial evaluation blood is obtained for a complete blood count, electrolytes, calcium, phosphorus, glucose, creatinine, blood gases, liver function studies, prothrombin and partial thromboplastin times, ammonium levels, and a toxic screen. In some children, neuroimaging studies are indicated to investigate structural causes of coma (e.g., subdural and epidural hematoma, cerebral edema, brain tumors, and cerebral abscess).

The primary goal of *treatment* is to identify the specific cause of the coma and to correct the problem in a safe and controlled fashion. The use of **invasive intracranial pressure monitoring** should be considered for any infant or child who is suspected of having increased intracranial pressure. Neurologic outcome is improved if the intracranial pressure can be reduced and maintained at 15 mm Hg or less and if the cerebral perfusion pressure (= mean arterial pressure − mean intracranial pressure) is above 50 mm Hg. Raised intracranial pressure may be lowered by sedation and pharmacologic paralysis, mechanical hyperventilation, or osmotherapy with IV mannitol or furosemide.

HEAD INJURIES
(*NELSON TEXTBOOK*, SEC. 20.57)

Accidents are the major cause of morbidity and mortality in children beyond 1 yr of age, and head trauma is the injury most responsible for death. In children, automobile, bicycle, and motorcycle accidents, falls, and nonaccidental trauma (i.e., child abuse) account for a significant number of head injuries in children.

SKULL FRACTURE

A skull fracture in association with head trauma does not necessarily imply injury to the underlying brain. Approximately one third of all children with a history of head injury have radiologic evidence of a skull fracture, but most of these children are intact neurologically at the time of examination and remain free of sequelae.

The most common skull fracture is *linear and nondepressed.* It does not, as a rule, interfere with the function and integrity of the brain, and the outcome in most cases is excellent. *Basilar skull fractures* are associated with bloody discharge from the middle ear or Battle sign. Cranial nerve palsies may occur, particularly in the facial and auditory nerves. CSF otorrhea or rhinorrhea and bacterial meningitis may complicate a basilar skull fracture. *Depressed skull fracture* must be treated surgically if a neurologic deficit results or a compound wound is present.

CONCUSSION

This is defined as a brief but variable and reversible alteration in the level of consciousness associated with transient paralysis of reflexes and amnesia for the events immediately surrounding the injury. During the acute phase of concussion there is loss of tone, flaccidity and areflexia, dilation of the pupils, and brief apnea. Cortical blindness may follow a concussion. Full recovery usually occurs within hours.

SUBDURAL HEMATOMA

This is a collection of bloody fluid between the dura and cerebral mantle. Head trauma produces subdural hematomas by rupturing bridging cortical veins that drain the cerebral cortex. Abused infants who are repeatedly and forcibly shaken are particularly susceptible to this type of head injury.

Infants may present with a bulging anterior fontanel and an enlarged head circumference. The eyes may show a "setting-sun" position as a result of increased intracranial pressure. Retinal or subhyaloid hemorrhages are present in 50% of cases. Focal or generalized seizures may occur.

The CT scan is diagnostic. If there is severe underlying brain injury, such as contusion and intracerebral hemorrhage, the prognosis for recovery is poor.

EPIDURAL HEMATOMA

This results from bleeding into the extradural space from rupture of the middle meningeal artery or a tear in the dural veins owing to direct trauma to the region of the temporal bones. The hematoma often enlarges rapidly and may cause herniation of the temporal lobe, leading to coma, ipsilateral dilation of the pupil, complete third-nerve paresis, and contralateral hemiparesis. The CT scan is diagnostic. Prompt surgical evacuation is indicated.

SEVERE HEAD INJURY

Major insults to the brain may result from contusion, particularly to the frontal lobes or inferolateral portion of the temporal lobes, a penetrating injury, the presence of an intracerebral hemorrhage, and diffuse axonal injury caused by cerebral edema. Initial signs associated with a poor prognosis include fixed and dilated pupils, apneic breathing, decorticate posturing, and a modified Glasgow Coma Scale score of less than 5.

TREATMENT

Cerebral edema is a major complication of head trauma and is the most common cause of death in the first few days after an accident. The management of increased intracranial pressure is discussed above.

Surgical management of head injuries includes the repair of depressed skull fractures and evacuation of hematomas producing a mass effect. Infants with subdural effusions should not undergo percutaneous subdural taps routinely unless the hematomas are large and symptomatic.

Seizures may complicate a head injury and can occur following relatively minor trauma. Seizures that develop within minutes or a few hours of head trauma are frequently brief and do not require long-term anticonvulsants. Convulsions that develop within 24–48 hr of the injury are classified as early post-traumatic seizures and result from cerebral edema, petechial and hemorrhagic lesions, or a penetrating wound. Late post-traumatic seizures tend to develop within 2 yr of the initial insult and are more likely to occur if the original trauma to the brain was severe and the dura disrupted.

PROGNOSIS

The most important determinant of neurologic and intellectual recovery is the duration of coma. If the child survives the immediate consequences of the head injury and recovers from coma within 14 days, the likelihood of normal or near-normal cognitive and neuromotor function is extremely favorable. However, infants less than 2 yr of age with major brain trauma have a uniformly poor prognosis compared with older children.

NEURODEGENERATIVE DISORDERS OF CHILDHOOD
(*NELSON TEXTBOOK*, SECS. 20.58–20.68)

The hallmark of a neurodegenerative disease is progressive deterioration of neurologic function with loss of speech, vision, hearing, or locomotion, often associated with seizures, feeding difficulties, and impairment of intellect. In general, diseases primarily affecting white matter show prominent upper motor neuron signs, whereas those primarily affecting gray matter show a predilection for seizures. Many of these diseases result from specific genetic and biochemical defects. For conditions in which the specific enzyme defect is known, prevention by prenatal diagnosis is possible.

SPHINGOLIPIDOSES

Gangliosidoses

Gangliosides are glycosphingolipids, normal constituents of neuronal and synaptic membranes. Abnormalities in catabolism result in accumulation of the ganglioside within the cell.

GM$_2$ GANGLIOSIDOSES. These are a group of autosomal recessive disorders that consist of several subtypes, including Tay-Sachs disease (TSD), Sandhoff disease, and juvenile GM$_2$ gangliosidosis.

TSD is most prevalent in the Ashkenazi Jewish population and has a carrier rate of approximately 1:30. Infants have marked "startle" reaction to noise. By 6 mo of age there is lag in developmental milestones, and by 1 yr of age the child loses the ability to stand, sit, and vocalize. Early hypotonia develops into progressive spasticity, and relentless deterioration follows with convulsions, blindness, deafness, and retinal cherry red spots in almost all patients. Macrocephaly results from accumulation of GM$_2$ gangliosides in the brain. Children usually die by 3–4 yr of age. A deficiency of hexosaminidase A is found in tissue and lymphocytes of patients with TSD.

Deficiencies of hexosaminidase A and B are found in *Sandhoff disease*, which is similar to TSD in the mode of presentation. Children usually die by 3 yr of age.

KRABBE DISEASE (Globoid Cell Leukodystrophy). Krabbe disease (KD) is a rare autosomal recessive disorder that is due to a deficiency of the lysosomal enzyme galactocerebroside β-galactosidase. There is destruction of myelin as a result of the inability to metabolize galactocerebroside in oligodendrogliocytes. KD presents during the first few months of life with excessive irritability and crying, hyperpyrexia, feeding problems, vomiting, and failure to thrive. Generalized seizures may appear early in the course. Rigidity and opisthotonus and visual inattention resulting from optic atrophy become apparent as the disease progresses. During later stages of the illness, blindness, deafness, areflexia, and decerebrate rigidity constitute the major physical findings. Most patients expire by 2 yr of age.

METACHROMATIC LEUKODYSTROPHY (MLD). MLD is an autosomal recessive disorder characterized by a deficiency of arylsulfatase A activity. This leads to accumulation of cerebroside sulfate within myelin sheath of the CNS and peripheral nervous system.

Late infantile MLD is the classic form, with onset between 1 and 2 yr of age. Initially the child appears clumsy and hypotonic. Deep tendon reflexes are absent or diminished and optic atrophy is present. During the next several months the child can no longer stand, and a deterioration in intellectual function becomes apparent. The speech is slurred and dysarthric, visual fixation is diminished, and nystagmus is present. A progressive decorticate posture develops and death occurs by 5–6 yr of age. Nerve conduction velocities are significantly reduced. CSF protein is elevated. CT images of the brain indicate diffuse symmetric attenuation of the cerebellar and cerebral white matter.

NEURONAL CEROID LIPOFUSCINOSES

These are a group of autosomal recessive neurodegenerative diseases characterized by storage of an autofluorescent substance within neurons and other tissue.

Infantile type (Haltia–Santavuori) begins toward the end of the 1st yr of life with myoclonic seizures, intellectual deterioration, and blindness. Optic atrophy and brownish discoloration of the macula are evident, and cerebellar ataxia is prominent. Death occurs at approximately 10 yr of age.

Late infantile (Jansky-Bielschowsky) is the most common type. It presents with myoclonic seizures between 2 and 4 yr of age in a previously normal child. Dementia and ataxia are combined with progressive loss of visual acuity and microcephaly. Retinal pigmentary abnormalities, optic atrophy, and a subtle brown pigment in the macular region are found. Electron microscopic examination of the storage material in the skin or conjunctival biopsy shows curvilinear bodies or "fingerprint profiles."

Juvenile type (Spielmeyer–Vogt) is characterized by progressive visual loss and intellectual impairment beginning between 5 and 10 yr of age. Funduscopic changes are similar to those for the late infantile type. Myoclonic seizures are not as prominent as in the late infantile type, but dystonic posturing is marked during the late stages of disease. Ultrastructural abnormalities of skin biopsies are present in most cases.

ADRENOLEUKODYSTROPHY

Classic adrenoleukodystrophy is an X-lined recessive disorder with onset between 5 and 15 yr of age. Early symptoms include academic deterioration, behavioral disturbances, gait abnormalities, and generalized seizures. Upper motor neuron signs and ataxia predominate in the late stages. Hypoadrenalism characterized by abnormal skin pigmentation is present in approximately 50% of cases. CT scans and MRI studies of patients indicate periventricular demyelination beginning posteriorly, which advances progressively to the anterior regions of the cerebral white matter. Death occurs within 10 yr of onset.

MISCELLANEOUS CAUSES OF NEURODEGENERATIVE DISORDERS

Pelizaeus–Merzbacher Disease

This X-linked recessive disorder is characterized by nystagmus and roving eye movements with head-nodding during infancy. Ataxia, choreoathetosis, spasticity, and optic atrophy develop. Death occurs in the 2nd or 3rd decade. There is loss of myelin as a result of a defect in the function of the oligodendroglia. The CT scan shows ventricular dilation in the late stages.

Alexander Disease

Alexander disease is a rare disorder that causes progressive macrocephaly during the 1st yr of life. Pathologic examination of the brain features the deposition of eosinophilic hyaline bodies (Rosenthal fibers) throughout the brain beneath the pia mater. Degeneration of the white matter that is most prominent in the frontal lobes is detectable by neuroimaging scans. The child develops progressive loss of intellect, spasticity, and unresponsive seizures causing death by 5 yr of age.

Menkes Kinky Hair Disease

Menkes disease is an X-linked recessive disorder of copper metabolism. Symptoms begin during the first few months of life and include hypothermia, hypotonia, and generalized myoclonic seizures. Pili torti (twisted hair), mental retardation, and optic atrophy are constant features. Serum copper and ceruloplasmin levels are low because of a defect in copper absorption and transport across the gut.

Rett Syndrome

This is a disorder of unknown etiology that occurs exclusively in female children and has an incidence of 1:15,000. Development proceeds normally until 1 yr of age, when regression of language and motor milestones and acquired microcephaly become apparent. An ataxic gait or fine tremor of the hand is an early neurologic finding. A peculiar sighing respiration, with intermittent apnea, repetitive hand-wringing movements with a loss of purposeful use of the hands, and autistic features also develop. Generalized tonic–clonic convulsions occur in the majority of cases. After the initial period of neurologic regression, the disease process appears to plateau.

VASCULAR DISORDERS
(*NELSON TEXTBOOK*, SECS. 20.69–20.73)

ARTERIAL THROMBOSIS

Thrombosis of the internal carotid artery may result from blunt trauma caused by a fall on a pencil or a stick in the child's mouth. The injury produces a tear in the intima of the vessel wall, which may lead to the formation of a dissecting aneurysm. The thrombus may break off and embolize. The onset of symptoms may be delayed up to 24 hr following the accident, with a stuttering but progressive flaccid hemiplegia, lethargy, and aphasia if the dominant hemisphere is involved.

Collagen vascular diseases, particularly lupus erythematosus and polyarteritis nodosa, frequently produce cerebral symptoms and signs resulting from vasculitis and thrombosis.

Basal arterial occlusion with telangectasia, or *Moyamoya disease*, has a characteristic angiogram. Children present with intermittent episodes of transient ischemic attacks coupled with progressive neurologic signs and severe disability.

Occlusion of small distal arteries is associated with diabetes mellitus, neurofibromatosis, sickle cell disease, homocystinuria, and IV drug abuse.

VENOUS THROMBOSIS

Bacterial meningitis may cause thrombosis of the superficial cortical and deep penetrating veins, leading to hemiplegia. *Severe dehydration* during infancy may cause thrombosis of the superior sagittal sinus as a result of hyperviscosity and sludging of blood.

INTRACRANIAL HEMORRHAGE

Arteriovenous malformations result from the failure of normal capillary bed development between arteries and veins during embryogenesis. They may rupture, causing an intracerebral hemorrhage. Arteriovenous malformations typically are located in the cerebral hemispheres but also may be located in the cerebellum, brain stem, or spinal cord. An **arteriovenous malformation of the vein of Galen** during infancy may cause high-output congestive heart failure as a result of shunting of large volumes of blood.

Cerebral aneurysms usually are asymptomatic in children.

EMBOLISM

Cardiac causes of cerebral embolisms include arrythmias, myxoma, and bacterial endocarditis that results in a mycotic aneurysm. Air emboli may complicate surgery, and fat emboli occur with fracture of long bones. Septic emboli may seed in the cerebral vessels and evolve into an area of cerebritis or cerebral abscess. In children over 2 yr of age, a *brain abscess* also may be a complication of embolization resulting from congenital heart disease with right-to-left shunt.

BRAIN TUMORS IN CHILDREN
(*NELSON TEXTBOOK*, SECS. 20.74 AND 20.75)

EPIDEMIOLOGY

Brain tumors are second only to leukemia as the most prevalent malignancy in childhood. Infratentorial tumors are more prevalent in the pediatric age group.

CLINICAL MANIFESTATIONS

Generally, there are two distinct patterns of presentation: symptoms and signs of increased intracranial pressure or focal neurologic signs. Tumors located within the posterior fossa primarily produce symptoms and signs of increased intracranial pressure as a result of obstruction of CSF pathways. Headaches, vomiting, papilledema, ataxia, diplopia, and head tilt are features of posterior fossa tumors. Supratentorial tumors are more likely to be associated with focal abnormalities, including hemiparesis, long-tract signs, and focal seizures.

INFRATENTORIAL TUMORS

The *cerebellar astrocytoma* is the most common posterior fossa tumor of childhood and has the best prognosis. These tumors tend to be cystic and have a mural nodule of solid tumor. The tumor causes hydrocephalus by obstructing the aqueduct of Sylvius or fourth ventricle. The treatment is surgical resection, and the 5-yr survival rate approaches 90%.

The *medulloblastoma* is the next most common posterior fossa tumor in the pediatric age group and is the most prevalent brain tumor in children less than 7 yr of age. Medulloblastomas grow rapidly to fill the fourth ventricle or invade the adjacent cerebellar hemisphere. Children less than 4 yr of age have a poorer prognosis than older patients. All patients are treated with surgical extirpation and irradiation. Irradiation is directed to the entire neuraxis because of the propensity for medulloblastomas to seed to remote sites. The expected 5-yr survival rate for children with a small tumor without dissemination is 70%. In children with a large tumor, chemotherapy in addition to surgery and irradiation results in a survival rate of approximately 45%.

Brain stem gliomas are the third most frequent posterior fossa tumor in children. Diffuse infiltrating tumors of the brain stem are found to be anaplastic astrocytomas. The symptoms and signs result from invasion and destruction of cranial nerve nuclei and the pyramidal tracts. The most common cranial nerve symptoms include diplopia and facial weakness. The primary treatment is irradiation. The mean 5-yr survival rate is approximately 20%. Hyperfractionated radiation therapy and chemotherapy also are being studied.

SUPRATENTORIAL TUMORS

The *craniopharyngioma* is the most common supratentorial tumor in children. The tumor may be confined to the sella turcica or it may extend through the diaphragma sella and compress the optic nerve system, pons, or third ventricle, producing hydrocephalus and papilledema. The tumor consists of solid and cystic areas that have a tendency to calcify. With complete or near-complete removal, 75% of patients experience no further recurrence. Endocrine disorders, including diabetes insipidus, hypothyroidism, and growth hormone and adrenocortical deficiency, may develop postoperatively.

Optic nerve gliomas present with decreased visual acuity and pallor of the disks. The tumors are primarily low-grade astrocytomas, and approximately 25% of patients have associated neurofibromatosis. Most centers follow these patients and resort to surgery, radiation, or chemotherapy when progression into the optic chiasm or hypothalamus is documented. Radiotherapy in older children with chiasmic/hypothalamic gliomas results in a 10-yr survival rate of almost 90%.

Astrocytoma and related glial tumors (ependymoma and oligodendrogliomas) have a less favorable prognosis when located in the cerebral hemisphere compared with the cerebellum. Clinical features include complex partial seizures or subtle upper motor neuron signs. Low-grade astrocytomas are treated with surgical excision and have a 50–80% 5-yr survival rate. High-grade astrocytomas are treated with surgery, radiation therapy, and chemotherapeutic regimens, resulting in a 5-yr survival rate of approximately 50%.

Tumors that arise in the region of the pineal gland cause pressure on the quadrigeminal plate and produce **Parinaud syndrome,** consisting of paralysis of conjugate upward movement of the eyes. Radiosensitive germinoma has a 5-yr survival rate greater than 75%. Some tumors (e.g., pinealomas) are resistant to radiation and are more likely to respond to chemotherapy, whereas others, such as teratomas, may be treated exclusively by surgery.

DIAGNOSIS

The MRI is the best tool for the delineation of brain tumors in children because of its fine resolution and multiplanar capabilities.

SPINAL CORD DISORDERS IN CHILDREN
(*NELSON TEXTBOOK*, SECS. 20.76–20.81)

SPINAL CORD TUMORS

In children, spinal cord tumors account for approximately 20% of neuraxial tumors. *Intramedullary tumors,* mostly low-grade astrocytomas, arise within the substance of the cord and grow slowly by infiltration, usually in the cervical region. *Extramedullary, intradural tumors,* such as neurofibromas, ganglioneuromas, and meningiomas, tend to be benign and arise from neural crest tissue. *Extramedullary, extradural tumors* characteristically consist of a metastatic lesion, particularly neuroblastoma, sarcoma, and leukemia.

Intramedullary tumors may cause sphincter disturbance and segmental lower motor neuron signs. Extramedullary tumors often present with back pain, paresthesias, and possible weakness. Extramedullary tumors that grow rapidly will cause compression on the spinal cord, leading to flaccid paraplegia and sphincter disturbance. Prompt diagnosis and surgical management are necessary to prevent irreversible damage to the cord.

Many spinal cord tumors can be totally and safely resected. Surgical removal of benign extramedullary tumor is associated with a good prognosis. For extramedullary metastatic neuroblastoma that presents with paraplegia, immediate radiation therapy is indicated.

SPINAL CORD TRAUMA

Common causes of spinal cord injury include traumatic breech deliveries, extensive shaking of the abused child, automobile and diving accidents, falls from playground equipment, and congenital defects such as the underlying vertebral abnormality in Down syndrome. A *severe cord injury* may present with **spinal shock,** consisting of flaccidity, areflexia, and loss of sensation. This may persist for up to 4 wk and is replaced by spasticity, hyperreflexia, and extensor plantar responses.

TETHERED CORD AND DIASTEMATOMYELIA

A *tethered cord* results when a thickened rope-like filum terminale persists and anchors the conus at or below the L2 level.

Diastematomyelia, a division of the spinal cord into two halves by the projection of a fibrocartilaginous or body septum, may coexist with a tethered cord. Midline skin lesion, including lipoma, cutaneous hemangioma, tuft of hair, hyperpigmentation, or a dermal pit, are common. Infants may have asymmetric growth in a foot or leg. Abnormal bladder function, progressive scoliosis, and diffuse lower extremity pain are common findings in the child. MRI study is diagnostic. Surgical management halts the progression of neurologic signs.

SYRINGOMYELIA

Syringomyelia is a cystic cavity within the spinal cord, which may or may not communicate with the CSF pathways. Communicating syringomyelia is frequently associated with the Chiari type I malformation, whereas the noncommunicating syrinx is complicated by cord tumors, trauma, and arachnoiditis.

Loss of pain and temperature sensation with preservation of light touch may be seen. Progressive enlargement of the cavity may impinge on the anterior horn cells and corticospinal tracts, resulting in muscle wasting of the hands, areflexia in the upper extremities, and upper motor neuron signs in the lower extremities. The MRI is the study of choice. Decompression of the foramen magnum and the upper cervical vertebrae is recommended when the syrinx is associated with a Chiari type I anomaly.

TRANSVERSE MYELITIS

Transverse myelitis is characterized by the abrupt onset of progressive weakness and sensory disturbances in the lower extremities. This may be due to cell-mediated autoimmune response, direct viral invasion of the spinal cord, or an autoimmune vasculitis. The legs are weak and flaccid. A sensory level is present, usually in the midthoracic region. Sphincter disturbances are common. Flaccidity gradually evolves to spasticity. The CSF shows moderate lymphocyte pleocytosis and a normal or slightly elevated protein. There may be residual deficits, including bowel and bladder dysfunction and weakness in the lower extremities.

19

NEUROMUSCULAR DISORDERS

The term *neuromuscular disease* refers to disorders of the motor unit. The motor unit consists of: (1) a motor neuron in the brain stem or anterior horn of the spinal cord, (2) its axons, (3) the neuromuscular junction, and (4) all muscle fibers innervated by a single motor neuron.

EVALUATION AND INVESTIGATION
(NELSON TEXTBOOK, SEC. 21.1)

CLINICAL MANIFESTATIONS

In general, the distribution of weakness in myopathies is proximal and that in neuropathies is distal. Deep tendon reflexes are generally lost in neuropathies and in motor neuron diseases and are diminished but preserved in myopathies. Fasciculations of muscle, best seen in the tongue, are a sign of denervation. Sensory abnormalities indicate neuropathy.

Generalized hypotonia and developmental delay are the most common presenting signs of neuromuscular disease in infants and young children. A prenatal history of decreased fetal movements and intrauterine growth retardation often is found in patients who are symptomatic at birth.

LABORATORY FINDINGS

Serum Enzymes

Serum creatine phophokinase (CPK or CK) is characteristically elevated in muscular dystrophies. However, in many diseases of the motor unit CK is not elevated.

Nerve Conduction Velocity

Slowing of the motor and sensory nerve conduction velocities (NCVs) is seen in various neuropathies.

Electromyography

Characteristic electromyographic (EMG) patterns may distinguish denervation from myopathic involvement. The specific type of myopathy usually is not diagnosed.

Muscle Biopsy

The muscle biopsy is the most important and specific diagnostic study of muscle. Neurogenic and myopathic processes can be distinguished. Specific myopathies and specific enzymatic deficiencies may be determined.

DEVELOPMENTAL DISORDERS OF MUSCLE
(*NELSON TEXTBOOK*, SECS. 21.2–21.10)

Congenital myopathies are a group of disorders in which distinctive morphologic and histochemical abnormalities are found. Many are reminiscent of stages in the embryologic development of muscle and may represent aberration of development. These disorders share many phenotypic features. Most congenital myopathies are nonprogressive, although some patients show slow clinical deterioration.

MYOTUBULAR (CENTRONUCLEAR) MYOPATHY

Pathogenesis

The morphologic appearance of myofibers in this disorder is similar to that of the fetal muscle during the myotubular stage of development at 8–15 wk of gestation. A row of central nuclei lies within a core of cytoplasm; myofibrils form a cylinder around this core.

Clinical Manifestations

Decreased fetal movements are perceived in late gestation. At birth, affected infants have a thin muscle mass involving the axial, limb-girdle, and distal muscles; severe generalized hypotonia; and diffuse weakness. Respiratory efforts may be ineffective. Infants have a poor suck and swallow and facial weakness. Deep tendon reflexes are weak or absent.

Laboratory Findings and Diagnosis

CK is normal. The EMG usually is normal or shows minimal nonspecific myopathic features in early infancy. NCV is usually normal. The electrocardiogram is normal. Muscle biopsy is diagnostic at birth. Muscle fibers are small and have centrally placed nuclei.

Genetics

X-linked recessive is the most common mode of inheritance. Autosomal dominant and autosomal recessive forms are rarer.

Prognosis

About 75% of severely affected infants die within the first few months of life. Survivors have major physical disabilities and remain severely hypotonic.

NEMALINE ROD DISEASE

Pathogenesis

Nemaline rods are rod-shaped inclusion-like abnormal structures within muscle fibers. They consist of excessive Z-band material with an ultrastructure similar to that of normal Z-bands.

Clinical Manifestations

Severe infantile and juvenile forms are known. Generalized hypotonia and weakness in bulbar and respiratory muscles are present. *Infants* have a poor cry, weak suck, and dysphagia. The head is dolichocephalic. High-arched palate or cleft is present. Infants may be very weak at birth, and some die in the neonatal period. In the *juvenile* form, patients are ambulatory and are able to perform most daily tasks. Weakness is nonprogressive but patients have more difficulty over time.

Laboratory Findings

Serum CK is normal. Muscle biopsy is diagnostic, showing nemaline rods.

Genetics

Autosomal dominant and autosomal recessive forms are well documented. An X-linked dominant form may occur in girls.

CENTRAL CORE DISEASE

This autosomal dominant disease is characterized by central cores within muscle fibers that lack myofibrils and organelles. Infantile hypotonia, proximal weakness, and muscle wasting are typical features. The weakness is nonprogressive and usually is not severely disabling. Congenital dislocation of the hips and skeletal deformities are common. This disease is associated with malignant hyperthermia, and special precautions should be taken before anesthesia. CK is normal. Muscle biopsy is diagnostic.

ARTHROGRYPOSIS

Arthrogryposis multiplex congenita (AMC) is not a disease but a descriptive term that signifies multiple congenital contractures. It may be due to neurogenic and myopathic processes. Neurogenic causes include infantile spinal muscular atrophy and Pena–Shokeir and Martin–Walker syndromes. Myopathic causes include congenital myotonic dystrophy and other congenital myopathies.

MUSCULAR DYSTROPHIES
(*NELSON TEXTBOOK*, SECS. 21.11–21.18)

Muscular dystrophies are distinguished from other neuromuscular diseases by the (1) primary myopathy, (2) genetic basis for the disorder, (3) progressive course, and (4) degeneration and death of muscle fibers at some stage in the disease.

DUCHENNE MUSCULAR DYSTROPHY

Duchenne muscular dystrophy, an X-linked disorder, is the most common hereditary neuromuscular disease. The incidence is 1:3,600 liveborn male infants.

Clinical Manifestations

Duchenne muscular dystrophy rarely is symptomatic at birth. Walking may be accomplished at a normal age, but hip girdle weakness may be evident as early as the 2nd yr. Gower sign and a hip waddle is apparent by 5–6 yr of age. There is enlargement of the calves (pseudohypertrophy). Cardiomyopathy, mild intellectual impairment, kyphoscoliosis, and contractures are seen. Progressive weakness occurs, and affected boys usually are nonambulatory by 12 yr of age. Death occurs by the late teen years.

Laboratory Findings

Serum CK is markedly elevated (15,000–35,000 IU/L). The EMG shows myopathic features.

Diagnosis

Muscle biopsy is diagnostic and shows dystrophic changes (i.e., scattered degenerating and regenerating myofibers, foci of mononuclear inflammatory cell infiltrates, and endomysial connective tissue proliferation).

Genetic Etiology and Pathogenesis

Molecular genetics of Duchenne muscular dystrophy reveal that there is a deletion at the breakpoint of the Xp21 gene, which encodes for a protein of sarcolemmal membranes called *dystrophin*. Dystrophin is absent in the muscle of patients with Duchenne muscular dystrophy. The exact function of dystrophin not known. A new mutation occurs in 30% of patients.

Treatment

There is no medical cure for Duchenne muscular dystrophy. Corticosteroids have been tried with mixed results. Myoblast transfer is a new experimental approach to treatment, but its success is not established.

BECKER MUSCULAR DYSTROPHY

Becker muscular dystrophy is similar to Duchenne muscular dystrophy but has a later onset and follows a slower, more protracted course. Patients are ambulatory until age 16 yr or later. Death occurs in the mid- or late 20s. Becker muscular dystrophy has X-linked recessive transmission. There is a mutation of the Xp21 gene as in Duchenne muscular dystrophy, but there is a different phenotypic expression.

MYOTONIC MUSCULAR DYSTROPHY

Myotonic dystrophy (Steinert disease) has an incidence of 1:30,000. It has an autosomal dominant inheritance with varied expressivity. The defective gene has been isolated to chromosome 19, but the gene has not been identified.

Clinical Manifestations

SEVERE NEONATAL FORM. The severe neonatal form may occur in infants born to mothers with myotonic dystrophy and is characterized by impaired swallowing and sucking, facial weakness, and multiple joint contractures. About 75% of severely affected neonates die within the 1st yr.

JUVENILE FORM. In usual clinical forms there is facial weakness, hypotonia, and a characteristic facial appearance, consisting of an inverted V-shaped upper lip and scalloped, concave temporalis muscles. Weakness is mild in the first few years. The juvenile form is characterized by distal weakness and atrophy, facial diplegia, and myotonia (slow relaxation of muscle after contraction). As the child grows older, cataracts, frontal baldness, intellectual dullness, and gonadal atrophy may become apparent. Cardiac dysrhythmia may occur.

Laboratory Findings

Classical myotonic discharges on EMG (high-frequency, repetitive discharges that have a "dive-bomber" quality) are seen in most children but may be absent during infancy. Serum CK is normal or mildly elevated. Muscle biopsy shows many fibers with central nuclei and selective atrophy of type I fibers.

LIMB-GIRDLE MUSCULAR DYSTROPHY

This is a group of progressive hereditary myopathies that affect the muscles of the hip and shoulder girdles. Most cases are of autosomal recessive inheritance. The onset is in middle to late childhood or adult life. There is a slow rate of progression, and patients usually are confined to a wheelchair by 30 yr of age.

FACIOSCAPULOHUMERAL MUSCULAR DYSTROPHY

This is a group of disorders with weakness in the muscles of the face and shoulder girdles. It has an autosomal dominant inheritance. The onset is in childhood to adult life, and it is slowly progressive.

CONGENITAL MUSCULAR DYSTROPHY

This is a group of disorders with onset in neonatal period, manifesting with diffuse hypotonia and contractures. It has an autosomal recessive inheritance. *Fukuyama type* is associated with brain malformation and severe cardiomyopathy. Serum CK is moderately elevated. The EMG shows nonspecific myopathic features. Muscle biopsy is diagnostic.

ENDOCRINE AND METABOLIC MYOPATHIES
(NELSON TEXTBOOK, SECS. 21.19–21.27)

STEROID-INDUCED MYOPATHY

Both natural Cushing disease or exogenous corticosteroid administration may cause progressive proximal weakness, increased serum CK, and a myopathic EMG. Muscle biopsy may be necessary for diagnosis.

POTASSIUM-RELATED PERIODIC PARALYSIS

Episodic weakness or paralysis known as *periodic paralysis* is associated with transient alteration in serum potassium, usually hypokalemia but occasionally hyperkalemia. This disorder has an autosomal dominant inheritance. During the attacks, the child is unable to move and gradually recovers muscle strength during the next few minutes or hours.

GLYCOGENOSES

Glycogenosis II (Pompe Disease)

Pompe disease is due to an autosomal recessively inherited deficiency of acid maltase. In the *infantile form,* there is severe generalized myopathy with diffuse hypotonia and weakness. Massive cardiomyopathy and hepatomegaly are characteristic. CK is greatly elevated. Muscle biopsy reveals vacuolar myopathy and deficiency of acid maltase. Death occurs in infancy or early childhood.

Glycogenosis V (McArdle Disease)

This is an autosomal recessive disorder resulting from a deficiency of myophosphorylase. It is characterized by exercise-induced cramps, weakness, myoglobinuria, and elevation of serum CK. Strength is normal in between attacks.

LIPID MYOPATHIES

Muscle Carnitine Deficiency

This disorder is due to an autosomal recessively inherited defect in the transport of dietary carnitine across the intestinal mucosa. Carnitine is the obligatory carrier of long- and medium-chain fatty acids into the muscle mitochondria. The course resembles progressive muscular dystrophy, with generalized proximal myopathy. The onset is in late childhood or adolescence. Serum CK is mildly elevated. Muscle biopsy shows lipid-filled vacuoles and nonspecific changes suggestive of muscular dystrophy. *Treatment* includes large doses of carnitine and diet low in long-chain fatty acids.

Systemic Carnitine Deficiency

This is an autosomal recessive disorder resulting from impaired renal and hepatic synthesis of carnitine. Clinically, there is progressive proximal myopathy. Muscle biopsy changes are similar to those of muscle carnitine deficiency, but the onset is earlier. Children may have Reye-like episodes, with hypoglycemia, metabolic ketoacidosis, and encephalopathy. Low serum and tissue carnitine levels are found. *Treatment* with L-carnitine improves maintenance of glucose.

INFLAMMATORY MYOPATHIES
(*NELSON TEXTBOOK*, SECS. 21.28–21.33)

DERMATOMYOSITIS

Dermatomyositis is a nonhereditary multisystem disease that produces progressive weakness. Clinical manifestations include: (1) proximal weakness that progresses for weeks or months with myalgia and muscle tenderness; (2) greatly elevated serum CK; (3) myopathic changes on EMG; and (4) muscle biopsy showing degeneration and regeneration of muscle fibers, intramuscular inflammation, and *perifascicular atrophy*. Dermatologic lesions include violaceous heliotropic rash, later involving the extensor surfaces of the fingers, elbows, and knees. *Treatment* includes corticosteroids and immunosuppressive agents.

DISORDERS OF NEUROMUSCULAR TRANSMISSION
(*NELSON TEXTBOOK*, SECS. 21.34–21.37)

MYASTHENIA GRAVIS

Myasthenia gravis is due to a defect in neuromuscular junction transmission. There is a decreased number of available acetylcholine (ACh) receptors as a result of circulating receptor-binding antibodies. It is a nonhereditary, autoimmune disorder.

Clinical Manifestations

In *juvenile myasthenia gravis,* ptosis and extraocular muscle weakness are early signs. Dysphagia and facial weakness may occur. Limb-girdle muscles also may be involved. Rapid fatigue of muscle is characteristic.

Transient neonatal myasthenia gravis is due to placentally transferred anti-ACh receptor antibodies when the mother has myasthenia gravis. Clinical findings include respiratory insufficiency, inability to suck or swallow, and generalized hypotonia and weakness. After the antibodies disappear, the infants have normal strength.

Laboratory Findings and Diagnosis

The EMG is specific, with decremental response to repetitive nerve stimulation in affected muscles. Anti-ACh antibodies may be present in serum. An enlarged thymus may be seen, but thymomas are rare in children with myasthenia gravis. The edrophonium (Tensilon) test may show improvement in muscle strength and fatigability.

Treatment

Cholinesterase-inhibiting drugs are the primary therapeutic agents. Corticosteroids, thymectomy, and plasmapharesis also are used. In transient neonatal myasthenia gravis, infants require short-term treatment with cholinesterase inhibitors.

OTHER CAUSES OF NEUROMUSCULAR BLOCKADE

Infantile Botulism

This disorder results from the ingestion of *Clostridium botulinum* spores that germinate in the intestinal tract and release a toxin. *Clinical manifestations* include ileus, constipation, pupillary dilation, bilateral ptosis or external ophthalmoplegia, and apneic spells. Generalized hypotonia and weakness then develop and may progress to respiratory failure. *Diagnosis* can be made by recovery of the bacterium and the toxin from feces. EMG with repetitive stimulation may show evidence of neuromuscular junction blockade.

DISORDERS OF MOTOR NEURONS

Spinal Muscular Atrophies

Spinal muscular atrophies (SMA) are a group of degenerative disease of the motor neurons that begin in fetal life and continue to be progressive in infancy and childhood. Most cases show autosomal recessive inheritance.

CLINICAL MANIFESTATIONS

Severe Infantile Form (Werdnig–Hoffmann Disease, SMA Type 1). Infants with Werdnig–Hoffmann disease have severe hypotonia, generalized weakness, thin muscle mass, areflexia, fasciculations of the tongue, and facial weakness. Infants lie flaccid with little movement. More than two thirds die by 2 yr of age as a result of respiratory failure.

Juvenile Form (Kugelberg–Welander Disease, Type 3). Affected individuals may appear normal in infancy. There is progressive proximal weakness, particularly in the shoulder girdle. Patients are ambulatory and may live into middle adult life. Fasciculations may be seen in muscles, particularly in the tongue.

LABORATORY TESTS AND DIAGNOSIS. In SMA, motor NCVs are normal but the EMG shows evidence of denervation. Muscle biopsy reveals a characteristic perinatal denervation pattern. At autopsy, extensive neuronal degeneration and gliosis in the anterior horns of the spinal cord and brain stem motor nuclei are found.

HEREDITARY MOTOR-SENSORY NEUROPATHIES
(*NELSON TEXTBOOK*, SECS. 21.38–21.45)

The hereditary motor-sensory neuropathies (HMSN) are a group of inherited, progressive diseases of the peripheral nerves.

PERONEAL MUSCULAR ATROPHY (Charcot-Marie-Tooth Disease, HSMN Type I)

This is the most common inherited neuropathy, with a prevalence of 3.8:100,000. It has an autosomal dominant inheritance with 83% expressivity.

Clinical Manifestations

The onset is in late childhood or early adolescence. The peroneal and tibial nerves are most severely affected. "Storklike" legs occur as a result of wasting of muscles of the anterior compartment. Progressive bilateral weakness of dorsiflexion of the ankle lead to eventual foot drop. Patients develop pes cavus deformities as a result of denervation of intrinsic foot muscles. The disease is slowly progressive throughout life. There is sensory involvement of large myelinated fibers, with proprioceptive and vibratory sense abnormalities. Peripheral nerves often are palpably enlarged. Deep tendon reflexes are absent distally.

Laboratory Findings and Diagnosis

Motor and sensory NCVs are greatly reduced. Muscle biopsy shows evidence of denervation and reinnervation. Sural nerve biopsy is diagnostic, showing reduced large- and medium-sized myelinated fibers and *onion-bulb formation* resulting from proliferated Schwann cell cytoplasm surrounding the axons.

PERONEAL MUSCULAR ATROPHY, AXONAL TYPE (HSMN Type II)

This is clinically and genetically similar to HMSN type I, but the rate of progression is slower and the disability is less. Sural nerve biopsy reveals axonal degeneration rather than demyelination.

TOXIC NEUROPATHIES
(*NELSON TEXTBOOK*, SEC. 21.46)

Many chemicals, toxins, heavy metals, and drugs are capable of causing peripheral neuropathy. Antimetabolite drugs, such as vincristine, produce an axonal polyneuropathy.

GUILLAIN–BARRÉ SYNDROME
(*NELSON TEXTBOOK*, SEC. 21.50)

Guillain–Barré syndrome is a postinfectious polyneuropathy that causes demyelination in nerves. Paralysis follows a nonspecific viral infection by about 10 days. Weakness begins in the lower extremities and progressively involves the trunk, upper limbs, and finally the bulbar muscles (*ascending paralysis*). Respiratory insufficiency may result. Deep tendon reflexes are lost, usually early in the course.

Children with this syndrome have a good prognosis, with spontaneous recovery beginning by 2–3 wk. Most regain full strength, although some are left with residual weakness. Autonomic nerves also may be involved, resulting in lability of blood pressure and cardiac rate and postural hypotension.

CSF protein is elevated to more than twice the upper limit of normal, with fewer than 10 white blood cells/mm^3. Motor NCVs are greatly reduced, and the EMG may show evidence of acute denervation.

Treatment includes respiratory support, if needed, and plasma exchange or intravenous gamma globulin.

20

DISORDERS OF THE EYE AND EAR

PEDIATRIC OPHTHALMOLOGY
(*NELSON TEXTBOOK*, SECS. 22.1–22.17)

EXAMINATION OF THE EYE

All children should undergo complete examination of the eyes in the first years of life because these years are essential to normal ocular development. Examination should begin with assessment of the external structures and proceed to an assessment of the pupils, extraocular movements, and alignment. Ophthalmoscopic examination of the fundi should be performed next, followed by evaluation of the visual acuity and visual fields. Biomicroscopy (slit lamp examination) and tonometry may be performed by trained personnel.

External examination includes gross estimates of orbital symmetry followed by assessment of the lids, lashes, lacrimal apparatus, conjunctiva, and sclera. The size and symmetry of the pupils should be assessed for proper direct and consensual reactions to light and accommodation. Ocular motility and alignment should be assessed by having the child follow an object in all directions of gaze.

Funduscopic examination is best performed after pupillary dilation with short-acting mydriatics, such as tropicamide or phenylephrine. Assessment should include examination of the macula, disk, and major retinal vessels.

Visual field examination typically is performed using confrontation techniques with finger counting in each of the quadrants, although more accurate methods are available.

Visual acuity is best measured by the standard Snellen chart, although completion of this examination is impossible in young or noncompliant children. In these cases, retinoscopy may provide reliable objective estimates of visual acuity, using different diopters to bring the retinal vessels into focus. Most term infants are born functionally hyperopic (farsighted); their retinal vessels usually are brought into focus using a convex, positive-numbered lens on the ophthalmoscope. Premature infants often are born myopic (nearsighted); their retinal vessels usually are brought into focus using a concave, negative-numbered lens on the ophthalmoscope. The greater the refractive abnormality, the greater the number of the lens required to bring the retinal vessels into focus.

ABNORMALITIES OF REFRACTION

Normal visual acuity requires the refraction and focus of parallel rays of light on the retina. There are three main types of deficiency in visual acuity: hyperopia, myopia, and astigmatism.

Hyperopia results from conditions in which the parallel rays of light come to focus posterior to the retina. Such conditions include a short anteroposterior diameter of the eye, posterior dislocation of the lens, or a deficient refractive power of the cornea or lens. Hyperopic patients may display disinterest in close activities, such as reading a book. In an effort to change the curvature of the lens, the ciliary muscle and the adductor muscles of the eye are stimulated. Although this may better bring objects into focus, such accommodative effort may lead to esotropia (see below). Correction of hyperopia is provided by convex lenses.

Myopia results from conditions in which parallel rays of light come to focus anterior to the retina. Such conditions include a long anteroposterior diameter of the eye, anterior dislocation of the lens, or heightened refractive power of the cornea or lens. Symptoms of myopia include frowning or squinting, with disinterest in distant activities, such as reading the blackboard. The degree of myopia tends to increase with age. Concave lenses are used in treatment.

Astigmatism most commonly is due to irregularity in the curvature of the cornea, leading to differences in visual acuity in various meridians of the eye. Symptoms include frowning, squinting, and headaches. Cylindric or spherocylindric lenses may be used in therapy.

DISORDERS OF VISION

Amblyopia

This is subnormal visual acuity despite correction of refractive errors. It usually results from prolonged sensory deprivation or improper ocular alignment. It may be unilateral or bilateral. Causes of sensory deprivation include cataracts and uncorrected anisometropia (a significantly different refractive state in one eye compared with the other). Fixed strabismus also may lead to a tendency to suppress the image of the deviated eye. If left untreated, amblyopia may result.

Patients are most susceptible to amblyopia in the first months and years of life. Successful management requires prompt diagnosis and intervention.

Treatment is based on provision of the clearest possible image to the retina (removal of a cataract, correction of refractive errors) and forced stimulation of the amblyopic eye (patching the good eye).

Other Disorders

Other disorders of vision include *amaurosis* (partial or total loss of vision), *nyctalopia* (night blindness), and *diplopia* (double vision).

ABNORMALITIES OF THE PUPILS AND IRIS

Iris

There are a number of different abnormalities of the iris. *Aniridia* is characterized by hypoplasia and may be associated with Wilms tumor. *Coloboma* is a developmental abnormality in the shape of the iris that may occur as an isolated defect or as part of a syndrome. *Heterochromia* refers to variation in color between or within the irises. *Lisch nodules* of the iris may be a sign of neurofibromatosis.

Pupils

Disorders of the pupils are equally varied. *Anisocoria* refers to an inequality in the sizes of the pupils and may be due to a variety of causes. A dilated pupil most commonly is due to purposeful or accidental instillation of a cycloplegic agent, although trauma, infection, dysautonomia, and increased intracranial pressure with impending transtentorial herniation should be considered. Miosis, ptosis, and enophthalmos are characteristic of Horner syndrome (oculosympathetic paresis).

Leukocoria is the term used to describe a white pupillary reflex on ophthalmoscopic examination. The finding of leukocoria requires complete ophthalmologic examination in an effort to treat the underlying problem and prevent amblyopia. The differential diagnosis includes cataract and retinoblastoma.

DISORDERS OF EYE MOVEMENT AND ALIGNMENT

Strabismus

Strabismus refers to a dyscoordination of conjugate gaze such that there is improper alignment of the visual axes. There are two main types of strabismus, *heterophoria* and *heterotropia*. The former refers to a gaze preference or latent tendency toward malalignment that is only apparent under certain conditions. The latter refers to persistently visible malalignment. Phorias and tropias may be further described by the prefixes, *eso-, exo-, hyper-,* and *hypo-,* depending on the visual quadrant to which the eye deviates (eso = medial, exo = lateral, hyper = up, hypo = down).

CLINICAL TYPES. Strabismus may be due to a number of different conditions that most commonly fit into one of three catagories: paralytic, nonparalytic, and accommodative. *Paralytic strabismus* is uncommon in childhood and may herald serious underlying disease. The affected eye is tonically deviated. In an effort to avoid diplopia, the patient may close one eye or turn his or her head in an effort to compensate for the affected muscle. *Nonparalytic strabismus* is more common in children and includes the infantile tropias. They are best treated by surgery. *Accommodative esotropia* is seen in children with hyperopia who attempt to increase visual acuity by contracting the ciliary muscle. Because this muscle and those leading to adduction are both stimulated by cranial nerve III, esotropia results. This condition is best corrected with convex lenses.

ASSESSMENT.   Strabismus is easily assessed in the pediatrician's office using the Hirschberg test and the cover–uncover test. The **Hirschberg test** assesses the symmetry of the reflection of a light source on the cornea. With the patient staring at a distant target, the **cover–uncover test** looks for gaze deviation when the eyes are sequentially covered and uncovered. The eye with a tropia will move to focus on the target when the fixating eye is covered. The eye with a phoria will deviate when covered and will move to focus on the target when it is uncovered.

TREATMENT.   Treatment of strabismus involves correction of any defects in visual acuity and optimization of alignment. Intervention is especially important in a child with a persistant, unilateral strabismus because the risk of amblyopia is high.

DISORDERS OF THE LIDS

Ptosis exists when the upper eyelid droops below its normal level. Ptosis may be congenital or acquired. It may occur in isolation or as part of more widespread disease. Acquired ptosis may be due to any disease causing third-nerve palsy, including myasthenia gravis, infant botulism, trauma, inflammation, or tumors. If persistent, cosmetic surgery may be required.

Lagophthalmos occurs when there is incomplete closure of the lid. It may be paralytic, spastic, atrophic, or accompanying proptosis or buphthalmos. Exposure of the eye leads to dessication, abrasion, and ulceration of the cornea. Treatment involves protection of the eye with artificial tears.

Blepharitis is an inflammatory condition of the lid margins that usually is due to seborrhea or infection with *Staphylococcus aureus*. The former should be treated with cleansing and scale removal, with concurrent treatment of disease on the scalp. Treatment for the latter involves the use of topical antibiotics. Pediculosis may affect the eyelashes, mimicking blepharitis.

A **chalazion** is a painless, granulomatous lesion affecting the meibomian gland. It appears as a chronic, firm, nontender nodule in the lid. Treatment may include warm compresses or surgical excision.

A **hordeolum** is an infection of the eyelid usually caused by *S. aureus*. The infection typically involves the glands of Zeis or Moll and appears as a painful furuncle on the lid margin. The meibomian glands also may be infected, mimicking a chelazion. Treatment includes warm compresses and topical antibiotics. Recurrence is common.

DISORDERS OF THE LACRIMAL SYSTEM

Dacryostenosis refers to blockage of the nasolacrimal duct. It usually is due to congenital obstruction and presents with persistent tearing (epiphora). Erythema, maceration of the skin, and mucopurulent drainage commonly complicate dacryostenosis. Conservative management includes massage of the nasolacrimal duct, good hygeine, and, possibly, topical antibiotics. Persistent blockage should be treated with surgical probing of the duct, usually performed in the 1st yr of life.

Dacryocystitis may complicate dacryostenosis and appears with erythema and pain overlying the nasolacrimal duct structures. Antibiotic therapy is indicated.

DISORDERS OF THE CONJUNCTIVA

Conjunctivitis

This is a common disorder in pediatrics that may be due to viruses, bacteria, allergens, irritants, toxins, and systemic diseases.

Viral conjunctivitis is the most common of these. It is usually bilateral and is marked by erythema with a watery discharge. Associated viral symptoms may be present. No therapy is necessary.

Bacterial conjunctivitis may complicate viral upper respiratory infection. It may be unilateral or bilateral and is marked by erythema and a purulent discharge. Common pathogens include *S. aureus, Haemophilus influenzae,* pneumococci, and streptococci. Gonococci and *Chlamydia* are important causes in the newborn period. Generally, therapy consists of topical antibiotics and warm compresses, although infections with gonococci and *Chlamydia* require systemic therapy.

Allergic conjunctivitis often accompanies allergic rhinitis. It may be seasonal. Symptoms include itching, tearing, and conjunctival edema. Allergen avoidance, cold compresses, and decongestant drops may afford relief to patients.

Other Disorders of the Conjunctiva

Other disorders of the conjunctiva include *hemorrhage,* which commonly is seen after birth trauma, sneezing, or with bleeding diatheses. Pingueculum, pterygium, dermoid cysts, and dermolipomas present as *masses* affecting the conjunctiva. *Symblepharon* is a cicatricial adhesion that typically follows chemical conjunctivitis or Stevens–Johnson syndrome.

ABNORMALITIES OF THE CORNEA

Corneal lesions may be congenital or acquired. Of the acquired lesions, those most commonly seen in pediatrics are due to trauma or infection. *Corneal abrasions* follow minor trauma and lead to pain and watery eye discharge. Diagnosis usually is made by fluorescein staining and examination. Therapy consists of topical antibiotics and patching of the eye with the lid closed in an effort to reduce sloughing of the new epithelial cells.

Herpes simplex infection causes a dendritic keratitis that also may be seen with fluorescein staining. Symptoms include erythema, pain, photophobia, tearing, and blepharospasm.

Therapy includes specific antiviral agents by a topical or systemic route.

Corneal ulcers may follow trauma and may be caused by various organisms. Infections due to *Pseudomonas aeruginosa* and *Neisseria gonorrhoeae* are particularly damaging to the cornea. Fungal infections are associated with contact lens use. Manifestations include corneal haze, injection, pain, photophobia, and blepharospasm. It is estimated that corneal ulceration is responsible for 10% of the blindness in the United States; systemic and topical therapy should be used in an effort to save the eye.

ABNORMALITIES OF THE LENS

Cataract

The most common disorder of the lens, a cataract is an opacification of the lens. It may be congenital or acquired, unilateral or bilateral. Cataracts prevent rays of light from reaching the retina and may result in amblyopia if not corrected.

Congenital cataracts may be isolated findings or part of systemic disease. Isolated congenital cataracts most commonly are inherited as an autosomal dominant trait, although other modes of transmission do occur. More commonly, congenital cataracts are associated with congenital infections. They also may be a manifestation of metabolic disease such as galactosemia.

In *childhood*, cataracts are most commonly due to trauma. They also may be a symptom of metabolic diseases, such as diabetes mellitus, Wilson disease, and the mucopolysaccharidoses and mucolipidoses. They also are associated with drugs, especially corticosteroids.

Treatment of cataracts includes removal of the severely affected lens, followed by correction of the resultant aphakic refractive errors with spectacles. Lens replacement may be appropriate in some patients.

Ectopia Lentis

This is a less common disorder in which the lens is not in its normal position. Symptoms include refractive errors or diplopia. Ectopia lentis may be congenital or acquired, with trauma being a major cause. It also has been associated with some systemic disorders, such as Marfan syndrome, homocystinuria, and Weill–Marchesani syndrome. Treatment is individualized and may include surgical removal of the lens.

DISORDERS OF THE UVEAL TRACT

The uveal tract may be subject to inflammatory, traumatic, and toxic damage. *Clinical manifestations* include pain, photophobia, lacrimation, and hyperemia. Anterior uveitis is commonly traumatic or associated with systemic diseases, such as pauciarticular arthritis, Kawasaki disease, and sarcoidosis. Posterior uveitis most commonly is associated with congenital infection. *Treatment* may include antibiotics, corticosteroids, and cycloplegic agents.

DISORDERS OF THE RETINA

The most common disease of the retina seen in children is **retinopathy of prematurity** (ROP). In this disorder, there is altered angiogenesis of the retina. Although hyperoxia is the most commonly associated factor, the lower the birth weight and the sicker the infant the greater the risk of ROP.

ROP is classified into five stages:

Stage 1—a demarcation line separating the vascularized from the avascularized retina
Stage 2—growth of this demarcation line into a ridge
Stage 3—deposition of extraretinal fibrovascular tissue
Stage 4—partial retina detachment
Stage 5—total retinal detachment

ROP is progressive in 10% of patients; in the remainder there is spontaneous arrest and regression. Patients at risk for ROP should be followed with sequential examinations, commencing in the second month of life. Progressive cases may be treated with cryotherapy in an effort to stop progression. Retinal reattachment procedures have had variable success. The benefit of vitamin E in this disease is controversial.

Progressive degenerative diseases of the retina include retinitis pigmentosa, hypertensive retinopathy, and diabetic retinopathy. Retinal changes may occur with a variety of metabolic diseases, such as the mucopolysaccharidoses, the sphingolipidoses, and the gangliosidoses. Retinoblastoma is the most common primary intraocular tumor of childhood. Trauma may lead to hemorrhagic changes of the retina as part of the shaken baby syndrome.

ABNORMALITIES OF THE OPTIC NERVE

Optic nerve hypoplasia may occur alone or with other abnormalities. It may be the principle feature of septo-optic dysplasia of de Morsier, in which other structures normally found in the midline of the brain may be abnormal. In addition to visual defects, patients with septo-optic dysplasia may experience seizures, diabetes insipidus, and hypopituitarism.

Papilledema occurs with increased intracranial pressure. Common causes include intracranial tumors and hemorrhage, obstructive hydrocephalus, certain metabolic diseases, and cerebral edema resulting from trauma, toxins, or infection.

Optic neuritis describes any inflammation of the optic nerve with attendant impairment of function. It may be due to toxins or demyelinating disease, or occur as part of a viral or bacterial infection. The process usually is acute and may be unilateral or bilateral. Symptoms include rapid loss of vision and pain on palpation. Corticosteroids may reduce visual impairment in certain cases.

DISORDERS OF THE ORBIT

Orbital cellulitis is an acute bacterial infection of the orbit usually caused by *H. influenzae*, *S. aureus*, group A streptococci, and the pneumococci. The most common cause of orbital cellulitis is direct extension of a paranasal sinusitis, although infections from other contiguous structures or due to bacteremia also are seen. Manifestations include proptosis, edema, limitation of extraocular movements, and decreased visual acuity. Hospitalization and intravenous antibiotics are indicated therapy because the potential for complications is great.

Although the same bacteria also may cause **periorbital cellulitis,** in this latter disease eye movement and visual acuity are not impaired. Periorbital swelling, however, may preclude complete clinical examination. In these cases, diagnosis is made by computerized tomographic scan or magnetic resonance imaging of the orbit. Parenteral antibiotic therapy is warranted because of the invasive nature of the causative bacteria.

THE EAR
(*NELSON TEXTBOOK*, SECS. 22.18–22.25)

EXAMINATION OF THE EAR

There are eight prominent *signs and symptoms associated* with disease of the ear and temporal bone: otalgia, otorrhea, hearing loss, swelling, vertigo, nystagmus, tinnitus, and facial paralysis.

Examination begins with the assessment of other structures of the head and neck that may be associated with diseases of the ear, such as cleft palate, nasal polyps, or stigmata of craniofacial syndromes. The examination continues with assessment of the external auditory meatus and surrounding structures before proceeding to otoscopic evaluation.

Otoscopic evaluation should include visualization of the external auditory canal and tympanic membrane before attempting pneumo-otoscopy. The normal tympanic membrane has a lucent, ground-glass appearance; a blue or yellow hue usually indicates middle ear effusion. Opacification of the tympanic membrane usually is due to thickening or effusion. **Pneumo-otoscopy** should be attempted with both positive and negative pressure application. Decreased compliance on positive pressure insufflation usually is seen with a bulging eardrum. Decreased compliance with negative pressure insufflation usually is seen with a retracted eardrum. Both are indicative of eustacian tube dysfunction.

HEARING LOSS

Moderate to severe hearing loss occurs in 0.5–1:1,000 live births, with the prevalence increasing to 1.5–2:1,000 children under the age of 6 yr. Hearing loss can be peripheral or central in origin. Peripheral causes include those that are *conductive* (in which there is physical impediment of sound transmission through the external or middle ear) or *sensorineural* (in which there is damage or maldevelopment to the structures of the inner ear). Central deafness originates proximal to the eighth cranial nerve.

Hearing loss may be congenital or acquired. It may be due to genetic or nongenetic causes. Examples of *congenital-genetic causes* of deafness include familial deafness, which usually is autosomal recessive, and deafness associated with myriad congenital syndromes, such as Waardenburg, Pierre Robin, Treacher Collins, and the trisomies. *Acquired-genetic causes* of deafness include Alport syndrome, neurofibromatosis, and Hunter–Hurler syndrome. *Congenital-nongenetic causes* of deafness include intrauterine infection, exposure to radiation, or exposure to ototoxic drugs. *Postnatal-nongenetic causes* include bacterial meningitis, ototoxic drugs, trauma, otitis media, and noise exposure.

Because hearing is essential to good language development, children with suspected hearing loss should be evaluated as early as possible. Infants in the intensive care nursery often are screened for hearing loss prior to discharge. Other children must be screened in the pediatrician's office, with suspicion most often based on delayed speech or parental concern. Audiologists use tympanometry and a variety of age-appropriate methods of audiometric examination to assess hearing.

CONGENITAL MALFORMATIONS

Congenital malformations of the ear include preauricular pits and skin tags, both of minor functional significance. *Congenital stenosis* or atresia of the ear may lead to conductive hearing loss. Surgical repair should be attempted in cases in which functional improvement may be gained with surgery (otherwise normal otic and neuroanatomy).

INFLAMMATORY DISEASES

External Otitis

External otitis, or "swimmer's ear," results from infection of the external auditory canal. It usually is associated with periods of excessive moisture or dryness in the canal. It may follow excessive cleaning with removal of protective cerumen. Bacterial species responsible for external otitis include *P. aeruginosa, Enterobacter aerogenes, Proteus mirabilis,* and *Klebsiella pneumoniae.* The fungi *Candida* and *Aspergillus* often are implicated.

Clinical manifestation of external otitis include pain, itching, conductive hearing loss, and serous or purulent secretions. On physical examination, purulent otorrhea, edema, and erythema of the canal are seen. *Differential diagnosis* includes furunculosis, cellulitis, dermatoses, herpes simplex infection, and otitis media with a perforation.

External otitis is *treated* with topical otic preparations containing antibiotics and corticosteroids. Although the corticosteroids may be sufficient to control pain in some patients, others will require oral analgesics.

Otitis Media

After upper respiratory infections, otitis media is the second most common illness of childhood. Infants and young children are at highest risk for otitis media; those who are diagnosed with otitis media in the 1st yr of life are at risk for recurrent or chronic disease. Boys are affected more commonly than girls. Native Americans, children of lower socioeconomic class, and children with craniofacial abnormalities such as cleft palate also are at increased risk.

PATHOGENESIS. Eustachian tube dysfunction is the critical event in pathogenesis. Otitis media commonly follows upper respiratory infection in which there is edema of the eustachian tube, leading to its blockage. Other antecedent conditions that lead to blockage of the eustachian tube include allergic rhinitis, nasal polyps, and adenoidal hypertrophy. After stasis of middle ear secretions, contamination of the middle ear typically occurs by reflux, aspiration, or insufflation during sneezing, crying, or nose blowing.

ACUTE OTITIS MEDIA. This presents with fever, otalgia, and hearing loss. Examination usually reveals a hyperemic, opaque, bulging tympanic membrane with poor mobility. Organisms responsible for acute otitis media are *S. pneumoniae*, nontypeable *H. influenzae*, and *Moraxalla catarrhalis*. Diagnosis usually is based on clinical examination. *Treatment* of acute otitis media is 10 days of an oral antibiotic effective against these bacteria. Choices include amoxicillin, erythromycin–sulfasoxazole, trimethoprim–sulfamethoxazole, cefaclor, cefuroxime, and cefixime.

Patients diagnosed with otitis media should be reassessed 2 wk after institution of therapy. If there has been resolution of erythema and there is no evidence of eustacian tube dysfunction, no further therapy is warranted. Partially treated infections should receive another course of antibiotics.

PERSISTENT MIDDLE-EAR EFFUSIONS. These commonly are treated with (1) another course of antibiotics, (2) decongestants and/or antihistamines, (3) systemic corticosteroids, or (4) prudent waiting and re-evaluation in 6 wk. None of the above therapies has proven more beneficial than the others in well-designed case–control studies.

RECURRENT OTITIS MEDIA. This may result from the inability to clear middle-ear effusions or as distinct acute events. In the former case, patients may benefit from prophylactic daily doses of amoxicillin or sulfonamides in an attempt to maintain the sterility of middle-ear secretions. If this therapy is not effective in preventing recurrence, **myringostomy tubes** should be considered. Distinct recurrences without chronic effusion should be treated similarly to any acute otitis media.

CHRONIC SEROUS OTITIS MEDIA. This may be a silent complication of acute disease or may present as decreased auditory acuity, "fullness" in the ear, tinnitus, or vertigo. Management of these patients is controversial. One of the most popular treatments is antihistamines and/or decongestants, both of which have been shown to be ineffective. Corticosteroids have been advocated by some. A prolonged course (up to 30 days) of antibiotics probably is the most appropriate therapy, because bacteria may be isolated from 65% of patients with chronic effusion. If the effusion lasts for more than 3 mo, it is unlikely to resolve spontaneously, and myringotomy with or without tube placement should be performed. Concurrent adenoidectomy may be of benefit in some children.

COMPLICATIONS. These may be suppurative or nonsuppurative. The most common nonsuppurative complication is acute **mastoiditis,** in which the patient may have swelling, erythema, and tenderness over the mastoid bone. The pinna may be displaced outward. The patient may appear toxic. Diagnosis usually is made clinically. Treatment includes antibiotics and surgical mastoidectomy in an effort to prevent further suppurative complications. **Intracranial suppurative complications** are uncommon and include meningitis, extradural abscess, subdural empyema, brain abscess, and lateral sinus thrombosis. **Nonsuppurative complications** of otitis media include perforation, cholesteatoma, and tympanosclerosis.

Hearing loss is the most common complication of otitis media. It may be transient or permanent. Middle-ear effusion commonly leads to transient hearing loss, which remits with restoration of eustachian tube patency. Although the scientific data for understanding the relationship of otitis media and permanent hearing loss is far from complete, several studies have shown an association between early otitis media and permanent hearing deficits.

OTHER DISEASES OF THE EAR AND TEMPORAL BONE

Traumatic injuries of the ear and temporal bone include hematoma of the pinna, frostbite, foreign bodies, fractures, and acoustic damage. Benign tumors of the ear and temporal bone include osteoma and polyostotic fibrous dysplasia. Malignant tumors include eosinophilic granuloma, rhabdomyosarcoma, and leukemia.

21

THE SKIN

MORPHOLOGY AND EXAMINATION
(*NELSON TEXTBOOK*, SECS. 23.1 AND 23.2)

PRIMARY LESIONS

macule: an alteration in skin color that cannot be felt

papule: a palpable solid lesion smaller than 0.5–1 cm in diameter

nodule: a palpable solid lesion larger than a papule

tumor: larger than a nodule and varying considerably in size and consistency

vesicles: raised, fluid-filled lesions less than 0.5 cm in diameter; large lesions are bullae, and pustules contain purulent material

wheals: flat-topped, palpable lesions of variable size and configuration, dermal collections of edema fluid

cyst: a circumscribed, thick-walled lesion located deep in the skin, covered by normal epidermis, and containing fluid or semisolid material

SECONDARY LESIONS

These include scales, ulcers, excoriations, fissures, crusts, and scars.

The *Wood lamp* transmits ultraviolet light and is used mainly to detect superficial fungal lesions in the dark by fluorescence.

KOH preparation is a rapid, reliable method to diagnosis fungal lesion; the *Tzanck smear* is used to detect herpes simplex, varicella, herpes zoster, and eczema herpeticum.

Immunofluorescence studies of skin punch biopsies may detect tissue-fixed antibodies.

PRINCIPLES OF THERAPY
(*NELSON TEXTBOOK*, SEC. 23.3)

Acute weeping lesions respond best to wet compresses, followed by lotions or creams. Dry, thickened, scaly skin responds best to an ointment base. Gels and solutions are most useful for the scalp and other hairy areas.

TRANSIENT LESIONS OF THE NEONATE
(*NELSON TEXTBOOK*, SEC. 23.4)

Most entities are common, benign, and transient and usually do not require treatment. These include sebaceous hyperplasia, milia, sucking blisters, cutis marmorata, harlequin color change, salmon patch, mongolian spots, erythema toxicum, and transient neonatal pustular melanosis.

DEVELOPMENTAL DEFECTS
(*NELSON TEXTBOOK*, SECS. 23.5–23.8)

CUTANEOUS DEFECTS

Skin dimples, redundant skin, or *accessory tragi* may occur in normal children or be associated with dysmorphologic syndromes.

Preauricular sinus tracts and pits may become infected.

Branchial cleft and thyroglossal cysts and sinuses may contain aberrant thyroid tissue as well as mucinous material, and they may become infected. Excision is indicated.

Aplasia cutis congenita usually occurs on the scalp, but developmental absence of skin may occur anywhere. In addition to the possible need for surgical coverage, hemorrhage and infection require treatment.

ECTODERMAL DYSPLASIAS

Hypohidrotic (anhidrotic) ectodermal dysplasia consists of hypohidrosis, anomalous dentition, hypotrichosis, and facial dysplasia. Inability to sweat may result in fever, and maldeveloped secretory glands in the respiratory tract predispose to purulent rhinitis, horseness, dysphonia, and recurrent respiratory tract infections. Lacrimation is defective. In some variants the nails are severely affected.

VASCULAR LESIONS

Port-wine stain (nevus) is present at birth and consists of mature dilated dermal capillaries. These nevi vary tremendously in size and may be part of the *Sturge–Weber* or other syndromes. Therapies vary from cosmetic coverage to laser excision.

Hemangiomas are the most common tumor of infancy and usually are sporadic. Many regress spontaneously; other may respond to corticosteroids, interferon-α, radiation, or surgery.

Capillary hemangiomas (strawberry nevus) are bright red, protuberant, compressible, sharply demarcated lesions that usually appear within the first 2 mo of life. Most resolve spontaneously.

Cavernous hemangiomas are deeply situated, more diffuse, and ill-defined cystic or compressible lesions that may have a bluish hue. They often regress spontaneously. There is an association with various syndromes.

Kasabach–Merritt syndrome consists of a rapidly enlarging, usually solitary, large hemangioma, thrombocytopemia, and a consumption coagulopathy. This may be life threatening and requires specific and supportive treatment.

Disseminated hemangiomatosis is an often fatal condition consisting of widely distributed cutaneous and visceral hemangioma.

Klippel–Trenaunay–Weber syndrome is a port-wine nevus in combination with bony and soft-tissue hypertrophy, and venous varicosities.

Hereditary hemorrhagic telangiectasia (Osler–Weber–Rendu disease) is an autosomal dominant trait that may present with recurrent, often severe, epistaxis, resulting from mucocutaneous telangiectastic lesions. Cautery or surgery may be indicated.

CUTANEOUS NEVI
(*NELSON TEXTBOOK*, SEC. 23.9)

These lesions are characterized histologically by collections of well-differentiated cell types normally found in the skin. Hemangiomas are vascular nevi.

ACQUIRED PIGMENTED NEVI (Moles)

These are benign lesions. Biopsy is required to distinguish these nevocellular nevi from pigmented lesions arising from melanocytes and rare malignant lesions of nevocytes. They are classified as junctional, compound, or dermal depending on the location of the nevis cells in the skin. Most often they are not present at birth.

DYSPLASTIC NEVI

These occur sporadically and in a familial melanoma-prone setting, usually around puberty. Children in the latter group require frequent monitoring.

CONGENITAL PIGMENTED NEVI

These are present in about 1% of newborn infants and pose an increased risk of developing malignant melanoma. Sites of predilection are the lower trunk, upper back and shoulders, chest, and proximal limbs.

Giant congenital pigmented nevi are highly associated with leptomeningeal melanocytosis and malignant melanoma.

OTHER NEVI

There are a large variety of benign lesions.

DISORDERS OF PIGMENT
(*NELSON TEXTBOOK*, SECS. 23.10–23.12)

Generalized or localized alteration in skin color may result from absence of melanocytes, defective melanization of melanosomes, overproduction of melanin, or increased numbers of melanocytes. Developmental, inflammatory, or hormonal mechanisms may be involved.

HYPERPIGMENTED LESIONS

These may be benign, such as freckles; benign and associated with syndromes such as lentigines (Peutz–Jeghers syndrome) and café-au-lait spots (neurofibromatosis-1); or associated with multisystemic hereditary disorders (incontinentia pigmenti). Cutaneous inflammation may subsequently cause increased or decreased pigmentation, especially in dark-skinned children.

HYPOPIGMENTED LESIONS

A variety of forms of *oculocutaneous albinism* have been described.

Tuberous sclerosis, a multisystemic developmental disorder often associated with severe neurologic manifestations, often presents early with hypopigmented white leaf macules.

Vitiligo, sharply circumscribed depigmented macules, usually is benign.

VESICOBULLOUS DISORDERS
(*NELSON TEXTBOOK*, SEC. 23.13)

Many diseases are characterized by these lesions, which represent only a transient stage of the disease. Blisters localized to the epidermal layers are thin walled, relatively flaccid, and tend to rupture easily; subepidermal blisters are tense, thick walled, and more durable.

ERYTHEMA MULTIFORME

This acute, sometimes recurrent, inflammatory disease of skin and mucous membrane probably is due to a hypersensitivity reaction triggered by drugs, infections, or toxic substances.

Erythema multiforme minor is the most common type and is characterized by the diverse, changing morphology of abruptly appearing skin lesions, which usually are symmetric and appear in crops on extensor surfaces 1–2 wk after an upper respiratory infection. The vesicobullous lesions arise centrally within pre-existing macules, wheals, papules, or plaques.

Erythema multiforme major (Stevens–Johnson syndrome) is a serious systemic disorder involving at least two mucous membranes and the skin. Abrupt onset usually follows prodromal respiratory symptoms, and manifestations usually include conjunctivitis, uveitis, bullae and denuded skin (fluid loss), fever, chills, weakness, neutropenia, and anemia.

Treatment is local and symptomatic, and Stevens–Johnson syndrome often requires intensive care.

TOXIC EPIDERMAL NECROLYSIS

This severe hypersensitivity phenomena is triggered by many of the same factors responsible for erythema multiforme. There is widespread epidermal necrosis after blister formation, loss of large sheets of skin, fever, erythema, malaise, Nikolsky sign, and mucosal lesions. Dehydration, shock, and sepsis may occur. Management is similar to that for severe burns.

EPIDERMOLYSIS BULLOSA

Epidermolysis bullosa (EB) is a heterogeneous group of congenital inherited blistering disorders exacerbated by trauma and high environmental temperatures.

Epidermolytic EB, a nonscarring autosomal dominant disorder, usually is noted during the neonatal period, and secondary infection is the most serious problem.

Junctional EB is a life-threatening condition (septicemia) with large blisters usually present at birth. Mucous membrane involvement may be severe and there may be ulceration of the respiratory, gastrointestinal, and genitourinary epithelium. Intensive supportive therapy is required.

Dermolytic EB may occur sporadically as well as by dominant inheritance. Various types range from mild to severe disorders.

ACRODERMATITIS ENTEROPATHICA

This rare autosomal recessive disorder of zinc deficiency resulting from reduced intestinal absorption has an insidious onset, usually during the 1st yr of life. The vesicobullous, eczematous, and psoriasiform skin lesions are symmetrically distributed on the cheeks, knees, elbows, and perioral, acral, and perineal areas. Oral zinc therapy is effective.

PHEMPHIGUS

The *vulgaris* type usually first appears as painful oral ulcers. Subsequently, large flaccid bullae emerge on nonerythematous skin, commonly on the head and trunk. High-dose systemic steroids and immunosuppressive agents are effective.

The *foliaceus* type is characterized by more superficial blisters and the course generally is more benign.

ECZEMA
(*NELSON TEXTBOOK*, SEC. 23.14)

Generically, acute eczematous lesions are characterized by erythema, weeping, oozing, and the formation of microvesicles within the epidermis. Chronic lesions are thickened, dry, and scaly, with coarse skin markings (lichenification) and altered pigmentation. Many types occur, and pyoderma, insect bites, and a variety of dermatoses may become eczematized from scratching.

CONTACT DERMATITIS

The irritant form is more common than the allergic form in childhood but clinically may be indistinguishable from atopic dermatitis or allergic contact dermatitis. History and site are critical to diagnosis. *Treatment* includes removal of the irritant stimulus, bland protective agents, and sometimes topical steroids.

PITYRIASIS ALBA

These hypopigmented round or oval lesions are macular or slightly elevated patches with fine scales. *Treatment* with a lubricant or topical steroids is effective.

SEBORRHEIC DERMATITIS

This is a chronic inflammatory skin disease that occurs at all ages but may begin in the 1st mo of life and be a special problem in the 1st yr. *Cradle cap*, a diffuse or focal scaling and crusting of the scalp, may be the initial or only manifestation.

Greasy, scaly, erythematous, papular dermatitis, usually nonpuritic, may involve the face, neck, retroauricular areas, axillae, and diaper area. Lesions may be focal or spread to involve the entire body. Postinflammatory pigmentary changes are common in black infants.

Treatment includes antiseborrheic shampoo, topical steroids, 3% sulfur ointment, compresses, and antifungal agents.

PHOTOSENSITIVITY
(*NELSON TEXTBOOK*, SEC. 23.15)

Cutaneous reactions may be due to sunlight (250–800 nm) or, less commonly, to artificial light. Host factors play an important role, especially the protective effected of skin pigmentation (melanin). A variety of rare disorders are associated (Cockayne syndrome, Hartnup disease, Bloom syndrome, xeroderma pigmentosum).

SUNBURN

Acute reactions can be severe, and pain and inflammation may require cool tapwater compresses, shake lotions, and mild oral analgesia. There are long-term increases in risks of malignant melanoma and skin damage that argue for strong preventive measures of avoidance and sunscreens.

PHOTOTOXIC AND PHOTOALLERGIC REACTIONS

These reactions are due to a combination of exogenous agents and light and range from mild to severe. Steroid therapy may be required for brief periods.

PORPHYRIAS

These are acquired or inborn abnormalities of specific enzymes in the heme biosynthetic pathway. Clinical manifestations are diverse, but photosensitivity is a constant feature.

DISEASES OF THE EPIDERMIS
(*NELSON TEXTBOOK*, SEC. 23.16)

PSORIASIS

This chronic disorder may have its onset during childhood, including the neonatal period. Erythematous papules coalesce to form plaques with sharply demarcated, irregular boarders. A thick silvery or yellow–white scale then develops. Severe disease may require hospitalization, and *therapy* is palliative, including tar preparations, ultraviolet or natural sunlight, and topical steroids.

PITYRIASIS ROSEA

This is a benign common general eruption consisting of oval or round, slightly raised pink–brown, fine, scaly lesions (1 cm in diameter) that usually are preceded by a solitary, large (1–10 cm in diameter), annular lesion with a raised border of five adherent scales (herald patch). No treatment is necessary for the asymptomatic patient. For some, a bland ointment containing methanol and camphor is helpful for puritis.

ICHTHYOSIS
(*NELSON TEXTBOOK*, SEC. 23.17)

This group of inherited keratinizing disorders is characterized by scaling in distinctive patterns of distribution; some cause disfigurement.

HARLEQUIN FETUS

This rare autosomal recessive disorder may represent several different genotypes. Markedly thickened, ridged, cracked skin forms horny plates over the entire body, disfiguring the face and constricting the digits. Most infants die in the neonatal period from respiratory distress. Survivors have severe icthyosis.

COLLODION BABY

These infants are covered by a thick, taut membrane that is subsequently shed. There is facial disfigurement. Mortality and morbidity are due to cutaneous infection, aspiration pneumonia, or dehydration from transcutaneous fluid losses. *Treatment* is supportive.

X-LINKED ICHTHYOSIS

This disorder of males often presents at birth. Scaling is due to steroid sulfatase deficiency. Deep corneal opacities develop in later childhood. Skin hydration and emollients may limit disfigurement.

ICHTHYOSIFORM DERMATOSES

There are a number of rare but distinct syndromes involving the skin and other organ systems.

DISEASES OF THE DERMIS
(NELSON TEXTBOOK, SEC. 23.18)

GRANULOMA ANNULARE

This common disorder can be polymorphous. Typical lesions begin as erythematous, firm, flat-topped papulonodules that gradually enlarge to form ring-shaped plaques with a normal or slightly discolored central area (several centimeters in size), especially occurring on the dorsum of the hands and feet.) Spontaneous resolution may occur after months or years without residual changes. Steroids may hasten the resolution.

CUTIS LAXA

This congenital inherited disorder may make a newborn appear prematurely aged or it may present later in childhood. The skin hangs on pendulous folds, and general laxness may make the skin appear like an ill-fitting suit. Skin hyperelasticity and joint hypermobility are not present (as they are in Ehler–Danlos syndrome).

Involvement of the cardiopulmonary and gastrointestinal systems may result in a shortened lifespan. Affected children are normal at birth in all 10 types of the disorder, which are due to defects in collagen.

DISORDERS OF SUBCUTANEOUS TISSUE
(NELSON TEXTBOOK, SEC. 23.19)

These disorders usually are characterized by necrosis and inflammation. They may be a primary event or secondary to a variety of stimuli or disease processes. *Diagnosis* depends on the appearance and distribution of lesions, associated symptoms, laboratory abnormalities, and an appreciation of exogenous provocative factors. Disorders include corticosteroid atrophy, panniculitis, lipodystrophy, sclerema neonatorum, and subcutaneous fat necrosis.

DISEASES OF SWEAT GLANDS, HAIR, AND NAILS
(*NELSON TEXTBOOK*, SECS. 23.20–23.23)

MILIARIA (Prickly Heat)

Retention of sweat in ducts and pores of eccrine sweat glands occurs as a result of keratinous plugs. Leakage may produce an inflammatory response. Tidy superficial papulovesicles occur. *Treatment* consists of cooling, including antipyretics to reduce sweating.

HYPOTRICHOSIS AND ALOPECIA

The causes of these disorders are rarely congenital; most often they are due to infections, inflammatory dermatosis, drug ingestion, mechanical factors, endocrinopathies, or other systemic metabolic disturbances.

CUTANEOUS BACTERIAL INFECTIONS
(*NELSON TEXTBOOK*, SEC. 23.26)

IMPETIGO CONTAGIOSA

This superficial pyoderma is characterized by erythematous macules that rapidly evolve into thin-walled vesicles and pustules. The latter rupture, resulting in sticky, honey-colored crusts over a moist base. Infection may spread to other parts of the body, but usually it is an indolent, self-limited disease. Group A β-hemolytic streptococcus and *Staphylococcus aureus* are the most common etiologic agents.

Treatment is indicated to decrease morbidity and prevent spread to others. It may include local washing and compresses, topical antibiotics, and systemic antibiotics.

STAPHYLOCOCCAL SCALDED SKIN SYNDROME

This is caused by one or more exfoliative toxins produced by the infecting *S. aureus*. There may be a prodrome of malaise, fever, and irritability associated with exquisite skin tenderness, followed by generalized erythema, or the skin lesion may occur abruptly without preceding manifestations. The initial rash is macular, involving the face, neck, axilla, and groin. It extends rapidly and becomes bullous, with increased irritability and pain. Sheets of epidermis peel away, dry, and heal by postinflammatory desquamation.

Treatment with a systemic, semisynthetic penicillin-resistant antibiotic is indicated.

CUTANEOUS FUNGAL INFECTIONS
(*NELSON TEXTBOOK*, SECS. 23.27–23.29)

TINEA VERSICOLOR

This is a common, innocuous chronic infection that varies widely in color and is caused by *Pityrosporon orbiculare*.

DERMATOPHYTOSIS (Ringworm)

These disorders are caused by a group of closely related fungi with a propensity to invade the stratum corneum, hair, and nails. Secondary hypersensitivity skin reactions ("id" reactions) also occur as a result of these fungi.

Tinea capitis involves the scalp through infections of the hair shaft and surrounding skin. Oral griseofulvin microcrystalline treatment is indicated.

Tinea corporis involves the skin of the face, trunk, and extremities. The typical lesion (ringworm) starts as a dry, mildly erythematous, elevated, scaly papule and spreads centrifugally, clearing centrally. Topical antifungal agents are usually effective.

TINEA UNGNIUM

This involves the nail plate and is difficult to eradicate even with systemic antifungal agents.

CANDIDAL INFECTIONS

Candida albicans usually is the cause of childhood candidosis. Infections may be acute or chronic, localized or general. Widespread infection is a high risk for immunosuppressed patients. Local *treatment* for vaginal, diaper, intertrigenous, perianal, paronychea, and onychia variants usually is effective.

VIRAL INFECTIONS AND PARASITIC INFESTATIONS
(*NELSON TEXTBOOK*, SECS. 23.30 AND 23.31)

Warts are caused by DNA viruses of the papillomavirus group. A variety of therapeutic measures are effective in their treatment.

Scabies is caused by the itch mite, *Sarcoptes scabiei* var. *hominis* and usually is transmitted by direct contact with an infected person. An intensely pruretic eruption consists of wheals, papules, vesicles, and tread-like burrows with superimposed eczematous dermatitis. Treatment consists of application of 1% gamma benzene hexachloride cream or lotion to the entire body from the neck down. The entire family may need to be treated.

Pediculosis is an infestation with lice (pubic, head, or body). The body louse is also the vector for typhus, trench fever, and relapsing fever. Local treatments are indicated and vary somewhat depending on the type of lice.

ACNE
(*NELSON TEXTBOOK*, SEC. 23.32)

ACNE VULGARIS

Acne occurs almost universally during adolescence and frequently persists into adulthood. It is a self-limited inflammatory process involving the pilosebaceous unit.

Etiology and Pathogenesis

A mature sebum-producing sebaceous gland, bacteria, and lipids in sebum play a role in the inflammatory reaction.

Clinical Manifestations

Four basic lesions are open and closed comedones, papules, pustules, and nodulocystic lesions. Scars may be interspersed.

Treatment

There is no evidence that early treatment can prevent lesions, but it can ameliorate lesions and prevent scarring. Diet plays no significant role, but manipulation and greasy cosmetics and hair lotion should be avoided. Topical therapy with cleansing agents containing keratolytic compounds may be helpful (e.g., benzoyl peroxide and retinoic acid). CO_2 also has been used. Systemic therapy includes antibiotics (esp. tetracycline and erythromycin) and estrogen.

OTHER TYPES OF ACNE

Steroid acne responds to discontinuation of the drug.

Infantile acne usually is self-limited.

Acne conglobata is a chronic, progressive, inflammatory disease that may start during adolescence and may respond to corticosteroids, sulfones, or isotretinoin.

22

THE BONES AND JOINTS

ORTHOPEDIC PROBLEMS
(*NELSON TEXTBOOK*, SECS. 24.1–24.28)

Musculoskeletal diseases and injuries comprise about 10% of pediatric practice. Disease affecting bones, muscle–tendon units, and articular structures can be congenital or acquired, and either primary or secondary to a more generalized disorder. Orthopedic illness as well as injuries can be acute or chronic, and this differentiation can be immensely helpful to the clinician in diagnosis and treatment.

EVALUATION
(*NELSON TEXTBOOK*, SEC. 24.1)

Establishing an accurate diagnosis is very important in the approach to pediatric orthopedic problems. The history and physical examination are the most important tools, but appropriate imaging studies often are necessary, and sometimes selected laboratory studies can be helpful.

The *history* should include birth and development as well as the progression of symptoms such as pain and alteration of function. The *physical examination* should be both generalized and specific, focused by the history and presenting complaint. An astute clinician once said, "know what you're looking for."

The *orthopedic examination* can be simplified by the following directions: look, feel, and move. Observation is the first step: for posture, gait, spontaneous movement (or lack thereof), and symmetry between the two sides. Palpation for warmth, swelling, joint effusion, and areas of tenderness also is important. The examination of movement includes active and passive joint range of motion, strength, stiffness and often provocative maneuvers to test the integrity of ligamentous structures.

Among the various *imaging studies*, plain roentgenograms can serve as a valuable extension of the physical examination. Common indications include chronic bone or joint pain, any suspected fracture, limited range of motion, and suspected bone disease or infection. Bone scans (scintigraphy) can be helpful for early identification of subtle fractures (e.g., in child abuse), stress fractures, and osteomyelitis. Plain tomography and computerized tomography (CT) scanning are useful for bone lesions, and magnetic resonance imaging (MRI) is very good for the spinal cord and soft-tissue lesions. Ultrasonography is becoming increasingly useful in the diagnosis of (congenital) developmental dysplasia of the hip.

(See Table 24–3, *Nelson Textbook,* for a glossary of orthopedic terminology.)

FOOT AND TOES
(*NELSON TEXTBOOK,* SEC. 24.2)

The **flatfoot** has no longitudinal arch and is so common as to be considered normal in infants. It is pathologic when stiff and/or painful in older patients. The *vertical talus* deformity is the most severe form of flatfoot, seen in infants with stiff "rocker-bottom" feet. *Tarsal coalitions* typically present in late childhood with a stiff painful flatfoot and secondary peroneal muscle spasm. These severe forms of flatfoot usually require surgical correction. Milder forms often respond to simple stretching and alterations in footwear.

Pes cavus, or the high-arched foot, generally is more painful than flatfoot. It often is associated with neuromuscular disease, so a thorough work-up of this problem is important.

Clubfoot (congenital talipes equinovarus) is the fixed combination of ankle equinus, hindfoot varus, midfoot adductus, and medial rotation. The foot is small and stiff—it cannot be forced into the neutral position. Referral should be made early (less than 1 wk) for serial casting; surgery usually is done, if necessary, between 4 and 12 mo.

Metatarsus adductus is the most common congenital foot abnormality. It is diagnosed by noting a convexity of the lateral border of the foot and by noting the position of a heel bisector on the sole of the foot (Figure 22–1). When the foot is flexible, spontaneous correction can be expected by 6 mo.

Toe problems include syndactyly and polydactyly. Extra toes probably should be removed surgically, before the child

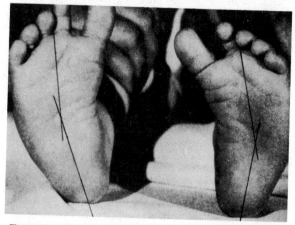

Figure 22–1. Metatarsus varus: A line bisecting the hindpart of the foot should pass through the 2nd toe or between the 2nd and 3rd toes. (From Behrman RE [ed]: Nelson Textbook of Pediatrics, 14th ed. Philadelphia, WB Saunders Company, 1992, p 1695.)

walks, at 9–12 mo of age. Ingrown toenails are common in childhood and are preventable by keeping the corners square and not trimming the nails too short. When they are inflamed, gentle elevation and packing of a cotton pledget beneath the nail edge is indicated. *Shoes* should be worn for walking, to protect the sole of the foot from the ground. Therefore, shoes should not be "supportive" or "corrective"; rather, they should be flexible, flat, and comfortable.

ROTATIONAL PROBLEMS
(*NELSON TEXTBOOK*, SEC. 24.3)

In-toeing and out-toeing are common in infancy and early childhood. These torsional deformities almost always resolve spontaneously with growth.

Evaluation of patients with torsional problems should include observation of gait, posture, and alignment, and careful range-of-motion testing at the hips, knees, ankles, subtalus joints, and forefoot. In-toeing tends to be related to the feet in infancy (metatarsus adductus), the lower leg in toddlers (medial tibial torsion), and the hip in childhood (medial femoral torsion).

Surgical correction (derotation osteotomy) should be reserved for cases of persistent, disabling deformities at 8–10 yr.

ANGULAR DEFORMITIES
(*NELSON TEXTBOOK*, SEC. 24.4)

Bowlegs and Knock-Knees

Normal growth results in bowlegs (genu varum) from birth until 2 yr, followed by knock-knees (genu valgum) peaking at 3–4 yr and usually resolving by 6–10 yr. Pathologic causes of bowlegs (rickets, achondroplasia, Blount disease, and many others) should be considered in patients with short stature, nutritional problems, asymmetry, or severe or progressive deformities.

Helpful physical examination techniques include measurement between the medial femoral condyles with the medial malleoli touching for bowlegs, and vice versa for knock-knees. Roentgenograms can be helpful in the diagnosis of pathologic tibia vara (Blount disease), and "beaking" or other abnormalities of the proximal medial tibial metaphysis should prompt orthopedic referral. Referral of the 8–10-yr-old child with knock-knees should be made if the intermalleolar distance exceeds 7.5 cm.

LEG LENGTH DISCREPANCY
(*NELSON TEXTBOOK*, SEC. 24.5)

A leg length discrepancy (anisomelia) exists when one leg is greater than 1 cm longer than the other. This can be measured by: (1) placing blocks under the short leg and levelling the pelvis (by palpating the iliac crests with the patient standing); or (2) noting the distance from the anterior superior iliac spine to the medial malleolus with the patient supine. Roentgenographic methods of measurement are essential to confirm the diagnosis. The presentation usually is a complaint of abnormal (i.e., "vaulting") gait.

Treatment options are complicated, based on estimates of remaining growth and projected adult limb discrepancy. Both limb-shortening (osteotomy, epiphysiodesis) and limb-lengthening (osteotomy with grafting or externally applied axial distraction) procedures are available to the pediatric orthopedic specialist.

KNEE
(*NELSON TEXTBOOK*, SEC. 24.6)

Knee problems become more common in older children and adolescents, but a few knee problems are important in babies and young patients.

Hyperextension or Knee Dislocation

Congenital knee dislocation can be the result of in utero positioning or a malformation syndrome and is manifested by a knee that can be moved to 45 degrees or more of hyperextension. Physiologic hyperextension or *genu recurvatum*, with hyperextension of 10–15 degrees, is common in toddlers and young children.

Knee Flexion Contractures

These are seen in children with arthrogryposis and neuromuscular disorders and are best managed with passive range-of-motion therapy, splinting in extension, and, if severe, surgical hamstring lengthening procedures.

Popliteal Cysts (Baker Cysts)

These are firm, painless cystic lesions found on the posterior and medial part of the knee joint. Unlike those seen in adults, Baker cysts in children usually do not communicate with the knee joint and usually are not associated with an intra-articular injury. They should be transilluminated to ensure the diagnosis and left alone, because spontaneous resolution can be expected within 1–2 yr.

Patellofemoral Pain Syndrome

This is very common in active older children and adolescents, usually manifested by chronic activity-related anterior knee pain. Sometimes there is swelling and a feeling of "giving out." This is often a tip-off to recurrent patellar subluxation (usually lateral), an associated problem. Often malalignment, weak quadriceps, and a rapid growth spurt predispose the patient to this syndrome.

Physical examination findings are medial peripatellar tenderness, the patellar inhibition sign, and the apprehension test.

Treatment involves relative rest, anti-inflammatory medications, and active quadriceps strengthening (best done with the help of a physical therapist). Straight-leg raising should be emphasized, because bent-knee exercises may exacerbate the problems. Sometimes patellar-stabilizing knee sleeves can be helpful, and surgical realignment is rarely necessary.

Intra-articular Injuries

These include *articular fractures, meniscus tears,* and *ligament sprains.* Usually there must be a significant degree of trauma involved, and clinical manifestations include a variable amount of pain and tenderness, limited range of motion, and a bloody joint effusion (hemarthrosis).

Fractures are more likely in younger patients whose ligaments are relatively stronger than their bones. For example, the same mechanism of injury might cause an *anterior cruciate ligament tear* in an adolescent or adult, but a *tibial eminence fracture* in a child.

Meniscus tears are rare in children, but sometimes a *diskoid lateral meniscus* is the cause of meniscal symptoms such as clicking, locking, or limited range of motion. A *medial patellar plica* can cause activity-related pain and snapping in the anteromedial aspect of the joint. Arthroscopy can be both diagnostic and therapeutic for these two conditions.

Osteochondritis dissecans is a condition of subchondral bone necrosis and often fragmentation, seen in both children and adolescents with chronic knee pain and stiffness. Any articular surface can be involved, but the lateral aspect of the medial femoral condyle is the most common site. Conservative treatment usually is indicated, but large (>1 cm), persistent or painful lesions should be referred for arthroscopic or open surgical treatment.

Osgood–Schlatter disease, or traction apophysitis of the tibial tubercle, is commonly seen in active, growing children. The combination of rapid growth and relative overuse leads to pain, tenderness, and swelling at the insertion of the patellar tendon. Roentgenograms can rule out other lesions, but are not required to make the diagnosis. Treatment consists of relative rest (reducing exacerbating activities), stretching, and sometimes a knee sleeve or counter-force straps.

HIP
(*NELSON TEXTBOOK*, SECS. 24.7–24.11)

The hip is a vulnerable joint, and many adult hip problems originate in childhood. It is common for symptoms of hip disease to be referred to the thigh and knee because of the dual sensory distribution of the obturator nerve. Important elements of the physical examination include stance and gait, posture, alignment and leg length, palpation, and full range-of-motion testing.

Developmental (Congenital) Dislocation of the Hip

Developmental dislocation of the hip (DDH), formerly called congenital hip dysplasia, affects 0.5–2% of all newborn infants. Since untreated DDH is known to cause both functional disabilities in childhood and degenerative arthritis in adults, the hips of all infants should be examined regularly.

The Ortolani and Barlow tests (Figure 22–2) should be mastered by all pediatric practitioners. Roentgenograms are not helpful until 2–3 mo of age, when the femoral head begins to ossify, but, with skilled personnel, ultrasonography can be helpful in the neonatal period.

Treatment focuses on maintaining reduction of the femoral head in the acetabulum until it is stable. This usually requires the use of a Pavlik harness for 4–6 wk and is best managed by a pediatric orthopedist.

Legg–Calvé–Perthes Disease

This is idiopathic avascular necrosis of the femoral head, seen predominantly in males between 4 and 8 yr of age. Presentation usually is with the insidious onset of limping, stiffness, and mild hip, thigh, or knee pain. *Diagnosis* is made radiographically, and bone scanning (showing decreased uptake) may be necessary early in the disease process.

Treatment is complicated, and may involve casting, bracing and/or surgery. The *prognosis* is fair at best (better if detected early), and many patients require hip replacement surgery in adult life.

Toxic Synovitis

Sometimes called transient synovitis of the hip, this is a common, self-limited, mild inflammatory arthritis of the hip seen in 3–6-yr-old children. It is crucial to differentiate this condition from septic arthritis or osteomyelitis, in which higher fevers, toxicity, increased pain, and guarding are seen. Septic arthritis must be treated urgently with surgical drainage and parenteral antibiotics, but toxic synovitis resolves within 7–10 days with nothing but rest and occasionally anti-inflammatory medications.

Slipped Capital Femoral Epiphysis

This occurs in adolescents during the growth spurt, and it represents a stress fracture through the proximal femoral growth plate. It can be acute or chronic, and patients usually complain of groin pain, a limp, decreased range of motion, and a shortened leg on the affected side. *Diagnosis* is made radiographically, and *treatment* is surgical.

SPINE
(*NELSON TEXTBOOK*, SECS. 24.12–24.22)

Spine problems can be congenital or developmental, and they may be static or progressive. Congenital deformities

$\longrightarrow$

Figure 22–2. *A*, The newborn child is laid on her back with the hips and knees flexed, and the middle finger of each hand is placed over each greater trochanter. *B*, The thumb of each hand is applied to the inner side of the thigh opposite the lesser trochanter. *C*, In a doubtful case the pelvis may be steadied between a thumb over the pubis and fingers under the sacrum while the hip is tested with the other hand. *D*, Limitation of abduction is an early sign of congenital dislocation of the hip. Note the restriction in abduction of the right leg. (From Behrman RE [ed]: Nelson Textbook of Pediatrics, 14th ed. Philadelphia, WB Saunders Company, 1992, p 1706.)

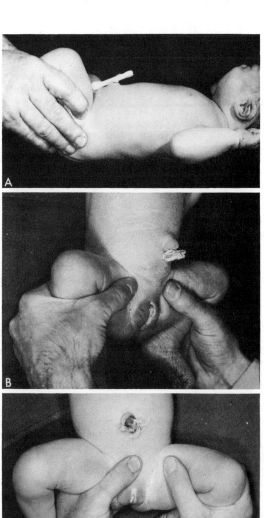

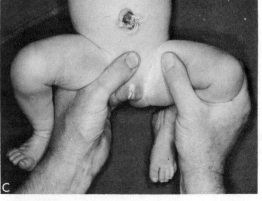

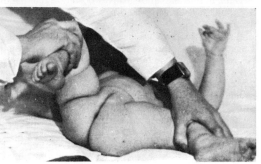

usually stem from anomalous vertebral development in terms of shape and segmentation, producing such lesions as *spina bifida occulta* and hemivertebrae. *Spinal dysraphism* is the general term encompassing all congenital spine anomalies. Most common and most severe are myelomeningoceles (spina bifida), which involve a variable degree of neurologic dysfunction (see *Nelson Textbook,* Sec. 20.5). Two other relatively common anomalies are diastematomyelia (a sagittal division of the spinal cord) and the *tethered (fixed) cord syndrome,* usually associated with a *lipomyelomeningocele.* These latter problems usually present with orthopedic foot deformities, leg pain, muscle spasm or atrophy, or bowel and bladder dysfunction.

Congenital Scoliosis

This is uncommon and is likely to involve fairly short, rigid, and progressive curves; therefore surgical therapy is usually required.

Idiopathic Scoliosis

This is fairly common, with a prevalence rate of 3–5% in school-aged children. It is more likely to be severe and progressive in females, especially in those who present early. Patients usually are picked up in school screening programs or by parents noting the asymmetry. Back pain usually is not a feature of idiopathic scoliosis and in fact is a rare condition, so this should arouse suspicion of another condition.

Physical examination should include careful observation and range-of-motion testing, as well as the forward bend test, looking for the commonly associated thoracic rotational deformity (rib hump). Roentgenograms of the entire spine define the location and severity of the curvature, as measured by the Cobb angle. Curves likely to progress measure greater than 30 degrees in preadolescent patients (bone age less than 12 yr). Curves of less than 20 degrees in skeletally mature adolescents rarely progress. For curvature between 20 and 30 degrees, patients should be followed carefully by physical examination and serial roentgenograms.

Orthotic treatment (e.g., the Milwaukee brace) should be started for curves of 20–30 degrees (depending on age and rate of progression). Surgical treatment with internal fixation may be necessary and can result in permanent correction.

Kyphosis

This is the normal curvature (convex posteriorly) of the thoracic spine, measuring 20–50 degrees in the sagittal plane. This can be exaggerated (hyperkyphosis) congenitally or in adolescents with *Scheuermann's juvenile kyphosis.* This disorder usually involves three adjacent thoracic or upper lumbar vertebral bodies, with anterior wedging of at least 5 degrees each. It is seen in 5–8% of adolescents (most common in active males) and usually presents with back pain and localized tenderness in pubertal patients thought to have poor posture. Physical examination should include back, hip, and knee range-of-motion testing and a side view of the forward bend test.

ORTHOPEDIC PROBLEMS / **465**

If lateral roentgenograms are normal, the diagnosis is *postural round back deformity*, a smooth and mobile convexity. However, treatment is similar, involving activity restriction (especially forward-bending activities), anti-inflammatory medications, stretching, and strengthening exercises to improve posture and achieve a "neutral spine." Severe cases in young patients require bracing and surgery.

Lordosis

This is the normal sagittal plane curve (concave posteriorly) of the cervical and lumbar spines. This often is found to be excessive in the lumbar spine in older children and adolescents. It often is associated with a hip flexion contracture, forward pelvic tilt, and weak abdominal muscles. Although usually asymptomatic in childhood, lumbar hyperlordosis can lead to overuse syndromes (e.g., facet synovitis syndrome) in active adolescents.

Spondylolysis

This is a fairly common problem that is related to lumbar hyperlordosis. It is a stress fracture of the pars interarticularis. In young patients (less than 8–10 yr of age), this can be acute and is best managed with relative immobilization (a Boston overlap brace), because bony healing may occur. In older patients, this can be managed with relative rest (avoiding esp. extension activities), anti-inflammatory medications, and stretching and strengthening exercises for posture improvement.

Spondylolisthesis

This also may cause an accentuated lumbar hyperlordosis. It consists of a forward slippage of one vertebral body on another. The diagnosis is made roentgenographically and is graded by the percentage of the vertebral body that is overriding. This usually can be managed conservatively (as with spondylolysis), but in young patients (less than 10 yr old) and in those with a progressive slip of over 25–50%, bracing or surgical fusion may be necessary.

Degenerative Disk Disease and Herniated Nucleus Pulposus

This may occur in older children and adolescents. A thorough neurologic evaluation, palpation, and dural tension signs (i.e., straight-leg raising) are indicated. Roentgenograms often are normal or show disk space narrowing; MRI is the imaging study of choice. Treatment need not be surgical, but should be managed by an orthopedist, physiatrist, neurologist, or other clinician familiar with the management of disk disease, which involves anti-inflammatories, physical therapy, and posture education ("back school").

Diskitis

This is an acute inflammatory process of the intervertebral disk space seen in young children with fever, vague back pain, and back stiffness. Roentgenograms may show disc space narrowing 10–14 days after the onset of disease, but the bone scan (showing increased uptake) will be positive early, and an MRI will show inflammatory swelling of the disk. Treatment consists of bed rest and anti-inflammatory agents. If a bacterial etiology is suspected, a 4–5-wk course of antistaphylococcal antibiotics is warranted.

Intervertebral Disk Calcification

This is a rare disorder of unknown etiology and usually is acute and self-limited. It may follow minor trauma or infection and is best treated symptomatically with relative immobilization (e.g., a cervical collar), rest, analgesics, and, if necessary, cervical traction.

Ankylosing Spondylitis

This often is seen in the lumbar spine and presents with back pain and limited range of motion (see Chap. 9).

NECK AND SHOULDER
(*NELSON TEXTBOOK*, SEC. 24.23)

Congenital anomalies of the cervical spine are uncommon and may produce cosmetic, mechanical, or neurologic problems.

Klippel-Feil syndrome is a congenital fusion of two or more cervical vertebrae, and often is associated with other congenital anomalies.

Sprengel deformity is a congenitally high scapula that is unilateral and sometimes associated with other orthopedic anomalies.

Atlantoaxial instability is common in Down syndrome and is due to laxity of the transverse ligament and abnormal odontoid process development. Because spinal cord compression may occur spontaneously in these patients, roentgenographic measurements should be taken and surgical fusion should be considered.

Torticollis (wryneck) is characterized by head tilt and lateral rotation. Most commonly, this is congenital *muscular torticollis* and is caused by a thickened, fibrotic contracture of the sternocleidomastoid muscle. This lesion always presents before 2–6 mo of age and resolves spontaneously in most patients. Gentle passive stretching may be of some benefit.

UPPER EXTREMITY
(*NELSON TEXTBOOK*, SEC. 24.24)

Upper limb problems generally are less common and less severe than those of the lower extremities in pediatric orthopedics. Uncommon congenital anomalies include *pseudoarthrosis of the clavicle* (usually unilateral, midshaft), *synostosis (fusion) of the elbow*, and *dislocation of the radial head*.

Congenital longitudinal deficiencies of the radius occur in 1:100,000 live births and often are associated with pancytopenia (*Fanconi syndrome*), thrombocytopenia (*TAR syndrome* with absent radius), or cardiac defects (*Holt–Oram syndrome*). In most of these, the thumb is absent or hypoplastic as well.

Madelung deformity involves the distal radial physis and results in bowing and radial displacement of the hand, analogous to that in Blount disease.

Syndactyly is the most common congenital anomaly of the hand. It consists of fusion or webbing of two digits and occurs in 1:2,200 live births. *Polydactyly* (extra digits) is slightly less common in general but much more common in males and blacks. It can be postaxial (little finger side) or preaxial (thumb side). Treatment for these and other congenital digital anomalies involves early (6–12 mo) surgery to improve hand function and appearance.

TRAUMA
(NELSON TEXTBOOK, SECS. 24.25 AND 24.26)

Musculoskeletal injuries in children are commonplace, but often difficult to diagnose because of lack of cooperation and variations of ossification in the immature skeleton. Important caveats to remember about pediatric fractures include the following:

1. Fractures are more likely in children than adults because their soft tissues (e.g., ligaments) may be stronger than their bones (e.g., growth plates).
2. Fractures tend to be more stable in children because of thickened periosteum, which often remains intact.
3. Fractures heal more quickly in children than adults, and angulation (but not rotational) deformities usually remodel with growth.
4. Fractures can be confused radiographically with ossification centers, but fracture sites are tender whereas ossification sites usually are not.
5. Growth disturbances may result from physeal fractures.
6. Multiple fractures in different stages of healing are specific for child abuse.

Evaluation and Initial Stabilization

Severely injured patients should be stabilized, with initial attention paid to life-threatening injuries, spinal cord injuries, cranial fractures, and limb-threatening injuries. Anyone suspected of having sustained a cervical spine fracture (i.e., vital sign instability, neck tenderness, or neurologic dysfunction) should be immobilized in a hard (Philadelphia) cervical collar until roentgenographic evaluation (including all seven cervical vertebrae) rules out an unstable fracture.

Hemorrhage from pelvic or long bone fractures can produce hypovolemic shock.

A *compartment syndrome*, consisting of tense swelling from hemorrhage into a tight fascial muscle compartment, may result in pain, pulselessness, paresis or paresthesias, and pallor. This emergency usually involves the lower leg or forearm and may require fasciotomy.

Roentgenograms are absolutely necessary for fracture diagnosis. Two views should be obtained (anteroposterior and lateral) and always should be interpreted in the clinical context (i.e., correlated with the site of tenderness). Fractures involving the growth plate should be assessed using the method of Salter and managed according to accepted orthopedic principles.

Common Fractures and Dislocations

CLAVICLE. *Clavicle fractures* occur in newborns (secondary to birth trauma) and older children (resulting usually from a fall onto the shoulder or outstretched arm). Treatment primarily is dictated by pain control, usually requiring no intervention in newborns and only a sling or clavicle (figure-of-eight) strap in older patients.

Acromioclavicular sprains and dislocations are relatively common in adolescents during contact sports. This injury stems from a fall onto the tip of the shoulders, resulting in pain, point tenderness, and painful range of motion (esp. horizontal abduction). Roentgenograms are necessary to grade the severity of the sprain and should be done with weights in the hands to magnify the degree of acromioclavicular separation. Treatment ranges from a simple sling to surgical reduction and internal fixation, depending on the grade of the injury.

HUMERUS. *Proximal humerus fractures* occur in 11–15-yr-old patients and frequently involve the growth plate. Treatment depends on displacement.

Supracondylar fractures are common in 5–8-yr-olds and often are complicated by associated neurovascular injury and growth deformities following healing. Treatment requires a long-arm cast for undisplaced and uncomplicated fractures, closed reduction and percutaneous priming for displaced fractures, or open reduction if neurovascular injury is suspected.

Lateral condylar and *medial epicondylar fractures* also are seen in children, and their treatment is complex; therefore, they are best managed by an orthopedic surgeon.

ELBOW. *Subluxation of the radial head* (nursemaid elbow) is the most common elbow injury in pediatrics. It usually is seen after a young child (less than 4 yr) is pulled by the hand, inducing a partial tear of the annular ligament. This results in pain (often poorly localized) and limited supination. Reduction often occurs spontaneously or by a radiology technician and easily can be accomplished with gentle supination under slight traction with the elbow at 90 degrees of flexion.

Complete *dislocation of the radial head* and *proximal radius fractures* sometimes are seen in older children and often require reduction (open or closed) by an orthopedist.

FOREARM. *Forearm fractures* are very common in children, especially torus (buckle) fractures of the distal radial or ulnar metaphysis. These nondisplaced or minimally displaced injuries are easily treated in a short-arm cast for 3 wk. Both-bone fractures are more complicated, requiring a long-arm cast and occasionally closed reduction by an orthopedist, depending on the degree of displacement.

WRIST AND HAND. Wrist, hand, and finger fractures also are fairly common. Injuries that require special consideration in management include:

Epiphyseal fractures of the distal radius (usually type II)

Scaphoid fractures (initial roentgenograms may be negative; repeat in 1 wk if snuffbox tenderness persists)

Ulnar collateral ligament avulsion injuries of the thumb ("skier's" or "gamekeeper's" thumb)

Metacarpal and *phalangeal fractures* (tendon function, growth plate, and articular involvement must be assessed)

PELVIS AND FEMUR. *Pelvic fractures, femoral neck fractures,* and *femoral head dislocations* are uncommon and usually are associated with major trauma (e.g., motor vehicle accidents). Fractures of the *femoral shaft* also stem from major trauma but also are seen in abused toddlers. Treatment involves immobilization in a spica cast or skin traction.

TIBIA. A fracture of the *tibial shaft* usually is spiral in a young child, and this "toddler's fracture" can result from surprisingly little trauma. The fibula usually is intact, and treatment involves an above-knee cast for 3–4 wk.

ANKLE AND FOOT. *Ankle sprains* are very common in active children and adolescents, usually on the lateral aspect, involving the anterior talofibular (and sometimes the calcaneofibular) ligament. Roentgenography can help to rule out distal fibula (or occasionally proximal fibula) fractures and avulsion fractures at the base of the 5th metatarsal. Treatment involves rest, ice, compression, and elevation in the short term, but active range-of-motion and lower leg strengthening exercises are important to prevent recurrences.

Tarsal and *metatarsal fractures* are uncommon except for the *Jones fracture* of the 5th metatarsal shaft, which must be differentiated from the normal epiphyseal plate. This injury is notorious for poor healing in adults, but usually heals with short leg casting for 4–6 wk in young patients.

SPORTS MEDICINE
(*NELSON TEXTBOOK*, SECS. 24.27 AND 24.28)

Sports participation can be very rewarding for children in a variety of ways, including physical fitness, psychosocial development, and self-confidence. Younger children should be allowed more opportunities for free play, and older groups of children benefit from more organized sports. Overzealous parents and coaches can contribute to both physical and psychological harm coming from too much sports involvement of children.

Preparticipation Health Evaluation

This should be focused on identifying specific conditions that place the patient at risk for injury (e.g., incompletely rehabilitated orthopedic injury) or death (e.g., hypertrophic cardiomyopathy) during sports competition. Also, conditions that might be made worse during sports (e.g., exercise-induced bronchospasm) should be evaluated. A screening history and physical examination are appropriate, and selected laboratory studies (e.g., electrocardiogram, chest roentgenogram, and echocardiogram for suspicious murmurs) or referrals may be indicated. At the completion of the evaluation (best done 6–8 weeks in advance of the season, clearance for sports should be sport specific and guided by accepted standards (see Tables 24–10 and 24–11, *Nelson Textbook*).

Overuse Injuries

These occur in highly driven athletes, especially in children who "specialize" early in their careers. Repetitive activities lead to microtrauma in specific, susceptible structures that respond with irritation, inflammation, and activity-related pain. Examples include osteochondrosis (e.g., Little League elbow, Osgood–Schlatter disease), tendinitis (swimmer's shoulder, achilles tendinitis), and stress fractures. Perhaps the most common overuse injury in adolescents is *patellofemoral pain syndrome*, stemming from repetitive activities involving knee flexion.

Stress Fractures

These represent the ultimate overuse injury, occurring when chronic repetitive forces at a specific site overwhelm the bone's reparative efforts, resulting in local dissolution of the bone. Usually this is seen after a sudden increase in activity and causes localized, activity-related pain and point tenderness over the bone. Roentgenograms typically are negative early, and a bone scan may be necessary to make the diagnosis. Treatment involves rest from exacerbating activities, but immobilization rarely is necessary.

Soft-Tissue Injuries

In sports, these include partial tears of ligaments (sprains), muscle–tendon units (strains), muscle contusions, skin abrasions, and lacerations.

Musculotendinous *strains* (pulls) occur within the muscle's normal range-of-motion plane, when antagonistic forces (e.g., gravity or momentum and active contraction of the muscle) exceed the tensile strength of the muscle–tendon unit. Ligamentous *sprains* are similar except that the forces are outside the affected joint's range of motion, and the ligamentous restraints of such abnormal motion are disrupted. Both mechanisms can result in avulsion, epiphyseal, or apophyseal fractures when the involved soft-tissue structure is stronger than its bony insertion point.

Both sprains and strains are graded I–III based on severity and require rest, ice, compression, and elevation for initial treatment. Nonsteroidal anti-inflammatory agents can help to decrease pain and inflammation. Some grade III sprains require surgery, but the most important part of treatment for all of these injuries is rehabilitation, the restoration of adequate motion and strength of the involved structures, before a gradual return to sports participation.

Head and Neck Injuries

These occur in high-speed contact and collision sports and consist of concussions, cervical spine fractures, nerve injuries (neurapraxia), and soft-tissue sprains and strains.

Concussions are graded I–V based on severity, and all concussions accompanied by post-traumatic amnesia (grades II or higher) put patients at risk for the *postconcussion syndrome* of difficulty concentrating, headaches, and irritability for several weeks. All players with concussions of grade III or higher should be held out of competition for 1 wk because of the possibility of a second injury causing the "second impact syndrome" of malignant cerebral edema, which can arise following a repeat injury.

Specific Sports and Associated Injuries

Certain sports are associated with characteristic injury patterns. Examples include:

gymnastics—spondylolysis bursitis (impingement syndrome)
baseball—medial epicondylitis ("Little League elbow")
ballet—snapping hip syndrome (can be medial or lateral)
wrestling—brachial plexus neurapraxias ("stingers" or "burners")
football—concussions, contusions, ligament tears, etc.
basketball—ankle sprains and achilles tendinitis
running—stress fractures, patellofemoral pain syndrome, and various forms of tendinitis, including the iliotibial band syndrome
skiing—ulnar collateral ligament sprains and avulsions, tibia fractures, and knee ligament (anterior cruciate) sprains.

GENETIC SKELETAL DYSPLASIAS
(*NELSON TEXTBOOK*, SECS. 24.29–24.58)

Developmental defects of the skeleton (dysplasias) are rare but often devastating disorders. Usually, they present at birth with disproportionate lengths of limbs and trunk.

Evaluation should include a careful growth history, family history, and physical examination, including precise measurements. Roentgenographic studies are essential, and sometimes pathologic studies (i.e., from bone biopsy specimens) are required.

Many of these syndromes are associated with immune deficiency, renal defects, and hearing impairment as well as other organ systems complications.

Management must include a precise diagnosis, evaluation and treatment of all complications, emotional support, and genetic counseling. Orthopedic goals should be to maximize mobility and minimize deformity.

DEFECTS OF THE GROWTH OF TUBULAR BONES AND/OR SPINE
(*NELSON TEXTBOOK*, SECS. 24.30–24.49)

Achondroplasia

Achondroplasia affects 1:25,000 newborns, causing short stature, short limbs (esp. the proximal parts), large head (occasional hydrocephalus), and delayed motor development. Lifespan usually is normal.

Hypochondroplasia

This form of short-limbed short stature usually presents at 2–3 yr of age, resembling achondroplasia but less severe.

Thanatophoric Dysplasia

This lethal disorder is similar to but more severe than achondroplasia. Hydrocephalus always is present, and the small, pear-shaped chest does not allow for sufficient pulmonary function to support life outside of the uterus.

Short Rib–Polydactyly Syndromes

Several distinct syndromes involve the association of polydactyly and short ribs. The narrow, dysplastic thorax that results from the short ribs is associated with pulmonary hypoplasia and varying degrees of respiratory distress. Most forms are lethal, but an exception is chondroectodermal dysplasia (Ellis–van Creveld syndrome).

Chondrodysplasia Punctata

This set of disorders, involving stippled calcification of the epiphyses and periarticular cartilage, includes Conradi disease and punctate epiphyseal dysplasia.

Epiphyseal Dysplasias

There are two major groups of syndromes characterized by flattened, fragmented, or irregular epiphyses: those with spinal involvement, the spondyloepiphyseal dysplasias (SED), and those without spinal involvement, the multiple epiphyseal dysplasias. Newborns with *SED congenita* have short-limbed short stature and many other skeletal deformities, and are diagnosed roentgenographically. *SED tarda* is X-linked recessive and presents at 5–10 yr of age with slowed spinal growth and kyphoscoliosis. *Kneist dysplasia* is an autosomal dominant condition associated with marked delay of epiphyseal ossification at the hips, progressive kyphoscoliosis, and joint limitations.

Diastrophic Dysplasia

Diastrophic dysplasia causes short-limbed short stature, severe clubfeet, joint contractures, and thumb deformities associated with dysplastic changes in auricular and tracheal structures.

Metatropic Dysplasia

In metatropic dysplasia, there are short extremities, bulbous enlargement of the joints, joint limitation, and progressive kyphoscoliosis.

Mesomelic Dysplasias

This set of disorders is hallmarked by shortening of the middle (mesomelic) portion of the limbs.

Cleidocranial Dysplasia

Cleidocranial dysplasia is manifested by hypoplasia of the membranous (flat) bones and, because of anterior clavicular involvement, can cause the shoulders to be low and set forward. Because of associated joint laxity, sometimes the shoulders can be apposed anteriorly.

Larsen Syndrome

This group of disorders involves marked hyperlaxity of the joints with multiple dislocations, especially of the hips, knees, and elbows. The lack of skin hyperlaxity differentiates Larsen syndrome from Ehlers–Danlos syndrome.

Otopalatodigital Syndrome

This syndrome is characterized by proportionate short stature, distinct facies, hand and foot abnormalities, and sometimes mental retardation.

Metaphyseal Dysplasias

Metaphyseal dysplasias typically spare the epiphyses and the spine, and the metaphyseal hypoplasia usually causes short-limbed short stature, bowing of the legs, and joint contractures.

Spondylometaphyseal Dysplasias

These syndromes involve the vertebrae and metaphyses of the long bones, typically presenting at 1–2 yr of age with growth retardation and abnormal gait.

Pseudoachondroplasias

This group of disorders are manifested by short-limbed short stature similar to that in achondroplasia, but with normal facies.

Trichorhinophalangeal Syndrome

This syndrome is characterized by mild short stature, typical facies, and abnormal cone-shaped epiphyses of the bones in the hands and fingers.

Osteochondrodysplasias with Anarchic Development of Cartilaginous or Fibrous Tissue

These heterogeneous conditions involve abnormally placed cartilage or fibrous elements causing skeletal deformity. Included are McCune–Albright syndrome (fibrous dysplasia with skin hyperpigmentation and precocious puberty); Trevor disease (dysplasia epiphysealis hemimelica); multiple cartilaginous exostoses; Langer–Giedion syndrome; and enchondromata. Exostoses are bony projections arising from the metaphyses of long bones, typically pointing away from the epiphyses. Enchondromata are cartilaginous, oval lesions within bone.

Surgical resection of either of these lesions should be considered for cosmetic deformity, neurovascular compromise, or malignant change, and is much more likely to be necessary with enchondromata than exostoses.

ABNORMALITIES OF DENSITY OR MODELING OF THE SKELETON AND CARTILAGINOUS TISSUE
(*NELSON TEXTBOOK*, SECS. 24.50–24.57)

Inherited Osteoporoses

Osteopenia means insufficiency of bone, and this is documented roentgenographically. *Osteoporosis* refers to the clinical condition resulting from osteopenia.

In childhood, this condition usually results from *osteogenesis imperfecta* (OI). At least four distinct genetic syndromes of OI (types I–IV) have been described. All are characterized by excessive bone fragility with bowing and frequent fractures, blue sclera, and variable degrees of hearing loss.

Type I—the most common, with fairly good (into adulthood) survival rates

Type II—usually fatal in the neonatal period (50% are stillborn)

Type III—associated with death during childhood

Type IV—the least severe, with features similar to type I but less scleral discoloration and hearing loss

Management of OI involves genetic counseling, family support, and aggressive splinting of fractures to minimize deformity.

Osteopetrosis, Pyknodysostosis, and Dysosteosclerosis

These disorders are manifested by a generalized increase in skeletal density.

Osteopetrosis ("marble bone disease") in its most severe form presents in early infancy with failure to thrive, hypocalcemia, and severe pancytopenia (due to crowding of the bone marrow cavities).

Osteopetrosis tarda (Albers–Schöenberg disease) presents in childhood or adolescence with similar but less severe involvement.

Pyknodysostosis has a postnatal onset, with short-limbed short stature, generalized hyperostosis, and short, broad hands and feet.

Dysosteosclerosis is similar but involves the vertebral bones predominantly and also causes problems with dentition.

Osteopoikilosis, Osteopathia Striata, and Melorheostosis

These disorders are usually asymptomatic and involve incidental roentgenographic findings of abnormal ossification.

Craniotubular Remodeling Disorders

Several distinct clinical entities have been described (all very rare) in which there are focal hyperostosis or modeling defects of various bones. The most important are *diaphyseal dysplasia*, in which the diaphyses (shafts) of long bones are involved, frequently with neuromuscular complications; and *craniodiaphyseal dysplasia,* in which hyperostosis of the skull leads to olfactory, hearing, and visual impairment.

Osteodysplasty

This is a group of familial disorders (Melnick–Needles syndrome) in which various bones are abnormally shaped.

Infantile Cortical Hyperostosis

This condition (also known as Caffey disease) presents in early infancy with fever, soft-tissue swelling over the jaws and face, and progressive thickening of both long and flat bones. Exacerbations and remissions commonly occur, but spontaneous regression can be expected after several years.

Marfan Syndrome (Arachnodactyly)

Marfan syndrome is an autosomal dominant disorder affecting 1:10,000 individuals, diagnosed by the combination of several distinct clinical features (primarily skeletal, cardiovascular, and ocular). Management should be focused on preventing complications, genetic counseling, and ophthalmologic, cardiologic, and orthopedic consultations. Prevention of aortic rupture by limiting maximal physical exertion when there is significant aortic root dilation is a priority. Longevity is decreased in Marfan syndrome, primarily as a result of cardiovascular complications.

ARTHROGRYPOSIS

Arthrogryposis multiplex congenita is a heterogeneous group of congenital disorders characterized by extreme stiffness of the joints and associated hypoplasia of muscle, bone, and periarticular soft tissues. Involved joints have either flexion contractures or ankylosis in extension. Therapy involves massage, passive stretching, and splinting to correct deformities. Most affected children are able to function adequately as adults.

METABOLIC BONE DISEASE
(*NELSON TEXTBOOK*, SECS. 24.59–24.74)

Bone is a dynamic organ, serving not only as the body's frame, the skeletal system, but also as a storage organ for calcium, phosphorus, and magnesium. Bone growth (including modeling and remodeling) is a hallmark of childhood and is influenced by hormonal, nutritional, and physical forces (i.e., gravity, weight-bearing, etc.). Any disruption in the metabolism of bone is referred to as a "metabolic bone disease," examples of which are discussed in the following sections.

RICKETS
(*NELSON TEXTBOOK*, SECS. 24.60–24.69)

The metabolism of calcium and phosphate is coordinated hormonally (by parathyroid hormone and calcitonin) involving the intestine (for absorption of dietary vitamin D, calcium, and phosphate) as well as the liver, skin, and kidneys (for conversion of vitamin D to its most active form and for excretion of calcium and phosphate). Abnormalities at any of these levels can be the cause of metabolic bone disease.

Rickets is unique to childhood, occurring whenever mineral (calcium and phosphorus) deficiency prevents the normal process of bone mineralization at the epiphyseal plate of growing bones. Classically, rickets has occurred when lack of sunlight interfered with the conversion of vitamin D to its active form, resulting in inadequate availability of calcium and phosphate at the epiphyses for proper bone formation.

Familial Hypophosphatemia (Vitamin D–Resistant Rickets)

This is the most common form of rickets in developed countries, and it is caused by an X-linked, dominantly inherited defect in phosphate and vitamin D metabolism in the kidney. Both vitamin D activation and tubular resorption of phosphate are impaired, resulting in hypophosphatemia. Clinically, there is exaggerated bowing of the lower extremities, a waddling gait, and short stature.

Diagnosis is confirmed by roentgenograms (metaphyseal widening and coarse trabecular bone) and laboratory studies (normal serum calcium, low serum phosphate, elevated alkaline phosphate, and elevated urine phosphate).

Treatment requires both oral phosphate supplements (0.5–4 g/24 hr) and vitamin D (dihydrotachysterol, 0.02 mg/kg/24 hr).

Vitamin D–Dependent Rickets

This disorder appears in infancy with features similar to those of familial hypophosphatemia, but the primary metabolic problem is hypocalcemia resulting from inadequate renal conversion of vitamin D to its active form. It can be treated with active vitamin D (1,25-dihydroxy vitamin D), in dosages of 1–2 μg/24 hr.

Hepatic Rickets

Rickets seen with liver disease is primarily related to malabsorption of vitamin D (a fat-soluable vitamin) as a result of inadequate bile salt secretion. Treatment is with high-dose vitamin D along with oral calcium supplements.

Rickets Associated with Anticonvulsant Therapy

The combination of phenobarbital and phenytoin is the most common cause, but all anticonvulsant medications have been shown to induce the development of rickets. This primarily is due to hepatic dysfunction in the conversion of vitamin D, stemming from the anticonvulsants' inducement of the cytochrome P-450 hydroxylation enzymes. Patients receiving long-term anticonvulsants should have serum levels of calcium phosphate and alkaline phosphatase checked periodically. Vitamin D and calcium supplements may be necessary.

Oncogenous Rickets

Hypophosphatemic rickets has been described with tumors of mesenchymal origin, resolving with resection of the tumor.

Rickets Associated with Renal Tubular Acidosis

Proximal renal tubular (RTA) has been associated with rickets primarily because of the hypophosphatemia that results from hyperchloremic metabolic acidosis and persistent alkaline urine, interfering with phosphate resorption. In distal (type I) RTA, bone dissolution occurs probably because the calcium carbonate of bone serves as a buffer against the persistent metabolic acidosis. *Therapy* for RTA requires bicarbonate to reverse the acidosis, but if rickets is seen with proximal RTA, oral phosphate and vitamin D supplements should be added.

Hypophosphatasia

This rare autosomal recessive disorder resembles rickets clinically and roentgenographically but is caused by an enzymatic defect in tissue-nonspecific alkaline phosphatase activity. Thus, the diagnosis is confirmed by a low serum alkaline phosphatase level. Childhood survivors of this condition may improve spontaneously as they mature. No specific therapy is available.

Primary Chondrodystrophy (Metaphyseal Dysplasia)

This rare disorder causes short stature and bowing of the legs related to abnormal metaphyseal bone growth, with normal serum calcium, phosphate, and alkaline phosphatase levels.

Idiopathic Hypercalcemia

Hypercalcemia can result from excessive ingestion of vitamin D or a familial renal defect and can cause failure to thrive, renal impairment, and osteosclerosis. *Williams syndrome* involves hypervitaminosis D (and secondary osteosclerosis) along with characteristic "elfin" facies, feeding problems, and mild mental retardation.

HYPERPHOSPHATASIA

This condition is characterized by elevation of the bone isoenzyme of alkaline phosphatase, causing growth failure, subperiosteal bone formation and bowing, and thickening of the diaphyses of long bones. This has been called juvenile Paget disease, because calcitonin may reduce the rapid bone turnover.

Fanconi Syndrome

Fanconi syndrome is a generalized renal tubular defect that is commonly idiopathic, but sometimes is secondary to certain genetic (e.g., cystinosis, galactosemia, Lowe syndrome, Wilson disease) or acquired (e.g., heavy metal or drug exposure) diseases. In any case, aminoaciduria, glysoruria, and phosphaturia develop, the latter being responsible for hypophosphatemic rickets, which should be diagnosed and treated as described above.

CYSTINOSIS

This inherited disorder is identical to Fanconi syndrome, with the additional finding of cystic deposition in various tissues (including the reticulo-endothelial system, renal tubular cells, cornea and conjunctiva, fibroblasts, and blood leukocytes). Prognosis and treatment are primarily related to the degree of kidney involvement.

OCULOCEREBRORENAL DYSTROPHY (Lowe Syndrome)

This rare X-linked disorder involves Fanconi syndrome (with secondary hypophosphatemic rickets), visual impairment (mostly from congenital cataracts and glaucoma), severe hypotonia, and mental retardation. The prognosis is poor and treatment is supportive.

RENAL OSTEODYSTROPHY

Children with chronic renal failure necessarily experience alterations in bone growth and remodeling related to impaired mineral (calcium and phosphate) metabolism. This can be related to both defective mineralization (osteomalacia) and excessive resorption (osteitis fibrosa).

Clinical manifestations of renal osteodystrophy include growth failure, bone pain, slipped epiphyses, bone deformities, and metaphyseal fractures.

Treatment involves controlling hyperphosphatemia, supplying adequate oral calcium, and supplementing vitamin D intake. Hemodialysis or chronic peritoneal dialysis may exacerbate or ameliorate the osteodystrophy. The primary goal of management should be to address the underlying renal disease.

23

MISCELLANEOUS DISORDERS

UNCLASSIFIED DISEASES
(*NELSON TEXTBOOK*, SECS. 25.1–25.6)

This varied group of disorders includes the sudden infant death syndrome (SIDS), amyloid diseases, sarcoidosis, progeria, the histiocytosis syndromes, and hemorrhagic shock and encephalopathy.

SUDDEN INFANT DEATH SYNDROME

The sudden and unexpected death of an infant, for causes that are not understood even after an autopsy, is the most common manner of death in the 1st yr following the neonatal period. Typically, SIDS occurs in an apparently healthy 2–3-mo-old infant put to bed without suspicion of a problem. It is a worldwide phenomenon with considerable ethnic and racial variation and a large number of associated genetic, environmental, and social risk factors that, unfortunately, do not permit identification of the particular infant who will suffer SIDS.

SIDS may have several etiologies, and multiple pathogenic mechanisms have been implicated, including:

immature or abnormal development of neurorespiratory
  control of respiratory pauses, leading to apnea
brain stem defects
carotid body defects
abnormal upper airway function and obstruction
hyperactive airway reflexes
cardiac abnormalities

Although home monitoring of high-risk infants for apnea and bradycardia is often employed, especially when a sibling has died of SIDS or there is a history of an apparent life-threatening event, this preventive intervention has not been shown to be effective.

ENVIRONMENTAL HEALTH HAZARDS
(*NELSON TEXTBOOK*, SECS. 26.1–26.19)

This diverse group of health problems includes radiation injury, food poisoning, chemical and drug poisoning, chemical pollutants, venom diseases, and bites.

FOOD POISONING

Inadvertent consumption of poisonous foodstuffs is a worldwide cause of illness.

Bacterial Food Poisoning

The major bacterial causes include *Salmonella*, staphylococci, and *Clostridium botulinum*.

Salmonella may contaminate usually innocuous foods that are improperly stored after cooking or eaten uncooked. Diarrhea, abdominal pain, vomiting, and often headache, chills, and fever occur 12–48 hr after ingestion. *Treatment* usually is only supportive, although antibiotics are indicated for bacteremia, meningitis, infants less than 3 mo with gastroentroitis, and immunosuppressed or chronically ill patients.

Enerotoxigenic strains of Staphylococcus may contaminate improperly stored or cooked or uncooked foods. Nausea, abdominal pain, vomiting, and diarrhea occur 1–8 hr after ingestion of the toxins. *Supportive treatment* is indicated.

Clostridium botulinum (botulism) may result in two syndromes: (1) ingestion of preformed toxin in contaminated food inappropriately cooked under anaerobic conditions leads to severe peripheral neurotoxicity, with paralysis resulting from blocking of presynaptic acetylcholine release; and (2) gastrointestinal colonization of ingested toxin-producing strains by an infant may produce weakness and apnea.

Nonbacterial Food Poisoning

This may occur from consumption of toxins in certain species of mushrooms, sprouted potatoes, and various seafoods. Manifestations may range from mild gastrointestinal upsets to severe gastrointestinal and systemic symptoms, including life-threatening central nervous system (CNS) abnormalities and shock.

CHEMICAL AND DRUG POISONING

Children 5 yr and younger are exposed to plants, household products, and medications; adolescents are exposed most frequently to medications and illegal drugs.

Principles of Management

The initial contact should provide basic information about the location of the patient, the clinical manifestations, age and weight, time of ingestion, past medical history, and the type, route, and amount of exposure. Triage to an appropriate facility is critical. Life support with a primary emphasis on cardiorespiratory care is essential because there are relatively few specific antidotes. However, simultaneous use of antagonists and life support measures are indicated for poisonings caused by carbon monoxide, cyanide, opiates, substances producing methemoglobinemia, and cholinergic agents. In general, efforts are directed at preventing absorption (by emesis, lavage, charcoal, and cathartics) or enhancing excretion (by forced diuresis, hemodialysis, and hemoperfusion over activated charcoal or resin).

Acetaminophen

Clinical manifestations may include:

  anorexia, nausea, vomiting, malaise, pallor, and diaphoreses (30 min to 24 hr)

  resolution of initial symptoms and onset of upper quadrant abdominal pain and tenderness; elevated bilirubin, prothrombin time, and hepatic enzymes; and oliguria (24–48 hr)

  severe liver function abnormalities and reappearance of anorexia, nausea, vomiting, and malaise (72–96 hr)

  death or resolution of hepatic dysfunction (4 days to 2 wk)

Potentially toxic plasma levels as determined by a nomogram are treated with N-acetyl-L-cysteine within 24 hr of ingestion. Supportive care is essential.

Salicylates

Clinical manifestations in young infants may be few other than dehydration, hyperpnea, and fever. Older children may demonstrate hyperpnea, vomiting, and progressive lethargy as the drug is distributed throughout the CNS. Tinnitus and deafness also may occur. Metabolic disturbances often occur and may be complex because of a combination of respiratory stimulus and metabolic acidosis. Hemorrhage and hypoglycemia are additional complications.

Supportive treatment includes management of dehydration and electrolyte and acid–base disturbances; alkalinization of urine; and, in severe cases, hemodialysis or peritoneal dialysis.

Hydrocarbons

A wide variety of chemical substances contain hydrocarbons, and many factors are involved in determining whether a particular exposure will produce systemic or local toxicity.

Clinical manifestations may include respiratory distress and pneumonia secondary to aspiration, fever, CNS depression, congestive heart failure, headache, vertigo, ataxia, and renal or hepatic damage.

Treatment may include emesis in patients who have comsumed a hydrocarbon whose primary toxicity is systemic, if there are no other contradictions to vomiting.

Cyclic Antidepressants

Clinical manifestations initially include tachycardia, pupillary dilation, dry mucous membranes, urinary retention, convulsions, lethargy, hallucinations, and flushing. Hypertension, convulsions, coma, and cardiac arrhythmias may occur with tissue saturation.

Treatment is directed at preventing absorption with activated charcoal and cathartics. Life support and antiarrhythmic and antiseizure drugs may be necessary.

Lead Poisoning (Plumbism)

In the United States, about 17% of children ages 6 mo to 6 yr have blood lead levels greater than 15 μg/dL. As sustained blood levels rise higher, children are at progressively ineased risk of neurobehavioral and cognitive deficits. The major sources of exposure include interior household dust, exterior surface soil, and old residential paints.

Most children are asymptomatic. Early symptoms include hyperirritability, anorexia, and decreased play activity. Sporadic vomiting, intermittent abdominal pain, and constipation suggest lead colic. The sudden onset of persistent vomiting, ataxia, impairment of consciousness, coma, and seizures indicate encephalopathy, which may progress to massive cerebral edema and increased intracranial pressure.

Treatment includes separation from the source of lead; chelation therapy; fluid, electrolyte, and seizure management; and general life support as indicated.

VENOM DISEASES AND BITES

Identification of the specific species is central to management of snake bites or poisonings from venomous marine animals. Only 200 of the 3,500 known species of snakes are poisonous.

The local and systemic manifestations of *poisonous snake bites* vary depending on the family of snakes and type of venom. Hypertension, shock, hemorrhage, and neurotoxicity with paralysis may occur. These bites require supportive care and specific antivenom.

The clinical manifestations of poisonings from *venomous marine animals* are remarkably similar, including immediate pain at the puncture site that spreads to involve the entire extremity, local ischemia, and cyanosis followed by edema, erythema, and necrosis. Systemic manifestations include pallor, nausea, vomiting, diaphoresis, and loss of consciousness. Treatment includes tourniquets, irrigation, control of pain, and general supportive care.

Coelenterate stings (hydroids, jellyfish, sea anemones, coral) may vary from mild to extremely painful. There may be both local signs of inflammation and systemic involvement, including fever, chills, weakness, nausea, vomiting, and even respiratory failure.

Mammalian bites are very common and require treatment of local damage, prevention and treatment of local infection, and prevention of tetanus and rabies. Follow-up for human immunodeficiency virus status may be indicated in some cases.

INDEX

Note: Page numbers in *italics* refer to illustrations; those followed by the letter t refer to tables.